A
OF RADIOGRAPHIC
EQUIPMENT

JEFF JOAQUIN
251 6876

A MANUAL OF RADIOGRAPHIC EQUIPMENT

SYBIL M. STOCKLEY MBE FCR TE

Formerly Principal, Ipswich School of Radiography
Ipswich, UK

Churchill Livingstone 🏛

EDINBURGH LONDON MELBOURNE AND NEW YORK 1986

CHURCHILL LIVINGSTONE
Medical Division of Longman Group UK Limited

Distributed in the United States of America by Churchill
Livingstone, Inc., 650 Avenue of the Americas, New York,
N.Y. 10011, and by associated companies, branches and
representatives throughout the world.

First published 1986
   Reprinted 1987
   Reprinted 1990
   Reprinted 1992
   Reprinted 1993

ISBN 0-443-02585-1

A catalogue record for this book is available from the
British Library.

Library of Congress Cataloging in Publication Data
Stockley, Sybil M.
   A manual of radiographic equipment.
   Includes index.
   1. Radiography, Medical — Equipment and supplies —
Handbooks, manuals, etc. I. Title. [DNLM:
1. Radiography — instrumentation. WN 150 S865m]
RC78.5.S86 1985   616.07'57'028   85–5741

The
publisher's
policy is to use
paper manufactured
from sustainable forests

Printed in Hong Kong
CPP/05

Preface

The aim of this book is to aid student radiographers in their understanding of the design and function of diagnostic X-ray equipment and the accessories they are required to use, so that they may:

- use the equipment more efficiently and effectively to produce the required radiographic image
- appreciate the need for safety in operation and in particular the reduction of X-ray dose
- understand the limitations of the equipment, recognise faults in the equipment and perform test procedures to check on equipment performance
- be able to select suitable equipment and room layout for the various classes of radiographic work.

The book covers the topics included in the DCR equipment syllabus which use X-radiation. It does not include descriptions of any specific manufacturer's equipment but does give, in simple terms, the principles underlying the operation of equipment. General explanations have been included to enable the student to understand and use manufacturer's equipment data sheets on particular units and accessories, so that they may select the most suitable equipment for a particular installation and then use the equipment to its full potential.

Some people may find my simplistic approach too basic but I hope that others will find the explanation and diagrams easy to follow and that this will encourage them to take an interest in the equipment around them, thus expanding their knowledge so that they are able to give sound advice to planners in the selection of new equipment.

Ipswich 1986   S.M.S.

Acknowledgements

It is impossible to name the many people who over the years have shared with me their expert knowledge, so I take this opportunity to record my gratitude to them for without their help this book might not have been written. I would nevertheless name my friend, Elizabeth Furnass, whose professional enthusiasm and training stimulated my interest in radiographic equipment from student days. I would also like to thank Jessica Denniss for her help in the preparation of the manuscript.

S.M.S.

Contents

PART | # ONE

The generation of
X-radiation

1

Introduction

To produce a high quality X-ray image, it is essential to produce a beam of X-radiation which can be closely controlled to give the exact quantity and quality of radiation required so that consistent results are obtained. It is also important to have safety devices

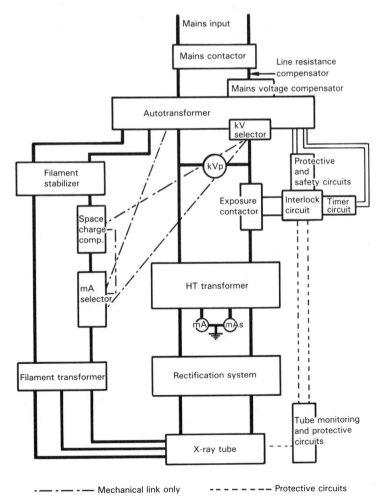

Fig. 1.1 Layout of the components of the electrical circuit of an X-ray generator.

which automatically prevent any hazard which could harm the person being examined, the operator or the equipment.

Central to the X-ray equipment is the source of radiation, the X-ray tube, and the generator supplying it with electrical power. Chapters 1–11 are concerned with the generation of X-rays and the parts of the equipment associated with this process.

Figure 1.1 is a block diagram representative of the layout of an X-ray generator and its controls. Each component shown in the layout is described more fully in the following chapters. Figure 1.2 shows the relationship of these components.

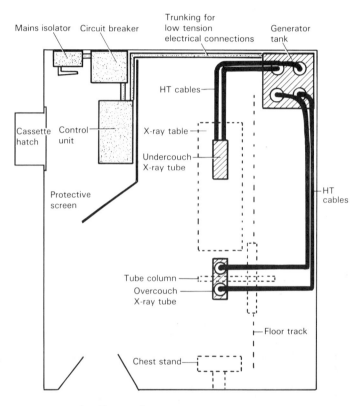

Fig. 1.2 Layout of the components of an X-ray unit.

2

The electrical supply

The four principal components to be considered are:

1. the generating system
2. the transmission system
3. local distribution
4. connection of an X-ray unit.

THE GENERATING SYSTEM

Power is generated by the Central Electricity Generating Board in its power stations. The energy source of this power is from:

a. gravitational energy obtained from water falling from a height, hydro-electric power.

b. thermal energy, heat is obtained by burning oil or coal or from nuclear reactions. The heat is used to convert water to steam.

The energy generated by both systems is used to rotate a turbine, which is connected to an electrical generator (Fig. 2.1).

The turbine is designed to rotate at 3000 revolutions per minute, hence the frequency of 50 Hz (50 cycles per second) of our supply in this country. Other European countries also have a 50 Hz supply but in other parts of the

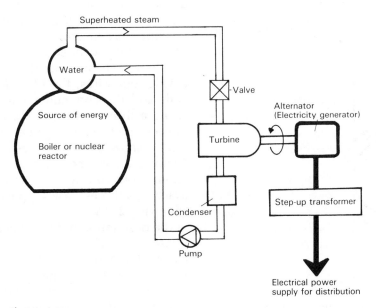

Fig. 2.1 The generating system.

world, principally the United States of America, generators produce a 60 Hz supply. Therefore care must be taken when referring to information on electrical equipment that 50 Hz is specified. The Central Electricity Generating Board is required to maintain the generator speed within very close limits as it is also required to maintain the generated voltage. The normal supply is 50 Hz at 240 V or 415 V phase-to-phase with a maximum permitted voltage variation of 6%. The voltage is quoted in r.m.s. value.

The generator

To make maximum use of the available energy the generator uses a three-phase system for production of the electromotive force. For easy understanding it is best to consider one phase (see Fig. 2.2). A coil of wire carried on a spindle is rotated at a constant speed (or frequency) of 50 Hz in an anticlockwise direction by a turbine through a uniform magnetic field. The magnetic field is produced by two opposing magnetic poles. As the coil rotates through 360° in the magnetic field, the coil cuts the lines of force produced by the magnetic field. The number of lines of force cut varies from zero when the coil is at right-angles to the field to a maximum when aligned with the field. When the coil has rotated through 180° the cutting of the magnetic field will be similar

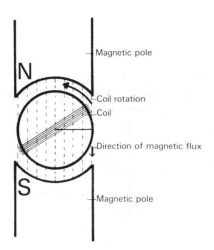

Fig. 2.2 Production of an electromotive force.

to the first half but in the opposite direction. Therefore the electromotive force will rise and fall as the rate of cutting increases and decreases changing its direction each half revolution, generating an alternating sinusoidal supply (Fig. 2.3).

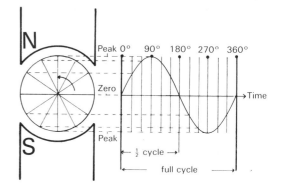

Fig. 2.3 Production of an alternating sinusoidal supply.

Examination of the waveform generated by a single coil shows that it is very inefficient, only giving its peak value twice in each revolution of the generator. This position is much improved by mounting not one coil but three symmetrically on the same spindle 120° apart (Fig. 2.4A). The generator will then produce three identical waveforms, each peaking twice during a revolution but with the peaks separated by the time taken for the spindle to rotate one-third of a revolution (120°). If one end of each coil is connected to a common point, the three coils become part of a single system having four wires, the three free ends of the coils and the common point. This system is called a three-phase system. If the waveform of each coil between its free end and the common point is plotted the result is as shown in Figure 2.4B. The common point is the neutral connection. Thus the Generating Board makes available a three-phase supply with each phase supplying 240 V.

The description of the generation of a three-phase supply has been greatly simplified to explain the basic principles of its operation. In practice it is the magnetic poles which rotate with the coils remaining stationary.

The advantages of a three-phase supply are:

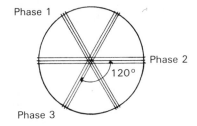

Fig. 2.4A Position of coils of a three-phase generator.

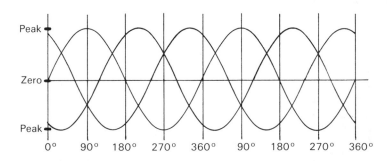

Fig. 2.4B Waveform from a three-phase generator.

a. more efficient use of the generator

b. smoother supply than that obtained from a single sinusoidal output

c. more economical use of conductors

d. simpler construction of all kinds of rotating electrical equipment because it has inbuilt 'phase rotation'.

THE TRANSMISSION SYSTEM

To supply the consumer, the electrical power generated by the Central Generating Board's comparatively small number of power stations is transmitted and distributed over very long distances. This is efficiently and economically done by linking all power stations to a National Grid and by drawing the supply for the consumer from the grid. The grid uses a network of electrical conductors carrying the three-phase supply and transformers designed to provide, in the most economical way, the electrical supply required by commercial and domestic users.

The **transmission system** (Fig. 2.5) provides for:

a. Transmission at a very high voltage. The voltage generated is stepped-up by a transformer at the power station. The National Grid transmits at 275 kV and 132 kV for long distance transmission, and even at 400 kV in some section of the system — the super grid. At the consumer end, the voltage is stepped down at a sub-station by a transformer to 33 kV and then down to 11 kV by a transformer for local distribution and finally by another transformer to 240 V which is the voltage provided in the U.K. for domestic use.

By using a high voltage the power is carried by a smaller current and as power losses are proportional to I^2R, where I is current and R resistance, the power loss is obviously much less if the current is small. It is also possible to reduce the cross-sectional area of the conductor without making the power loss unacceptable. The reduction in the cross-section area means a smaller amount of copper, the conducting material, is required to transmit the electrical power. This reduction will reduce the weight of the conductors which must be supported on pylons, cut the demand for the diminishing world reserve of copper and

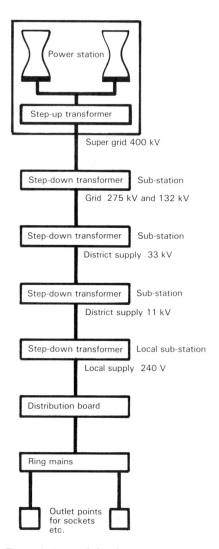

Fig. 2.5 Transmission and distribution system.

reduce the cost per mile of transmitting electrical power.

b. Carrying of a three-phase supply on a smaller number of conductors. Each phase has two wires from its generating coil, which are connected to the other two phases so that the three phases can be carried by four cables, one for each phase and a common neutral return cable. This method of connecting phases for transmission is known as Star connection (Fig. 2.6). Equipment requiring a three-phase supply is usually connected to the three phases by a Delta connection. An earth return

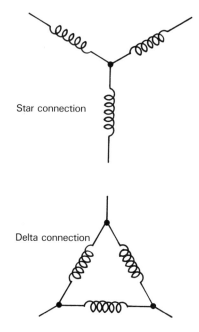

Fig. 2.6 Phase connection.

cable is also provided on the transmission lines.

LOCAL DISTRIBUTION

The hospital receives its supply from a substation, or in the case of power failure essential services are supplied from a local petrol or diesel driven generator.

Outlets for the supply are provided for each department. The department has its own distribution board from which is drawn the supply for the lighting circuit, the power circuit for the outlet sockets and in some sites, such as the X-ray department, permanent connections for equipment such as fixed X-ray units. To each distribution point the supply is brought by four cables, one from each phase and one for the neutral return cable. There is also one cable connected to earth.

The line voltage available at the outlet is 240 V or 415 V. These values are the r.m.s. (effective) values. The voltage, either single- or three-phase, is obtained by making suitable connections to the terminals on the distribution board. 415 V is used for X-ray equipment where the equipment is permanently fixed to the supply and never when a plug and socket connection for a mobile X-ray unit is required.

Figure 2.7 shows how the two voltages are obtained by connecting into the board. 240 V is obtained by attaching the equipment to any one of the phases and the neutral conductor. 415 V is obtained by connecting the equipment to two of the three phases. It might be expected that this method would give twice the single phase voltage but it must be remembered that one phase either lags or leads the other by 120°, therefore the potential difference can only be 415 V (240 × √3), as can be seen in Figure 2.8.

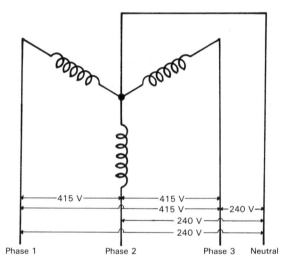

Fig. 2.7 Method of connection to provide 415 V or 240 V.

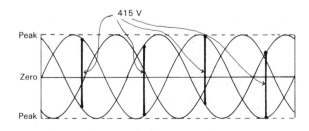

Fig. 2.8 Connection between two phases to give 415 V.

The electrical supply for an X-ray unit

An X-ray generator has unusual characteristics when considered as a load on the electrical supply system. Most loads draw their maximum currents for a relatively long time and the size of the cables required to supply them can be determined from data concerned with the heating effect of the current in the cables and the voltage drop arising over their length. But with X-ray generators the continuous current is quite small; except for the fraction of a second during which the radiographic exposure takes place when the current is very high indeed and during this time it is essential to maintain the actual supply voltage to the generator within certain manageable limits. The duration of this current is too short to be of significance in the heating of the cables, but the size of the cables has to be determined by the voltage drop requirements of the manufacturer of the unit. The voltage drop requirement is usually expressed in terms of the maximum impedance of the supply. Generally the major part of the impedance of a supply in a hospital is the resistance of the wiring system.

The electrical supply for an X-ray unit is obtained from the hospital's main distribution board, generally through one of its ring mains. If the unit is a major fixed unit, it will be supplied with large conductors so that they will not have an impedance greater than the manufacturer's specification. The mobile unit with its much smaller power requirement is supplied from a socket. This socket is connected to a power circuit supplied directly from a local distribution board or by a smaller ring main serving the ward or department. This ring is fed by one of the larger rings supplying a part of the hospital.

Once the voltage required by the X-ray unit is known, the maximum load which can be applied by the unit determines the maximum current drawn from the supply. In drawing this current through the feeder cables supplying the unit, power losses occur. The magnitude of these losses depend upon the impedance of the circuit, not just locally but through the the whole supply circuit right back to the generator. Therefore assessment of the load and acceptable loss has to be made at the planning stage, mains checked and conductors selected whose resistance is low enough to prevent the loss exceeding the X-ray manufacturer's acceptable level.

The impedance of cables of various cross-section and material is given in data sheets in ohms per metre. This allows the calculation of conductor size and type to be made once the length of run and the maximum acceptable impedance is known. For example, the impedance of the supply mains for a particular small major unit is 0.34 Ω. If this level of impedance cannot be achieved, it may be necessary for a new main to be installed, for if the power loss exceeds the maximum, the unit will never operate satisfactorily. As a double check after the X-ray power supply has been provided by the electrical contractor, the impedance is measured to make sure that it is acceptable before the installation of the unit commences. When equipment is to be fitted to existing mains the impedance is checked before the equipment manufacturer will agree to instal.

Therefore the main factors which must be considered when arranging the power supply for an X-ray unit are:

a. *Voltage of the mains supply* — when practical 415 V is preferred since the current drawn will be less than that needed with a 240 V supply.

b. *Resistance of the cables and their effect on the supply voltage to the unit.*

c. *Load current flow through the cable resistance* — the actual passage of current through the X-ray tube, a very high resistive load, will drop volts.

Therefore

(i) The voltage must satisfy the manufacturers supply requirements for the unit
(ii) The cables must have the specified current carrying capacity. This is normally stated in terms of fuse-rating.

In every part of the supply line, circuit breakers and fuses are introduced to operate should a current in excess of normal be drawn. This protects the equipment from damage through overheating and also protects

personnel. In hospital where an electrical power supply may be vital to life, a standby generator will automatically switch on should the normal supply to the hospital fail. An emergency generator will not be able to provide for all the needs of the hospital and may not be able to support a particular generator at all. Therefore it is essential that clear instructions are given on what can and cannot be used whilst on emergency power.

CONNECTION OF AN X-RAY UNIT

There are two methods of connecting an X-ray unit to its electrical supply from the hospital distribution board. These are by a:

1. permanently fixed connection for a static unit
2. temporary connection for a mobile unit.

Permanently fixed connection

The electrical mains supply is brought to a Mains Isolator box which is located in the X-ray room. In the box the cables from the X-ray unit are connected through a switch to the mains input cables. The supply for a major unit is drawn from two or three phases. It is normal in a large X-ray department to spread the load over the three phases. Without tools it is not possible to disconnect the unit from its supply. The isolation of the unit is through the switch in the isolator box.

Design and function of a typical mains isolator box

The function of this unit is to isolate the X-ray unit completely from its mains supply. The isolator breaks the continuity of supply simultaneously on all the live lines. The isolator is contained in an earthed metal box securely attached to the wall of the X-ray room within easy reach of the operator of the unit. The main supply cables from the hospital distribution board are brought to this box to be terminated on connector bolts. There are four terminal bolts, one for the conductor from each phase and one for the neutral return conductor. The bolts are mounted on a board of highly insulated material supported within the box so that the surrounding air increases the isolation from the metal casing. By providing all X-ray rooms with a three-phase supply on the connector bolts in the mains isolator box, any type of generator can be connected. In the past only the phases necessary for the type of generator selected were provided requiring costly rewiring and switch unit replacement when a single-phase unit was replaced by a three-phase unit.

Figure 2.9 shows how the live conductor from each phase of the mains supply is connected through a switch and fuse. The switch is specially designed to ensure that all three live lines are switched. The switch has three sets of blades which on closure make contact with three 'U'-shaped connector pieces. The blades and 'U'-shaped connector pieces are formed of thick copper to reduce the electrical resistance across the switch to a minimum. The blades are supported very firmly on a

thick rod of insulating material to ensure that the supply from each phase is isolated from the others, and to allow the switch to be operated manually with safety.

It is important that the switching action is very brisk once the handle has been operated, for any delay will increase the risk of arcing between the input and output side of the switch. Arcing causes distortion of the connecting surfaces through excess heat. Any distortion will cause the resistance across the switch to increase. A sharp action is provided by strong springs which operate as soon as the handle is turned. In some units the manually operated handle is replaced by a remote switching system which is more convenient. Electrical safety is increased by the introduction of an interlock switch in the remote control circuit which will switch off the supply to the unit once the box is opened.

The supply cables for the X-ray unit leave the box to be directly and permanently connected to the X-ray unit. Once connected the unit cannot be isolated from its supply except

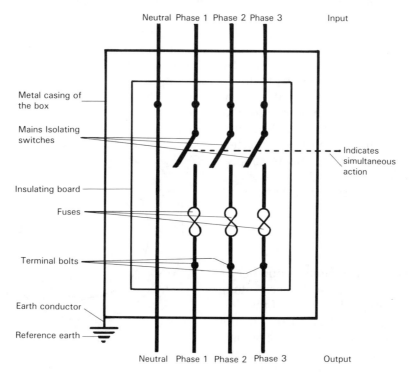

Fig. 2.9 Mains isolator box.

by the use of the isolator switch. There is never a plug and socket connection.

The earth connection on the mains isolator box is the main earth connection for the installation and must conform to prescribed safety standards. The earth continuity conductor attached to this connection must have a current carrying capacity at least equal to the largest current carrying conductor and the coupling of the conductor to the connection must also have the same current carrying capacity. For safety reasons, the coupling must require a tool for its disconnection. This earth connection is sometimes termed the 'Reference earth'.

Temporary connection for a mobile unit

Mobile units are connected by plug and socket to the 240 V domestic supply. The sockets are provided in many sites so that the X-ray unit or other electrical equipment has an electrical supply near to the place where the equipment will be used. The sockets are wired directly back to a hospital distribution board or into a ring main which supplies a number of socket outlets. A ring main is provided in most modern installations as it allows more flexible and economical use of the available supply. Whichever method of connection is provided, the circuit supplying the main is protected by a fuse or circuit breaker and in both cases the mains cable of the X-ray mobile unit terminates in a three-pin plug which can be inserted into any socket receiving the mains supply. The socket should be fitted with a switch so that before the plug is inserted or withdrawn, the supply can be switched off.

Ring main

A ring main is a circuit containing a number of separate sockets in series with each other around the circuit loop. The wiring of the ring is designed to carry the highest current that is expected to be drawn at any one time assuming that not all the sockets will be fully loaded at the same time and is fused accordingly. A typical ring circuit is protected by a fuse or cir-

cuit breaker rated at 30 A. Details of the design of fuses and circuit breakers are considered later in Chapter 9 where other safety devices are described.

Each piece of electrical equipment plugged into a socket must be protected by its own fuse. The value of the fuse selected must allow the normal current required by a piece of equipment to be drawn and also to protect the flexible cord connecting the equipment to the plug socket from overload current. If the total load on the ring main demands more than 30 A, the ring's own fuse or circuit breaker will operate to cut off the supply. Figure 2.10. shows how the sockets are supplied by the ring. Each ring has three conductor loops: a live line from a single phase, a neutral line and an earth line. When a socket is to be connected into the ring, a short length of wire from each line is bared of its insulating sheath and bent up so that part of the loop can be fitted into the appropriate terminal in the back of the socket.

In hospital installations, the earth in a ring main is not always a wire conductor, but may be the metal conduit (tubing) carrying the insulated live and neutral conductors or the copper sheath of the MICC (Mineral Insulated Copper Cable). The metal socket boxes are soundly connected to the metal conduit or copper sheath of the mineral insulated cable.

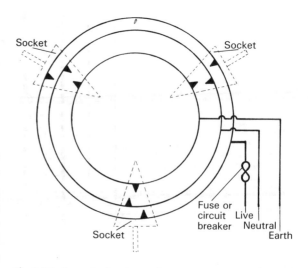

Fig. 2.10 Layout of a ring main.

This provides a very efficient, low resistance earth pathway. In addition it ensures that the conducting cables from the distribution board are carried within a strong rigid protective covering.

Design of a plug top (13 A)

The plug top is designed to give the maximum possible protection from electrical hazard. The standard plug top has three rectangular brass pins connecting with the three conductors supplying the socket (Fig. 2.11). The largest

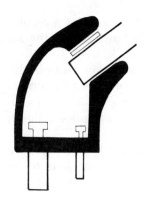

Fig. 2.12 'X-ray only' plug.

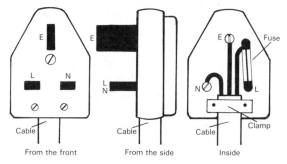

Fig. 2.11 3-pin plug (13 A).

and longest pin is in the apex of the triangular-shaped top and is the earth connection. As this pin is longer than the others, it ensures that it is the first to connect with its conductor when the plug top is pushed into the socket and the last to break its connection when the plug is removed. The insertion of the earth pin displaces a cover from the sockets for the other two pins. This prevents any child poking a metal object into the socket. The remaining two pins are aligned across the base of the triangle; one pin connects the live supply to the equipment through a fuse, while the other connects directly with the neutral return line.

'X-ray only' plug (Fig. 2.12). This plug is specially designed for use with mobile X-ray units. The arrangement of pins is similar to a standard plug, but there are a number of modifications necessary to suit its particular purpose. These are:

a. no fuse within the plug.

b. a top which is larger and more rounded to allow for the much thicker mains cable from

the unit to be connected with the terminals within it.

c. a much larger cable entry opening to accommodate the thicker cable required to supply a high-powered unit.

d. an insulated cover made of thick red plastic with larger fixing screws to withstand the strain of the thicker and heavier supply cable for the X-ray mobile unit.

e. a red plug to draw attention to its special and limited function with the words 'X-ray only' clearly scribed upon it. This is essential as the plug contains **no** fuse and can draw up to the full 30 A available from the ring.

Safety features provided by the design and method of manufacture of all plug and socket connections

These include:

a. a moulded insulating plastic cover which will not easily break.

b. a clamp to fix the cable within the plastic cover to prevent pulling strain on connections made with the terminals within the plug.

c. provision for the fitting of a fuse of appropriate value to suit the equipment connected through it and protect its flexible cable except for the 'x-ray only' plug.

d. a very good earth connection obtained by ensuring that the earth line is connected first and disconnected last because its connecting pin is longer than the other pins. The use of a larger and longer pin reduces the resistance between the connecting surfaces of the pin and socket. Its size also prevents it being inserted into one of the supply connections of the socket.

e. plastic sleeving around the top of the pins may be provided to protect any foolish person touching the live line with a metal lever being used to remove a tightly fitting plug from its socket.

f. large areas for electrical contact between the pins and their sockets to reduce the resistance at their junctions and to reduce heat production.

g. the shape and location of the pins makes it impossible for the plug to be put into the socket in any way other than when correctly orientated.

h. identification by initial letter of the pins provides yet another means of ensuring correct wiring.

i. secure fixing of the conductors to the pins inside the plug prevents detachment or loose connection.

j. firmly secured screws make it impossible to open the plug without a tool.

k. a shutter over the live and neutral pin socket which is only withdrawn when the plug's earth pin enters the socket.

l. a switched socket to allow the supply to be switched off before the equipment is connected or removed from the socket.

The mains cable of the X-ray mobile unit
The mains cable of the X-ray unit carries three conductors, each well insulated from the others and all three enclosed in a thick sleeve of insulating plastic. The thickness of the insulating covers of the conductors is dictated by the 240 V supplied to the X-ray unit. The thickness of the enclosing sheath is also controlled by the need to protect the contained conductors from mechanical damage. The conductors are colour coded to simplify their correct connection: brown for the live line, blue for the neutral and yellow/green for the earth. The cross-sectional area of the conductor is determined by the maximum current drawn by the unit, the length of the mains cable and the manufacturer's impedance specification.

The use of adaptors and extension leads is to be deprecated since:

a. the level of safety provided by the earth path is reduced by an additional break in its continuity, there being an increase in its resistance every time a junction is introduced.

b. any increase in the length of the cable increases the voltage drop and may affect the performance of the unit and make management of the unit more difficult.

Care in the use and observations to be made of the mains cable of a mobile unit and its plug and socket before, during and after the unit is used
a. The plug and mains cable must not be damaged by crushing beneath or between parts of the X-ray unit, nor must the cable be pulled tightly round structures.

b. The cable must not be allowed to become twisted or knotted.

c. The cable must never be strained by stretching it too far from the socket or by removing the plug from the socket by pulling on the cable.

d. The mains cable should be examined before use for any damage to its covering. If the contained conductors are exposed, the unit should not be connected to the mains supply.

e. The cable must be checked to see that it is securely clamped where it enters the plug top.

f. The plug must be examined to see that it is not damaged and that the cover and body are firmly screwed together. The plug top should be shaken and if it rattles, the plug should be opened by the maintenance engineer to check that all the conductors are firmly attached to their terminals. A rattle may well indicate that one of the terminals is loose, in which case it is very unwise to connect the unit to the mains supply.

g. The socket should be switched off before the plug is inserted into the socket, and the operator should examine the socket and not use it if there is any doubt about its condition.

h. If a pin(s) is found to be hot after an exposure has been made, this should be reported as it may indicate that an excessive current has been drawn, or more likely that the pin is making poor contact in the socket because the socket is worn and should be replaced.

Radiographers working in the Health Service are not permitted to undertake any electrical or mechanical repairs, but are required under the Health and Safety at Work Act to report any potential hazard and not use equipment which may cause harm to themselves or others.

3

The electrical circuit of an X-ray unit

HIGH VOLTAGE GENERATOR'S MAINS CONNECTION

The electrical supply for a fixed X-ray unit is obtained by connecting it to the output of a mains isolator unit and a mobile unit by a plug and socket. Both methods of connection have been described in Chapter 2.

In addition to the isolating units, all high voltage generators have their own isolator and protection against overload. The isolator of a portable or dental unit is a simple On/Off switch, but in the mobile or fixed unit a more sophisticated system is needed. The overload protection for a portable unit is a cartridge fuse or a thermal circuit breaker, but in a mobile or a fixed unit an electromagnetic circuit breaker is incorporated in the switch system. The introduction of an electromagnetic circuit breaker has many advantages over the simpler systems as it gives adequate protection for the low powered mobile unit from overload but is not sophisticated enough to protect a major unit from overload.

The level of protection required depends upon the technical demands made by the unit. Generally, the more highly rated the unit, the more elaborate must be the protection. Highly rated units are required to give heavy exposures and on occasions may be required to undertake rapid repetitive exposures. Under these conditions, the X-ray high voltage generator will draw very high currents, and to protect the high voltage generator from excessively high currents which can arise under faulty conditions, such as sudden massive breakdown of an X-ray tube or high voltage cable requires a system that is able to respond rapidly to the sudden excess currents which if allowed to pass might cause damage to the generator.

The additional features provided by an electromagnetic circuit breaker which are not provided by a simpler system include:

a. a quick and easy reset mechanism for use once the cause of the overload has been overcome.

b. a precise method of setting up the point at which the unit will operate to disconnect the unit.

c. a much quicker response to a heavy overload, but at the same time having a degree of tolerance to a harmless short-lived voltage surge.

d. the inclusion of a remotely operated On/Off switch in its circuitry increasing electrical safety for the operators.

The electromagnetic circuit breaker (Fig. 3.1) is housed in a wall-mounted metal box or within one of the high voltage generator sub-assemblies. The electrical supply for the unit passes through the box from the mains isolator to the control unit. Its function is to allow the operator to switch on the X-ray unit safely, and by the design of the unit act as an automatic circuit breaker should an overload occur.

The conductors supplying the unit are connected through two switches which are closed and kept closed by a solenoid. This solenoid forms part of a control circuit operated from the control panel. The operator completes this control circuit by pressing the Main On button. When this button switch is operated the solenoid is energised, which in turn closes the 'by-pass holding' contact in subsidiary circuit. The 'holding' contact is essential to the operation of the unit for it allows the operator to remove pressure from the On switch without causing the unit to switch itself off. Once

pressure is taken off the press-button it returns to its normal position ready to be used again.

When the operator pushes the Off button it breaks the continuity of the control circuit causing the solenoid to cease to hold the switches in the unit supply and the holding contact closed. The unit is then disconnected from its supply which can only be restored by operating the Mains On switch again. Examination of the control circuit shows that it is protected by a low-value fuse, normally a 5 A, and a key-switch to prevent any unauthorised

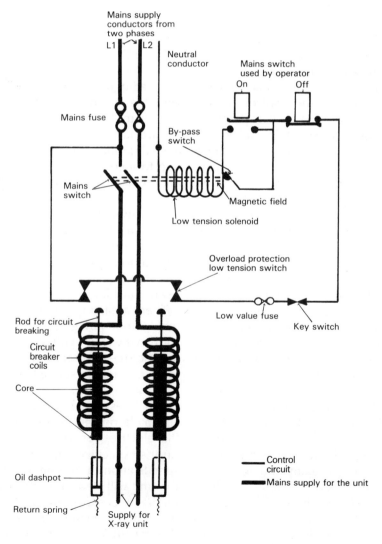

Fig. 3.1 Electromagnetic circuit breaker.

person using the unit. By means of the control circuit the operator remotely switches the 415 V supply for the unit. The control circuit is supplied with 240 V by connecting it between one phase of the mains supply and the neutral supply. Figure 3.1 shows the control circuit in a fine line and the unit supply in a bold line.

When the switches in the generator's supply are closed the X-ray unit is ready for use and comes under the control of other circuits which enable it to perform as required by the technique and is protected from damage to itself or personnel in contact with it. Figure 3.1 shows that the conductors leading to the unit are connected through the coils of the circuit breaker. Should an overload current occur, the excess current passing through the coils will, by magnetic attraction, draw the cores further into the coils causing the attached rods to break the contacts in the control circuit. The breaking of these contacts will interrupt the current through the solenoid coil in the control circuit with the result that there will be no magnetic field to hold the mains supply switches closed. When this occurs the supply to the unit will be cut off.

When a normal current is passing through the conductors the magnetic field is not strong enough to draw the cores in far enough to cause the control switches to be broken. In this way the unit is protected from an excess current. If the excess current is only the result of a very short-lived surge, the switches may not be broken as each core is connected to an oil dashpot which delays the action by a short time. The dashpot can be set to ensure the delay will not allow a current to pass which could do harm. If a very high current passes, the magnetic effect will be great enough to override any delaying effect of the dashpot. Once the high current ceases to pass through the coils the cores will be drawn out of the coils by return springs taking the rods back with them. The contacts on the remote switching circuit are no longer held apart and will close restoring the control circuit to its normal switched off position. The operator

can then switch the unit on again. Should the fault not be a transient one, the supply interrupting sequence will occur again making it impossible to use the unit until the fault causing the excess current is corrected.

It is important that the electromagnetic circuit breaker chosen to suit the particular generator is set to operate with an overload current slightly less than that needed to 'blow' the fuse. This allows the operator to reset the circuit breaker and continue to work without the delay or inconvenience, which occurs when an engineer has to be called to replace the fuse.

THE PROVISION OF A STABLE VOLTAGE INPUT FOR THE X-RAY UNIT

The radiographer requires the X-ray unit to generate X-radiation of a consistent quality and quantity every time the same set of exposure factors are selected. Without consistency the number of unsatisfactory radiographs due to incorrect exposure will be large, causing unjustifiable additional radiation of the patient, extra cost in materials and time for the examination to the Health Service. Variation in the mains input leads to changes in X-ray output. An examination of the effect of a change in mains input on mA and kVp will be undertaken after the autotransformer has been considered.

There are many factors which cause an incorrect output. Of great importance is the variation in the mains voltage supplied to the unit. If this source of variation can be overcome, there is at least a stable base-line on which the unit can function. To achieve this stable base-line it is essential that pre-installation checks are made on the mains supply to ensure that the electrical provision reaches the manufacturer's specification. If the manufacturer's specification cannot be reached, the output of the unit will never be satisfactory whatever remedial measures are introduced. Assuming the nominal mains voltage to the unit fulfils the manufacturer's requirements, there will still be variation in the input voltage to the unit. These arise as a result of:

a. the location of a mobile unit — different supply outlets will have different line (supply cable) impedance.

b. changes in voltage from the mains supply.

c. varying demands by other equipment drawing from the supply.

d. different load current drawn by the X-ray tube when a choice of tube currents is available.

Analysis of the voltage variation shows that it can be divided into three types based on the time span over which changes occur. These are:

a. the permanent voltage variation from the base-line due to the impedance of the line at the outlet point.

b. variations which last for a considerable part of the day.

c. rapid changes lasting for only a very short time, the result of sudden alterations in the load on the supply or sudden changes at the generator.

The effect of the radiographic exposure must also be allowed for; methods of overcoming variations derived from this source will be considered later. Permanent and slow changes from the base-line can be allowed for by arranging compensation as they occur and can take place in the intervals between radiographic exposures. The compensating devices are either manually or automatically operated up to the start of the 'prepare' stage of the radiographic exposure. Compensating devices operate by comparing the incoming voltage with a predetermined base-line or nominated voltage and then adjusting the outgoing voltage up or down until it is equal to the base-line voltage so ensuring a stable output.

A voltage compensating device can only allow correction over a fairly narrow range of voltage variation from about 5–10% above, to 5–10% below the normal base-line voltage

value. The base-line is set by the manufacturer of the equipment.

Line resistance compensation

The purpose of this unit is to bring the total line resistance value at the input point to a value specified by the manufacturer. With the total line resistance fixed at this value, it is comparatively simple to compensate for the voltage drop caused by the current drawn when the tube load is applied.

There are two types of line resistance compensators: a simple one for the permanently fixed unit and a more elaborate one for the mobile unit. The design and operating principles are set out below.

Line resistance compensation for a permanently fixed unit
This is generally a simple variable resistor which is connected in series with the X-ray circuit. Its value is adjusted until it modifies the outlet voltage to the base-line voltage. Once its value is set during the installation of the unit, there is no need for further adjustment. This compensator is placed within the unit, as there is no need for further access.

Variable line resistance compensation for a mobile unit
The situation is very different when the X-ray unit is mobile and can take its supply from many outlet points around the hospital, for each outlet will have a different voltage output, the result of different line resistance. To overcome the variation in supply it is necessary to allow a different resistance to be selected in the compensator. The line resistance at each outlet point is measured so that the value of the line resistance compensating resistor can be matched to the needs of the particular outlet socket. There are generally half a dozen resistance values which can be selected on the control panel. Each position on the selector is either labelled with the ward where it should be used, or, rather more

satisfactorily, the outlet socket is marked with the control position which should be selected. The selection may be by a rotating knob with connecting studs, or by a series of push buttons which allow the appropriate value of resistance to be placed in series with the X-ray unit circuit. Figure 3.2 shows a variable resistance compensator and indicates its position in the X-ray circuit. An alternative name for this compensator is a 'padding' resistor.

This compensator may not be found on old mobile units. The radiographer who uses such a unit will adjust the exposure factors to allow for any variation in X-ray output arising from the inability to compensate for the differences in line resistance at different main supply sockets. This empirical approach is fairly satisfactory with low output units but when higher output units having higher tube currents cause significant voltage drop on load, even the experienced radiographer will find it almost impossible to judge the effect of this on X-ray output correctly and will frequently produce radiographs which are not satisfactorily exposed.

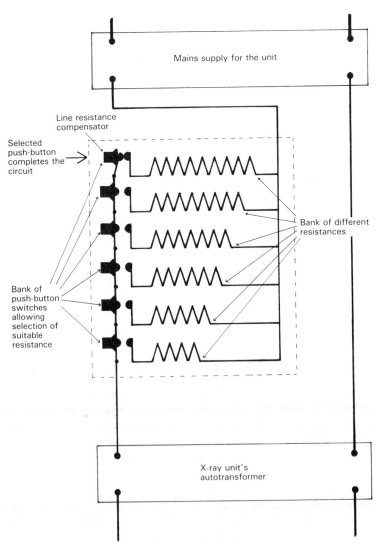

Fig. 3.2 Line resistance compensator.

Modern capacitor discharge units will not require a line resistance compensator as they have no critical line resistance requirements.

THE AUTOTRANSFORMER

After passing through the mains isolator and after correction by the line resistance compensator, the mains voltage is connected to the input side of the X-ray unit's autotransformer. This unit can be safely housed in the X-ray generator's control unit as its voltage is no greater than the mains supply.

It is a simple device performing a number of functions:

a. compensation for changes in the mains voltage.

b. provision of a voltage for the tube filament circuit.

c. provision of the primary voltage for the high tension transformer which can be altered to allow a change in the X-ray beam quality.

d. provision of a kVp meter compensator to make a prereading kVp meter read the on-load value.

e. provision of suitable voltages for the subsidiary circuits.

Each of these functions will be described in more detail later (pp 22–28), but first it is important to consider very briefly the design and operation of an autotransformer, and to list how this unit is superior to two other means which could have been used instead of an autotransformer.

Design and function of an autotransformer

The autotransformer's operating principle is self induction. It has one winding on a laminated closed core. The single winding is formed from shellac-coated copper wire, that has a comparatively large rectangular cross-section. The flat sides of the tape-like wire facilitates the connection of tappings (conductors) to many individual turns. In some modern units a small area on the top of the coil is cleared of the insulating shellac so that the copper is exposed and can connect with a fine carbon brush. This can be motor driven to a particular turn where electrical connection can be made, thus providing an alternative method of connection to the numerous tapping connections. For simplicity, the older system will be described.

The tappings are taken to terminals where they may act as a step-up or a step-down transformer. Figure 3.3 features a very simple autotransformer. The passing of a current through the turns between the input tappings will induce a flow of magnetic flux round the core. This magnetic flux will link with all the turns forming the coil. Assuming the autotransformer to be a 'perfect' transformer, the volts per turn will be equal to the quotient of the input voltage and the number of turns between the two tappings connected to the input supply. For example, if the input voltage is 400 V and there are 200 turns, the volts per turn will be 2. Therefore, if an output is taken from two tappings with 300 turns between them, the output voltage will be 2×300 V, 600 V — the unit has acted as a step-up transformer. On the other hand, if the output is connected across only 100 turns the output will be 2×100 V, 200 V, — a step-down effect. The range of voltage change in an autotrans-

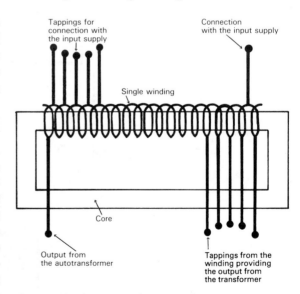

Fig. 3.3 Simple autotransformer to show its connections.

former is somewhat limited by its construction, normally the voltage cannot be reduced to less than a half or increased more than twice the original value. There are power losses in an autotransformer as in any other form of transformer but they are kept to as low a value as possible by the design and construction of the unit.

Value of an autotransformer
a. Relatively simple
b. Robust
c. Fairly small
d. Able to accommodate a large number of tappings on the input and output side

e. Operated by manual controls sited on the X-ray unit's control panel
f. Able to control the output of the high tension transformer by varying the voltage supply to the primary winding of the high tension transformer
g. Able to maintain the volts per turn ratio at a constant value when the input voltage varies over quite a wide range of values
h. Able to supply a number of circuits with a suitable voltage because of its multiple tappings.

In the X-ray circuit it would be possible to perform some of the functions of the autotransformer by:

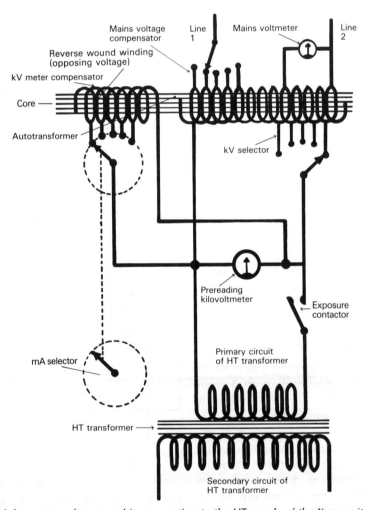

Fig. 3.4 Location of the autotransformer and its connection to the HT supply of the X-ray unit.

a double-wound transformer but this would be:

(i) much more expensive
(ii) much more difficult to vary the output because of the nature of the windings
(iii) more bulky.

a simple resistance control but this would :

(i) only allow the output to be reduced — no compensation for a low input mains voltage possible
(ii) use some of the available energy as the current would have to flow through the whole unit and not through only a proportion of the unit as in an autotransformer. Therefore, less energy is available for its principal use, the generation of X-rays.

Because of these disadvantages all X-ray units in use today have autotransformers.

Figure 3.4 shows the location of the autotransformer and its connection with the HT transformer in an X-ray unit.

Compensation for changes in mains voltage

Variations from the base-line mains voltage, which are comparatively long lived and occur between X-ray exposures, can be corrected by the autotransformer through its mains voltage compensator. The unit may be operated by the radiographer who is trained to look at a voltmeter for evidence of change and then take action to correct the change from normal. This procedure must continue until the exposure 'prepare' stage is reached. This method of control requires the radiographer to take her eyes off the patient being examined just at the moment when there is need for observation of the patient's phase of respiration, etc. Additionally, it relies on the radiographer's conscientious attention to detail which may not always be present. Therefore, automatic compensation is provided on most units, completely relieving the radiographer of any responsibility for manual operation of the compensator controls. In the text, the older manual method will be described as the principles are the same and then the modification allowing for automation will be added.

Manually adjusted mains voltage compensation

There are two essential parts to be considered:

1. the method of monitoring the input mains voltage so that the need for correction is apparent
2. the means of correcting the observed variation from the normal input mains voltage.

1. Monitoring — when the correct input voltage is applied across a known number of turns, a value of volts per turn can be calculated. This value will be constant for each turn, so if a voltmeter is connected across a fixed small number of turns this too will indicate a set value when the input voltage is correct. The meter does not need a numerical scale — it is sufficiently accurate, much quicker and easier to check whether the meter needle is sited between two lines or over a central coloured-band on the scale than it is to read a numerical value. Therefore, a mains voltmeter is connected between two tappings.

Figure 3.5 shows it connected one end to the same tapping as the input cable, L2 and the other end five turns away. For simplification of the diagram, the number of turns drawn in the diagram are many times fewer than in the actual unit, but using turns shown in the diagram and a normal value of 2 volts per turn, the mains voltmeter will read 2 × 5, 10 volts. The meter range is selected so that at 10 V the needle will register in the centre of the scale. Should the volts per turn fall, the needle will move from the centre to a lower value, or if the volts per turn rise above normal, the needle will move in the opposite direction. The radiographer having noticed the change adjusts the compensator until the needle returns to its correct position. A simple moving iron meter is satisfactory as the current passing through the meter is comparatively large and a fine degree of accuracy is not necessary.

2. Correction of variation from normal. For correction of a variation from normal, it is essential to maintain the correct volts per turn, since any supply drawn from the autotransformer will be dependant on this value. It is simple to correct a variation. The number of

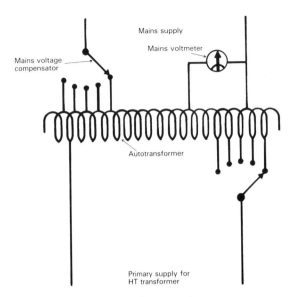

Fig. 3.5 Manually operated mains voltage compensator.

turns between the connecting points of the mains voltage supply has to be increased or decreased so that the standard volts per turn can be restored.

For example, if the normal base-line mains voltage of 400 V is connected across 200 turns, the volts per turn is 2; if the mains supply voltage drops to 380 V, the volts per turn will be 1.9 V, a change which will be observable on the mains voltmeter. The operator restores the value of volts per turn to 2 by decreasing the number of turns connected to 190, giving 380 V between 190 turns, the standard 2 volts per turn. If the mains voltage is in excess of 400, say 420, the number of turns must be increased to 210. Therefore, the compensator is a device allowing tappings from different turns to be connected.

In manual units the system used is generally a rotating knob selector, which makes connection through one of a number of stud terminals positioned around the border of the selector. The terminals receive conductors from the tapped turns of the autotransformer. The conductors from the tappings are long enough to allow the unit to be fitted on the control panel alongside the mains voltmeter

which indicates the necessity for correction of the unit. This is very convenient as the correction must be made immediately before the exposure takes place.

Automatic mains voltage compensator
The mains voltage compensator described above can be converted to an automatically controlled unit by exchanging the voltmeter for a voltage sensing device and the manually operated control for a motor driven device. The voltage sensing device samples the incoming voltage and compares the sample with an accurate reference voltage. The sample voltage, like the manual unit, draws its supply from the autotransformer. It has a fixed relationship with the mains input voltage and so will vary as the mains voltage varies.

If the sensing device finds a discrepancy between the sample voltage and the reference voltage, the compensating unit will automatically direct a motor to drive a carbon brush along the surface of the autotransformer winding to make contact with a particular turn which will give the correct turns ratio. The motor may drive the brush in either direction, connecting across more turns if the sensed voltage is high or across fewer if the voltage is low. The sensing-correction process is continuous, ensuring that any mains voltage variation is corrected at once, and continuing right up to the 'prepare' position before exposure.

Figure 3.6 illustrates the essential features of this automatic system and although there are many variations in the method of obtaining automatic compensation, they all work on the sense-correct system; it is the circuitry of the sensing device and the drive method that varies.

The radiographic effects of an incorrect mains voltage input
If the mains voltage supplying the unit is not at the prescribed value, the normal base-line value, there will be variation from the expected X-ray tube output, and the quantity of radiation generated will be affected as will the

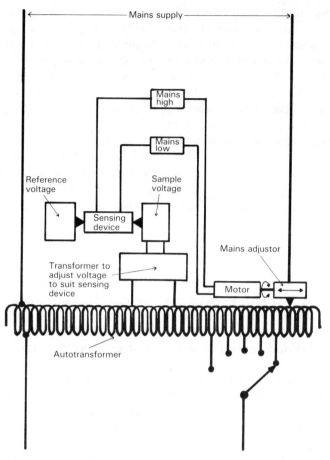

Fig. 3.6 Automatic mains voltage compensator.

quality of the beam. Other subsidiary and accessory circuits will also be affected which may have an indirect effect on the radiographic image. Therefore, there will be:

a. increased or decreased film density, due to a difference in the tube filament electron emission resulting in a larger or smaller number of X-ray photons being generated at the target. Since the electron emission by the filament is very sensitive to small changes in filament voltage (see p. 33), the filament circuit is provided with further stabilisation, but even with this additional unit which can only operate over a narrow range of voltage change, any mains voltage variation which goes uncorrected will be apparent on the radiograph.

b. increased or decreased subject penetration will arise if a mains variation is not corrected, although the magnitude of the change will not be great and in most instances the effect will not be observable in the radiograph. A calculation which will illustrate the effect of a voltage change on the resultant kVp can be seen on page 29. The alteration in the kVp is the result of the variation on the primary winding of the HT transformer which is reflected on the secondary winding output. Should the unit be provided with a pre-reading kVp meter, the radiographer will observe the low kilovoltage and correct it before making the exposure, so compensating for the incorrect setting of the mains voltage.

Provision of a voltage for the tube filament circuit

The supply for the X-ray tube filament circuit

is provided by connecting the circuit between two tappings from the autotransformer. The number of turns between the tapping is determined by the value of voltage required and the volts per turn value. In the text, when the filament circuit is considered, a value of 160 V has been selected as a reasonable value for this circuit in a modern unit. The full filament circuit will be considered as a separate section.

Provision of a supply for the primary winding of the HT transformer and the method of varying its value

In radiography it is necessary to vary the quality of the X-ray beam to provide optimum penetration of the subject. The quality of the beam depends upon the kilovoltage across the X-ray tube. The voltage is provided by the secondary winding of the HT transformer whose primary voltage is obtained from the autotransformer. Due to the need to vary the kilovoltage, a means of varying the supply to the primary winding is arranged by connecting to the autotransformer through a device, known as the kVp selector (see Fig. 3.7). This allows a connection to be made to any one of a series of tappings on the autotransformer. When the

selector is operated the number of turns between the points of connection, the tapping, is altered, providing a different voltage to the primary winding of the HT transformer, which is reflected in the secondary voltage. In this way it is possible for the operator to select a suitable kilovoltage to generate X-rays which will penetrate the organs under examination.

The kV selector unit may be a simple rotary unit or a bank of switches to which are brought conductors from a number of tappings on the autotransformer. In general units, the tappings allow a range of voltages from 50–150 V to be selected in steps of 2–2.5 kV. Selection of a particular voltage on the control panel connects the primary supply of the HT transformer through the tapping on the autotransformer which will, when stepped-up by the HT transformer, provide the selected voltage across the X-ray tube. It is important when a rotary control is used that the kilovoltage is not changed during an exposure, for each kV position has a discrete stud through which current passes during the exposure. If the kV selector is altered during the exposure, arcing will take place at the connection. The heat produced will distort the connecting surfaces and so increase the resistance at the switch, necessitating regular service if a fall off of X-ray production is not to be apparent in the radiograph.

In modern units this problem is overcome by using a control which drives a selector motor carrying a carbon brush along the autotransformer winding to make contact with the selected turn. Where fluoroscopy is provided in addition to radiography, the kVp selector is duplicated, providing one for selection of a radiographic kilovoltage and the other, which has a more limited range of kilovoltages for selection, for fluoroscopy. This duplication allows a radiographic exposure to be set whilst fluoroscopy continues, thereby enabling a radiographic exposure to be made immediately after fluoroscopy has ended.

kV meter compensation

In some units the kilovoltage selected is dis-

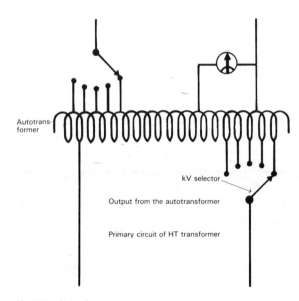

Autotransformer

kV selector

Output from the autotransformer

Primary circuit of HT transformer

Fig. 3.7 kV selector.

played by a voltmeter connected across the input for the primary winding of the HT transformer. The voltmeter is connected across the supply before the exposure switch so that it will record the selected kVp before the exposure takes place — hence its name of pre-reading kilovoltmeter. It can in addition record the actual voltage during the exposure. As there is a discrepancy between the voltage before the exposure and the voltage actually applied during the exposure, the radiographer must know the actual value during the exposure as this value governs the quality of the X-ray beam. The discrepancy between the two values is caused by the voltage drop which

occurs when the X-ray tube conducts.

The magnitude of the discrepancy is not fixed, so it will vary with a change in the tube current (mA) selected. Therefore a kV meter compensator (Fig. 3.8) is provided to make the necessary correction to the reading so that although the meter registers before the exposure, the value displayed is what it will be during the exposure. This is obtained by applying an opposing voltage on the meter before the exposure which will have the same effect on the meter's reading as the exposure load voltage drop occurring when the tube is conducting. The opposing voltage must be removed before the exposure takes

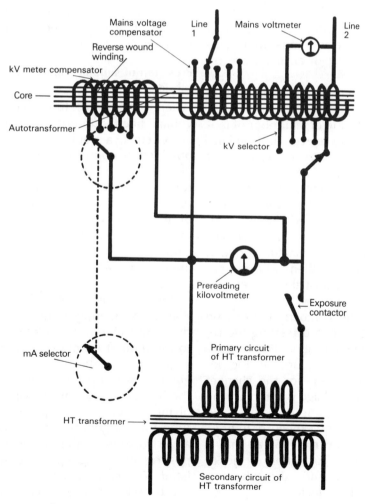

Fig. 3.8 kV meter compensator.

place; it is one of the actions that takes place automatically when the unit is brought up to 'prepare'.

The opposing voltage to be applied to the meter is obtained by winding a small extra coil on the autotransformer core. The important feature of this coil is that it is connected so that it opposes the voltage from the main winding of the autotransformer. The winding of this extra coil will have the same magnetic flux flowing through it as the main coil, but because the winding is in the reverse direction the electromotive force developed in the winding will have its polarity opposite to that of the autotransformer winding. If the compensator winding is also connected to the meter, its action on the meter is to oppose the needle movement caused by the supply from the autotransformer causing it to read less than the true value of the autotransformer output, simulating the effect of an exposure on the meter.

To allow for the effect of a change in tube current, one of the connections to the reverse wound coil is made to one of a number of tappings through a rotating selector unit linking it with the appropriate turn. The selection of the tapping is made by a linkage, often mechanical, with the mA selector, so that as a particular mA is selected by the radiographer, the correct position is selected on the compensator so that the reverse voltage reduces the indicated voltage to the actual on-load voltage. The radiographer, then, will observe the fall in voltage and adjust the kV selector to give the required value.

The efficiency of the compensator can be seen by the operator, since by setting the required kVp and then changing the mA selected, the kVp will drop, and if the kV selector is altered to correct for the change, then when the reverse voltage is removed the kVp will read the same value during the exposure as it read before the exposure. In practice a slight 'kick' on the meter is all that is generally seen. To avoid correction of the kV when setting up an exposure, the tube current, the mA should be selected first.

The prereading kV meter is a moving iron meter. It measures the voltage from the autotransformer that is to be applied to the primary of the high voltage transformer and to make the reading taken before any current is drawn to correspond to the value that will exist during the actual loading of the X-ray tube. As an example, assume that the X-ray tube is to be operated in the range of 50–150 kVp. This corresponds to r.m.s. values of 35–106 kV. If the ratio of the HV transformer is 1000:1, then the primary voltage required will be 35–106 $V_{r.m.s.}$, a range that is convenient for the autotransformer to provide. The prereading meter actually measures the primary voltage but its scale is marked in the corresponding values of the tube voltage, in this case 50–150 kVp. It is important to appreciate that this meter is not connected directly in the high voltage circuit.

Provision of suitable voltages for many subsidiary circuits

When the manufacturer has calculated the voltage needed to operate one of the subsidiary circuits, a stable voltage of this value is obtained by connecting the circuit to two tappings separated by the appropriate number of turns. The output will be stable as the volts per turn has been adjusted to the correct value by the mains voltage compensator. Examples of circuits supplied by the autotransformer include those for the tube stator, the timer, and interlock circuits.

Calculation of power used for an exposure

Before considering in detail circuits supplying the tube filament and the high voltage supply to the tube, it is important to be aware of the magnitude of the power used by a radiographic exposure and the effect of drawing the necessary current through the cables supplying the unit on the power available at the tube for the generation of X-rays. Therefore, as an illustration, the power used for two exposures on a single-phase unit will be calculated. The current drawn through the mains will be calculated for a mains supply of 415 V and 240 V. Finally, for a given line resistance value the voltage drop will be determined. To simplify the calculation, the efficiency of the system is taken as 100% whereas in practice this would be nearer 80%.

The determination of the true power used by an X-ray exposure is quite difficult to determine, but a simple convention is widely used for arriving at it. The convention is that power P is given by the following

$P = V \times I \times f$ watts

where V is the peak voltage in kV
I the average tube current mA
f is a factor depending on the type of rectification. A single-phase generator has an f factor of 0.74.

Example 1
Exposure: 70 kVp   800 mA
Using the convention $P = V \times I \times f$ watts
Power $= 70 \times 800 \times 0.74$ W
$= \dfrac{70 \times 800 \times 0.74}{1000}$ kW
$= 41.4$ kW

Current drawn when the mains voltage available is 415 V
Since Watts = Volts × Amps
Current $= \dfrac{41\ 400}{415}$ A
$= 100$A

Current drawn when the mains voltage is 240 V
Current $= \dfrac{41\ 400}{240}$ A
$= 173$A

Example 2
Exposure: 70 kVp   100 mA
Power $= 70 \times 100 \times 0.74$ W
$= 5.2$ kW

Current $= \dfrac{5200}{415}$ A
$= 12.5$A

You will see that the power in Example 1 is eight times that in Example 2. This is because power is proportional to tube current.

Considering the two examples using 415 V mains supply, the effect on voltage drop resulting from the two currents can be compared. A line resistance of 0.2 ohm is assumed.

Example 1   100 A   V = I R
                          V = 100× 0.2
                          V = 20.0
Example 2   12.5 A   V = I R
                          V = 12.5 × 0.2
                          V = 2.5

Example 1 drawing a current of 100 A causes a voltage drop of 20.0 V, whilst Example 2 causes a loss of only 2.5 V. It is obvious that when the mA is high the voltage drop will be greater and this will reflect on the kilovoltage considerably, therefore the meter reading compensator must be adjusted to suit the mA selected for in the second example the effect on the kilovoltage will be much less.

Further examination of the first example will show how advantageous it is to use the highest mains voltage available, in this example the two values are 100 A and 173 A. The 173 A will cause a much greater voltage drop than the 100 A which is the current drawn when 415 V is used. This effect has already been discussed earlier in the text when the mains voltage supply was considered.

Calculation of the effect of voltage loss on mA and kVp

Before leaving consideration of the autotransformer and its function, it is instructive to calculate the magnitude of the loss in kVp and mA output from an X-ray tube if there is no correction either manual or automatic of a low mains voltage

To illustrate the effect on kVp
Assume the normal base-line input voltage of 410 V and that the input tappings are separ-

ated by 820 turns of the autotransformer. The HT transformer has a ratio of 1:1000 and for the purpose of this calculation has no losses. The supply to the primary winding of the HT transformer is drawn from two tappings 120 turns apart.

First calculate the kVp applied to the X-ray tube when the mains voltage is at its correct value (410 V r.m.s.)

Input mains voltage   410 V r.m.s.
Volts per turn on autotransformer

$$\frac{410}{820} = 0.5 \text{ V per turn}$$

Primary voltage for 120 turns on autotransformer applied to the primary winding 120 × 0.5 V r.m.s. = 60 V r.m.s.

Secondary voltage from the HT transformer with a ratio of 1:1000 = 60 × 1000 V r.m.s. = 60 kV r.m.s.

The voltage applied to the X-ray tube is quoted in kVp. Therefore the voltage in this example is 60 kV r.m.s. × 1.414 = 85 kVP

Then repeat the calculation using the low input voltage of 400 V r.m.s.

Input mains voltage   400 V r.m.s.
Volts per turn on autotransformer 400 = 0.49 V per turn
Primary voltage from 200 turns on autotransformer applied to primary winding   120 × 0.49 V r.m.s. = 59 V r.m.s.

Secondary voltage from the HT transformer with a ratio of 1:1000 = 59 × 1000 V r.m.s. = 59 kV r.m.s.

The voltage applied to the X-ray tube is kVp for the low input mains is 59 V r.m.s. × 1.414 = 83.4 kVp

Therefore the difference in kVp resulting from the low input mains voltage, 2.5% low (400 V instead of 410 V) is 83.5 kVp instead of 85 kVp = 1.5 kVp

In practice, the small change in the radiographic image resulting from the drop in kVp will not be apparent but the importance of a correct setting of the mains input voltage will become obvious when the effect of a 2.5%

drop in the mains voltage is applied to the X-ray tube filament.

To illustrate the effect on mA
Every X-ray tube filament has its own characteristics so when calculating the value of the tube current generated, it is necessary to consult the manufacturer's data sheet for the particular X-ray tube insert, the particular filament within the tube and for the type of generator waveform that is supplying the tube.

Therefore, this example is worked through using the data for one particular filament. The filament voltage is obtained from the autotransformer by connecting between 320 turns using the same value of 0.5 V per turn with the mains voltage at its correct value. The filament is supplied through a step-down transformer of ratio 16:1. For simplicity, any resistance in the filament circuit has been disregarded as the purpose of this calculation is to illustrate the effect of setting the mains voltage incorrectly.

The filament circuit voltage obtained from the autotransformer is:

320 × 0.5 V r.m.s. = 160 V r.m.s.

After being stepped down by the filament transformer the voltage actually applied to the filament is:

$$160 \times \frac{1}{16} = 10 \text{ V}$$

The value of the filament current is obtained from the manufacturer's graph. The graph takes into account the filament characteristics. In the graph provided (Fig. 3.9) the 10 V gives a filament current of 5.05 A. When this value of 5.05 A is used in the second graph (Fig. 3.10) it can be seen that for 85 kVp a filament current of 5.05A will give a tube current of 550 mA. If the calculation is repeated using the reduced value of 0.4 V per turn, the result of a reduction in the mains voltage, the filament voltage is reduced to 9.8 V giving a filament current of 5.0 A which provides only 500 mA at 85 kVp.

Therefore, for a small loss of 2.5% on the mains input voltage, there is a 9% change in

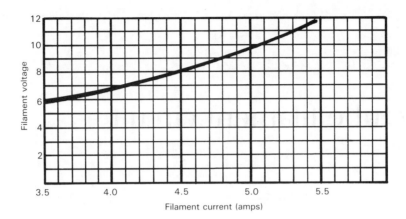

Fig. 3.9 Value of filament current obtained from various filament voltages (applicable to one particular focus).

mA output. This change will certainly be apparent as a loss in density on the radiograph, making the radiograph unacceptable. Hence the importance of compensation for mains voltage variation and stabilisation of the filament voltage, for without these, there can be no standardisation of radiographic density for a given set of exposure factors, especially as in normal working conditions a 5% voltage drop can be expected. If no voltage compensator is provided both the tube voltage and the tube current will be affected. A drop of 5% in the mains voltage will reduce the radiation emitted from the X-ray tube by 34%.

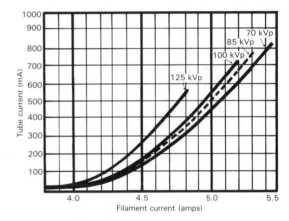

Fig. 3.10 Value of the tube current (mA) obtained from the use of various values of filament current at selected kilovoltages.

4

X-ray tube filament circuit

The X-ray tube filament is supplied by an electrical circuit whose main components are:

1. voltage stabilizer
2. space charge compensator
3. mA selector
4. filament transformer.

The block diagram (Fig. 4.1) shows the position of these components in the circuit, which will be considered separately.

The function of the filament circuit is to heat the filament to very exact temperatures so that the number of electrons freed by thermionic emission from the filament is just right to give precisely the tube current selected by the radiographer generating the required quantity of X-radiation. To fulfil this function the circuit must ensure that the number of electrons passing from the cathode to anode, comprising the tube current, are shielded from any external conditions and adjusted to accommodate any internal variations resulting from changes in exposure factors.

VOLTAGE SUPPLY FOR THE CIRCUIT

The voltage supply for the filament circuit is obtained from two tappings from the winding of the autotransformer. The output from the autotransformer is maintained at the correct value by the mains voltage compensator up to the point when the exposure enters the 'pre-

pare' period. Because of the need to provide a stable output during the actual exposure the voltage is further stabilised.

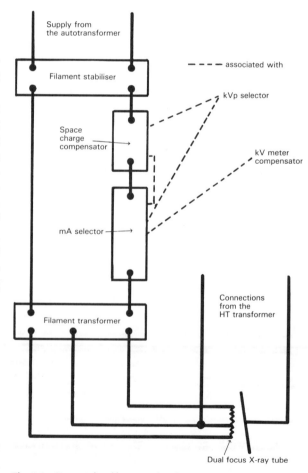

Fig. 4.1 X-ray tube filament circuit.

32

VOLTAGE STABILISER

The functions of the voltage stabiliser in the filament circuit are:

a. to correct any small change occurring during the radiographic exposure from the normal value of the voltage supply to the filament circuit.

b. to compensate for any change in mains frequency by adjusting the voltage supply to the filament to overcome the effect of the frequency change on the filament. It is not possible to alter the frequency which is fixed by the speed of rotation of the generator at the power station.

In most modern X-ray units there is an electronic voltage stabiliser. It is connected into the filament circuit immediately after the supply for the circuit is obtained from the autotransformer.

Electronic voltage stabiliser

This stabiliser is the unit of choice because it will perform both functions, compensating for variations in the voltage and frequency of the mains supply rapidly and automatically, so ensuring that there will be no evidence of voltage variation on the radiograph provided that the mains voltage compensator has been adjusted before the exposure sequence starts.

The principal component of the unit is a transducer which is a form of saturable reactor. The unit functions by monitoring the output from the transducer by sampling the output voltage and comparing this with a very accurately produced reference voltage. If comparison shows a discrepancy between the sample and the reference voltage, the unit automatically corrects the output by adding to or subtracting from the input voltage so that the output voltage is restored to its correct value. The monitoring by sampling and comparing with a reference voltage and correcting any discrepancy operates continuously.

Examination of Figure 4.2, the outline of the unit, shows that one of the input lines is wound round two limbs of a three-limbed

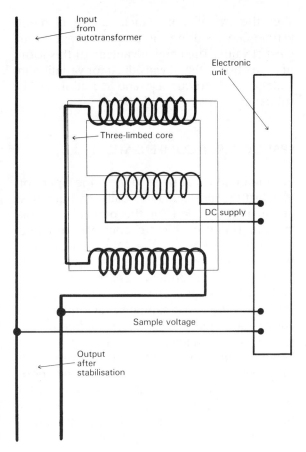

Fig. 4.2 Electronic voltage stabiliser.

core. Notice that the winding on one limb is in the opposite direction to the other winding so that the impedance produced by one winding is equal and opposite to that produced by the other. Therefore the impedance of one winding cancels out the impedance of the other. The unit corrects the output voltage by making the impedance of one coil differ from the other causing the output voltage to vary from the input by the magnitude of the altered impedance. Impedance can be varied by introducing an additional magnetic flux to the core by winding an additional coil on the centre limb of the core. The additional coil is provided with a DC supply from an electronic control unit. If the output is found to be incorrect by the sampling system, the electronic control adjusts the DC supply to the coil so varying the flux produced by it. This change in the value of flux will alter the overall impedance to the filament winding so restoring the output voltage to its correct value. The chief advantage of this form of regulation is that it will adjust for variation in voltage and frequency and additionally is robust and uses negligible power.

SPACE CHARGE COMPENSATION

In radiography it is necessary for the operator to select the most suitable quality and quantity of radiation needed for the particular examination. Therefore X-ray circuits are designed to ensure that when the kVp is increased, there is no increase in tube current, i.e. kVp and mA are independent of each other.

Up to 100 mA, it is only necessary to operate the X-ray tube in the saturated region because above saturation all the electrons freed from the heated filament are drawn across to the anode by the positive potential and even when this potential is increased, there are no more electrons available to be drawn across, so the tube current remains the same. Remember tube current (mA) is determined by the number of electrons passing from cathode to anode in one second. For tube currents above 100 mA there is some increase in mA for a rise in kVp, due to an increase in the number of electrons attracted to the anode by the increased potential. It is suggested that the high filament temperatures produce rather more electrons than are necessary for the selected current, but at low kV these extra electrons cannot escape from the depth of the focusing cup being held back by the electrons between them and the anode. When the potential on the anode is increased its attractive force overcomes the space charge effect of the interposed electrons and allows the extra electrons to pass to the anode increasing the mA.

Examination of Figure 4.3 shows how the tube current gradually rises as the kilovoltage increases. Therefore, if mA is to be really independent of kVp, a form of space charge compensation must be introduced to ensure that the tube current is unchanged whatever kVp is selected. The effect of the compen-

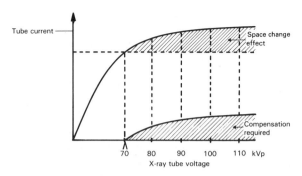

Fig. 4.3 Gradual rise in the tube current as the kilovoltage is increased and the value of compensation required to offset the effect.

sation must be arranged to increase gradually at the same rate as the tube current, so that when it is set against the tube current, the value of tube current produced is trimmed down to the selected value.

Design of a simple space charge compensator

Figure 4.4 outlines the circuit diagram of a simple space charge compensator, and shows the links which must be provided with the kV and mA selectors. The aim of the unit is to reduce slightly the temperature of the tube filament as the kV selected is increased so that the number of electrons released will be just enough to provide the mA even when the anode potential is increased. The temperature of the filament is governed by the filament voltage applied to it, so the unit operates by modifying the voltage applied to the filament of the X-ray tube.

To perform this function a small compensating transformer is used. Its secondary winding is in series with the filament circuit. The primary winding is connected to the 70 kVp tapping of the autotransformer (70 kVp is selected as it is this value of kV that is normally used as the base-line voltage for setting up X-ray units), and to the output of the kV selector unit.

If 70 kVp is selected, there will be no voltage difference between the two connections for the primary winding as their connections are made to the same tapping. With no potential difference across the primary, there will be no

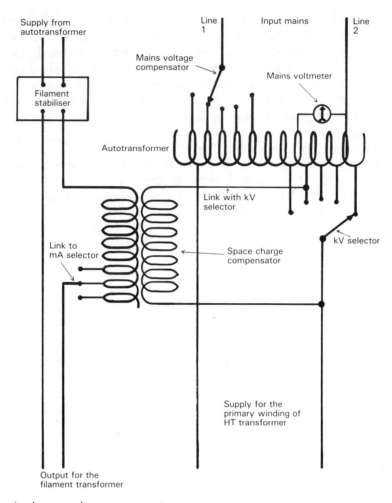

Fig. 4.4 Design of a simple space charge compensator.

current flow in the primary winding and so no e.m.f. developed on the secondary. Therefore there will be no effect upon the filament circuit supply. However, if the kVp selected is greater than 70 there will be a potential difference across the primary winding, a current will flow, an e.m.f. will be developed across the primary and this e.m.f., because of its winding will oppose the voltage of the filament circuit, so reducing its value. A reduction in the filament voltage supply will reduce the temperature of the filament and thus reduce the number of electrons freed by thermionic emission. This is just what is required to overcome the increase in tube current which will occur, and by this method any change in

selected kilovoltage will automatically modify the filament voltage to ensure that tube current is not allowed to vary as the kilovoltage increases.

Examination of Figure 4.4 shows that when the kV selector is moved to a setting below 70 kV, the polarity of the voltage applied to the compensating transformer is reversed causing the supply to the filament to be boosted rather than reduced.

The magnitude of the compensation necessary is not the same for different tube currents, since the space charge effect is greater as the overall number of electrons emitted increases. This is allowed for in this type of space charge compensator by adjusting the number of turns on the secondary winding of the compensating transformer. When a different mA is required an adjustment is made to the mA selector. This action not only selects the new mA but alters the number of turns on the space charge compensating transformer secondary winding by causing another tapping to be selected. The adjustment of the number of turns on the secondary winding alters the turns ratio of the transformer causing the induced e.m.f. to be altered. If more turns are selected the induced e.m.f. will be greater and this will result in a filament voltage reduction. This reduction is required when the selected mA is increased. Less turns will be required when the mA is reduced.

The outcome of space charge compensation is to ensure that the tube current is always at the selected value whatever kVp is applied and whatever the mA selected.

mA SELECTION

The magnitude of the tube current (mA) depends upon the number of electrons attracted across to the anode by the presence of a positive potential on the anode. As previously described the number of available electrons depends upon the level of thermionic emission from the filament. Therefore the various mA values which are available for selection are the result of the availability of different temperature settings for the range of mA values.

Filament temperature is controlled by the current passing through the filament and the resistance of the filament. The resistance of the filament cannot be changed since it depends upon the length and cross-sectional area of the wire, the material (tungsten) forming the helix and its temperature. The value of current is controlled by the resistance through which the current must pass and the potential difference, the voltage. In the filament circuit because the value of resistance is fixed, it is alteration of the filament voltage that varies the filament temperature and so the tube current, the mA.

The method of altering the voltage is to 'drop' some of the filament circuit voltage through a resistance and as a range of tube currents (mA) is needed, there must be a bank of resistances of different values providing the appropriate value to adjust the voltage to the correct value to give the desired mA.

Design of a radiographic mA selector

Figure 4.5 shows the layout of a typical radiographic mA selector supplying a single dual focus X-ray tube. There are two banks of resistances illustrated, one bank energises the filament for the fine focus and the other the filament of the broad focus. There is a different value of resistance for each value of mA so that each will 'drop' the filament voltage to the exact value needed to provide the precise filament temperature.

With use the emission of the filament helix alters and so to provide consistent mA values it must be possible to adjust the mA selector resistance values a little. Therefore each resistance comprises two resistances in series, with one of variable type so that the X-ray engineer may set up the mA values accurately by means of the mA meter. This process is undertaken with each routine service.

One resistance is selected at a time by a rotary form of selector or through one of a bank of push-button switches. The action of selection of an mA is automatically linked to the kVp selector switch, the kVp meter compensator and the space charge compensator. This linkage ensures that any change in mA will not alter the kVp selected.

To conserve the life of the filament, its temperature between exposures is kept at a low value — its 'standby' value — by energising the selected filament through a high resistance. Only when the unit goes into prepare is the supply route altered to it through the mA selector resistance and the filament raised to its correct value, sometimes spoken of as its 'boosted' value. Once the exposure is over, the circuit reverts to its pre-prepare position causing the filament temperature to reduce to its standby value.

It should be remembered that once the X-

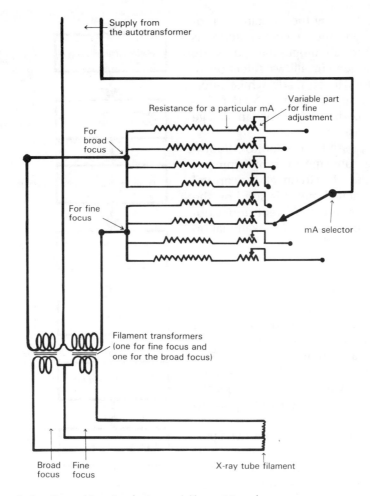

Fig. 4.5 Design of a typical radiographic mA selector and filament transformer.

ray unit is switched on, the filament, either broad or fine, in circuit is energised, so radiographers must switch off units when there is likely to be a delay before the next exposure. This will also help to reduce to a minimum the prepare time so that the filament is only at its boosted value for the shortest possible time. Care to apply these two rules will extend the life of the tube filament.

Design of an mA selector suitable for fluoroscopy

It is important that the unit is able to adjust the mA value as the fluoroscopic examination proceeds so that a standard image brightness is maintained when the examination ranges from

areas of high to low attenuation. The variation in attenuation arises when different areas of the body are scanned and different patient positions selected. Therefore a variable resistance is provided allowing a free choice of tube current over a very restricted range, from 0 mA to 3 mA which can be adjusted whilst the tube is conducting. This variable resistance is generally of a rotary type, either operated manually or automatically in response to a brightness sensing system.

The mA selector (Fig. 4.5) does not show this control as it would complicate the diagram unnecessarily. It is in parallel with the radiographic selector circuit; the choice between the fluoroscopic route and the radiographic route is made by a switch operated remotely by the person performing the examination, or automatically when the X-ray cassette is moved into place for a radiographic exposure. This parallel arrangement allows selection of radiographic factors to be made whilst fluoroscopy proceeds, so enabling a rapid radiographic record to be made of an image observed by fluoroscopy.

It is normally possible to monitor fluoroscopic and radiographic mA by a milliammeter connected into the HT circuit at its earthed centre point. The actual meter is sited on the control panel so that it can be kept under observation by the operator as the examination takes place.

FILAMENT TRANSFORMER

To raise the temperature of the filament helix to the required value to emit electrons it is necessary to pass a current of around 4–5 A. This value of current is provided by a step-down transformer, whose ratio is typically 16:1, thus reducing the filament supply to 4–5 A at 8–12 V.

Figure 4.5 shows the layout of the two step-down transformers and shows that two filaments in the same X-ray tube have a common connection, so that only three rather than four wires to the cathode are needed.

The primary windings are in series with the mA selector unit for the chosen focus.

The common lead from the secondary winding of the filament transformer is connected to the HT supply to cathode. As a result of this connection to high tension, it is essential that the filament transformer is housed with the high tension transformer in the high tension generator tank. Also for electrical safety, the insulation between the secondary and primary windings must be very great to ensure electrical isolation of the X-ray tube cathode's high tension from the mains input. Electrical isolation is therefore one of the filament transformer's functions and because of this makes it possible to provide direct manual operation of the control unit.

Figure 4.6 summarises by a block diagram

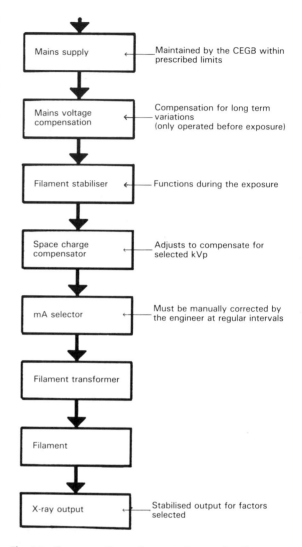

Fig. 4.6 Compensating units operating on the filament voltage.

the series of compensating units operating on the filament voltage ensuring the selected mA remains at the correct value despite any mains voltage variation or any change in kVp.

Without compensation the radiographic effect of:

a. *an increase in the mains voltage* — an over-exposed radiograph with increased density due to the increased quantity of radiation produced by the greater number of electrons emitted by the filament. The increase in electrons is caused by the increase in filament temperature resulting from the increase in filament current, the result of the voltage increase occurring in the mains supply.

    b. *decrease in the mains voltage* — an underexposed radiograph with decreased density due to less radiation generated by the release of fewer electrons by the lowered filament temperature due to a lower filament current resulting from a reduced mains voltage.

THE FILAMENT

The design and function of the actual filament is considered in Chapter 6 on the X-ray tube.

5

X-ray tube high tension circuit

A high tension supply is needed to cause the electrons freed by thermionic emission from the X-ray tube filament to be attracted to the tube anode. Without the presence of the positive potential on the anode the electrons will be unable to overcome the space charge present in front of the cathode to form the tube current, and if a high positive charge is not present on the anode, the freed electrons will not acquire sufficient kinetic energy to convert some of this energy to X-radiation on interaction with the tube target.

The high tension is provided by the HT transformer, a step-up transformer, with a ratio of 1:1000 or 1:500 depending upon the equipment manufacturer. Assuming a perfect transformer, a 1:1000 ratio means that for every 1 kV of potential difference at the X-ray tube, 1 V must be provided on the primary, i.e. 100 kVp requires a primary voltage of 100 V. It will be recalled that the voltage to the primary winding of the HT transformer is varied by the kV selector on the autotransformer. The application of the positive potential on the tube anode is dependent upon the closing of the exposure contactor. This is a switch sited in the primary HT circuit which will be discussed in Chapter 7 on exposure switching and timers.

Manufacturers aim for as near perfection as possible when designing the HT transformer by providing the most efficient and compact unit consistent with safety and loading requirements. A transformer efficency of 98% is

possible. The 2% loss is the result of the transformer copper and iron losses.

DESIGN AND CONSTRUCTION OF A TYPICAL HT TRANSFORMER

Figure 5.1 shows the layout of a typical HT transformer found in the HT generator tank of an X-ray unit.

The core is a laminated shell-type unit made of special iron alloy, called stalloy or permalloy. The laminated construction of the core

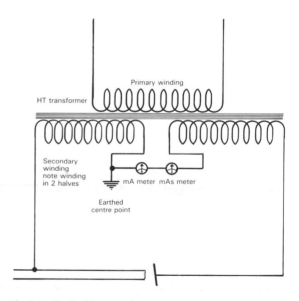

Fig. 5.1 Typical layout of an X-ray transformer. Note the earthed centre point.

will reduce Eddy currents; Eddy currents cannot pass freely from one layer to the next and the use of a special iron alloy reduces the hysterisis loss. These two features reduce the iron losses and the amount of heat developed within the core. The core is earthed to provide protection should there be a breakdown of the insulation between the windings and the core.

The windings — the secondary winding is wound over the primary winding to improve the efficency of the transformer by increasing the interlacing of the magnetic flux. Both primary and secondary windings are divided in half, one half mounted on one limb of the core and the other half on the second limb (Fig. 5.2). The centre point of the secondary winding is connected to earth, which provides symmetry, increased electrical safety and a position where the mA and mAs meters can be connected. It is important that the core and windings are electrically isolated from each other so the windings are wound on insulated cylinders. Between the inner primary winding and the outer secondary there is an earthed stress shield of thin copper so that in the event of insulation breakdown in a winding there is a low resistance path to earth (Fig. 5.3).

As the HT transformer is a step-up trans-former, it has a high current and low voltage input on the primary and a low current high voltage secondary output. It is necessary to reduce the copper losses which arise when a current is passed through the copper wire forming the winding to an acceptable level. Therefore the primary winding is formed from fairly thick wire so that its resistance is low despite the passage of a high current which in a major unit may momentarily reach 300 A, and as the voltage is to be stepped up, only about 100 turns of thick wire are necessary which will also reduce the resistance.

The secondary winding in contrast comprises some 100 000 turns giving around 1000:1 turns ratio. This will require a very great length of wire but as the current drawn through the secondary winding is very small, measured in milliamps, the winding can be formed of very thin wire which will occupy little space whilst still only offering acceptable resistance. The designer of the transformer specifies the gauge of wires to be used to ensure that the copper loss is kept within specified limits.

Insulation of the individual turns of the windings is provided by shellac coating the wire, which gives adequate insulation between adjacent turns since the potential difference between them is very small. To accommodate the number of turns needed for both primary and secondary windings, it is necessary to place one layer upon another and because the windings must be formed in the same direction each layer must start at the same end (see

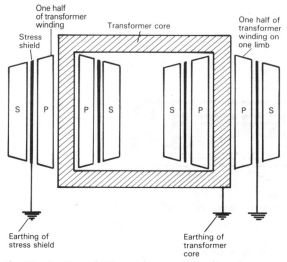

Fig. 5.2 Section of HT transformer. Note the primary and secondary windings are in two parts, one on each limb of the core. P= primary winding, S= secondary winding.

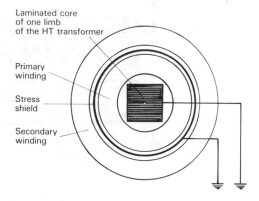

Fig. 5.3 Layout of the transformer windings around the central core.

Fig. 5.4). Therefore the potential difference between the coil in one layer and the one above is equal to the product of the number of turns in the layer and the voltage per turn. This value of potential difference requires greater insulation than the shellac coating so each layer of turns is separated from the one above and below it with a special grade of paper which is impregnated with oil during construction of the transformer. When the whole transformer is soaked in highly insulating vegetable oil, and then immersed in a tank full of this oil, a very high level of electrical safety is provided.

From a section through the coils (Fig. 5.4), it can be seen that the secondary winding is trapezoid in shape. This is necessary to ensure that the gap between the ends of the coil and the earthed core builds up as the voltage in-creases as layers of turns are added. In a unit with 150 kVp output, each half of the secondary winding can reach a maximum of 75 kVp. In addition to the gap, the ends of the paper interposed between each layer are folded up forming a progressively increasing thickness of insulating material.

Electrical connections — this type of transformer has a fixed turn ratio. It has only two input and four output connection points. The centre pair of secondary connection points allow the centre point of the winding to be earthed and the meters and occasionally other equipment to be connected at this low voltage point.

The HT generator tank

The HT transformer is placed in a metal tank

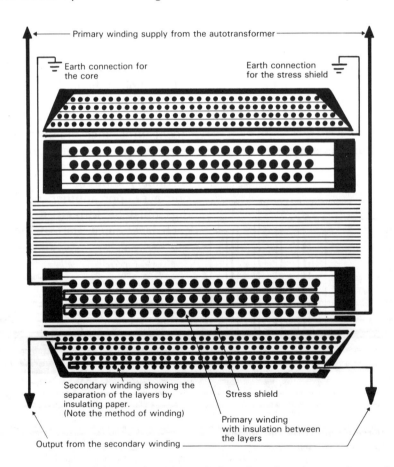

Fig. 5.4 Longitudinal section through HT transformer core limb to show the primary and secondary windings.

which also houses the other components operating at high tension, namely the filament transformers, rectifiers and the change-over switches which allow different X-ray tubes to be energised. If the unit has triode valves and capacitors in its secondary circuit, these will also be housed in the tank and if the unit is so old that it has valve rectifiers, their filament transformers will also be in the tank. All of the components generate heat which must be dissipated as efficiently as possible.

The tank, termed the HT generator tank, is filled with highly refined vegetable oil which acts as an insulator and aids the dissipation of heat. The size and layout of the components within the tank must be carefully planned to ensure that the separation of the components from each other and from the tank walls is sufficient to provide adequate electrical insulation. The gap separating the components is determined by the potential difference between the parts and the dielectric efficiency of the oil. Allowance has to be made for the reduction in dielectric efficiency which occurs as its temperature rises. In addition, the metal tank is well earthed by a copper tape of large cross-sectional area. The tank is covered with a well fitting lid, sealed to prevent entry of any material which would contaminate the oil and lower its insulation value.

Electrical connections for the components within the tank are made through cables entering the tank top. The low tension cables connecting components to the control unit and the autotransformer are of large cross section and protected from mechanical damage. The high tension cables linking the HT transformer secondary winding and the X-ray tubes are connected by highly insulated plug and socket junctions. Each tube supplied by the generator has its own pair of sockets fitted into the top of the tank, one for the anode and one for the cathode cable. The HT cable is terminated at each end with the same size and type of plug, so details of the plug and socket are given in the section on X-ray tubes (p. 63). The change-over switch is described on page 61. Figure 5.5 shows a section through the tank indicating the position of the contents of

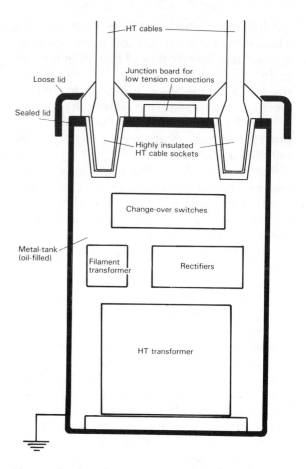

Fig. 5.5 Section of HT generator tank to show the location of its contents and their electrical connections.

the tank and the connecting sockets.

To improve the dissipation of the heat generated within the tank, air must circulate freely around the tank and nothing must be placed on top of the tank to prevent heat loss.

THE HT SUPPLY TO THE X-RAY TUBE

The electrical supply from the HT transformer is alternating. If this output is connected directly to the X-ray tube, the tube being a form of diode valve will allow current to pass across the tube when the anode is positive with respect to the cathode, so in only one half of each cycle of the supply will X-rays be produced. This is a most inefficient use of the available power.

Additionally, the X-ray tube must only be allowed to operate at very low power as there is a risk of an inverse flow of current in the half cycle with reversed polarity if the anode reaches a temperature sufficient to release electrons from its surface. This limits the use of self-rectification by the tube to very low powered units such as dental units and truly portable units.

Better use of the available electrical power and elimination of the risk of inverse current is obtained by re-routing the unused half cycle so that the polarity of the supply is reversed before it is applied to the tube. To re-route the supply to the X-ray tube the alternating supply provided by the secondary winding of the HT transformer is rectified to provide a direct supply. Rectification is obtained by the use of high tension solid state rectifiers placed in the secondary circuit.

After rectification the electrical supply received by the tube is pulsating. This pulsating waveform has a 100% ripple, where the voltage rises to a peak value and then drops to zero volts with each pulse. This waveform restricts the amount of time in each cycle when X-rays can be produced, since for much of the time the voltage across the tube is too low to give the electrons sufficient energy to generate X-rays when they interact with the target. To overcome this low level of X-ray, production methods of reducing the percentage ripple can be applied. The ripple may be reduced to zero by smoothing with a capacitor or reduced to 5% by a 12-pulse system or 10% with a 6-pulse unit. Reduction of the ripple, known as smoothing, not only increases the rate of X-ray production but increases the average energy of the X-rays produced. This allows any exposure time to be selected, something which cannot be done with a 100% ripple because exposure times must be restricted to the pulse frequency, multiples of 0.01 s with a 2-pulse unit.

X-ray generators are classified by their waveform and by their method of connection to the mains supply, either single or three-phase.

Before considering the circuits which will provide the various waveforms, the solid-state rectifier will be considered.

Design and function of a solid-state rectifier

The high tension rectifier is formed by linking in series many P-N junction diodes within a ceramic tube which has metal connecting caps at each end (Fig. 5.6). The rectifiers are available as a single 'stick' or as a series of short sticks mounted on a board and connected in series.

The material most commonly used in the construction of the solid-state junctions is silicon, with a small percentage of arsenic added to form the donor n-type material and gallium to form the acceptor p-type. Selenium was used but has been superceeded by silicon because silicon is less sensitive to alteration in temperature. From the characteristic curve of the current flowing through a P-N junction (Fig. 5.7), it can be seen that the current flows freely with a forward bias and is very restricted, virtually none with a reverse bias until breakdown point is reached. Notice that a P-N junction diode differs from its valve equivalent, the thermionic valve diode, having no saturation current.

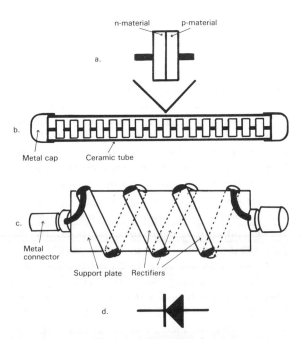

Fig. 5.6 HT solid state rectifier (a) N-P junction diode (b) solid state 'stick' rectifier made up from a series of N-P diodes (c) rectifier for use in an HT circuit, formed from a number of rectifiers linked in series (d) symbol for a solid state rectifier.

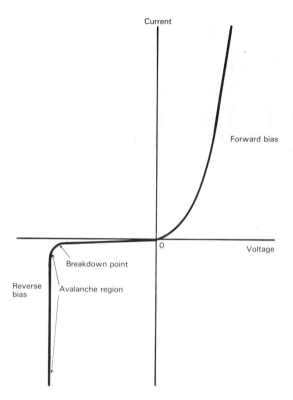

Fig. 5.7 Typical current curve flowing through a P-N junction.

Features of a silicon rectifier

a. Very reliable — will last the life of the X-ray unit

b. Low forward voltage drop, negligible for practical purposes and unchanging in value throughout its life

c. Very high resistance to reverse current

d. Will work at higher temperatures than selenium rectifiers.

The function of all types of rectifiers is to allow current to pass in one direction only, blocking any reverse current. The symbol of a solid state rectifier is shown in Figure 5.6.

Advantages derived from the use of solid-state rectifiers instead of the previously used thermionic valves

1. Much longer life, therefore more economical

2. More robust — no glass envelope to rupture

3. No heated filament needed, no valve filament transformers are required, therefore less heat generated in the generator tank

4. Much more compact and without the need for filament transformers the generator tank can be reduced in size and considerably lighter than the equivalent unit using thermionic valves.

SINGLE PHASE GENERATORS

The single-phase generator is supplied with 415 V obtained by connecting the unit between 2 phases, or if low-powered or a mobile between one phase and neutral. Both types are described as single-phase units. They have a single high tension transformer supplying the X-ray tube(s). The waveform across the tube is governed by the arrangement of the rectifiers and whether or not their pulsed output is smoothed by capacitors.

The capacity of the HT cables will smooth to a very limited extent the waveform but this is of no practical significance unless the cables are very long and the tube current extremely small. Other extrinsic factors will distort the waveform but this distortion may be disregarded although it is one of the reasons why two exactly similar units do not provide exactly similar output.

Five examples of single-phase units will be decribed in this section:

a. 1-pulse generator

b. 2-pulse generator

c. constant potential generator

d. medium frequency (high-pulse) generator

e. power storage generators.

1-pulse generator

A 1-pulse generator is the smallest single-phase generator. The waveform across the X-ray tube gives only 1 pulse in each AC cycle, because the tube can only pass current during half of the cycle; the other half is blocked by the tube itself, self-rectified. The unit may be described as a 1-pulse, half-wave rectified or self-rectified unit. Because of the low power

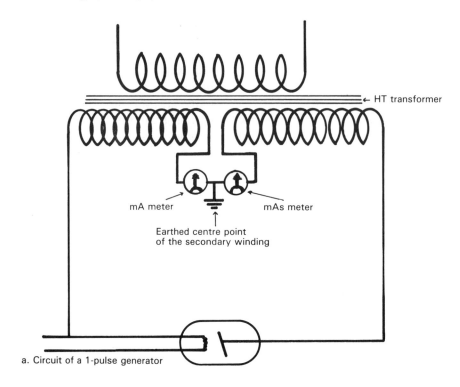

← HT transformer

mA meter

mAs meter

Earthed centre point
of the secondary winding

a. Circuit of a 1-pulse generator

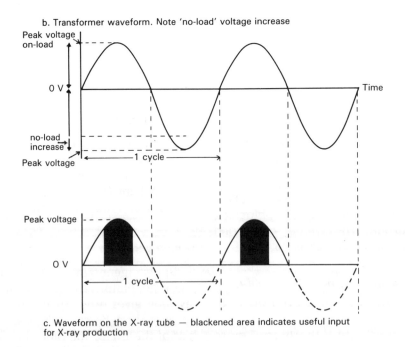

b. Transformer waveform. Note 'no-load' voltage increase

Peak voltage
on-load

0 V

Time

no-load
increase

Peak voltage

1 cycle

Peak voltage

0 V

1 cycle

c. Waveform on the X-ray tube — blackened area indicates useful input
for X-ray production

Fig. 5.8 A 1-pulse (self-rectified) generator.

the main use is for dental radiography or very small mobile units, although the mobile use will soon be phased out following the introduction of the power-storage units with their much higher X-ray production.

The voltage and current across the X-ray tube and the X-radiation output is shown in Figure 5.8c. The X-radiation pulse time is defined as the time between the first and last crossing of a line 75% of the peak value of the tube voltage by the International Electro-technical Commission. The pulse time represents the period during which useful generation is produced, although with a waveform having a ripple, the maximum energy of the X-ray photons only occurs for a fraction of time when the voltage is at peak value. Figure 5.8c includes an illustration of pulse-time.

In the circuit layout of a 1-pulse generator (Fig. 5.8a), rectification is provided solely by the X-ray tube.

The 1-pulse generator is inefficient, making no use of half of the available power, therefore to obtain the same amount of radiation the exposure must be twice as long as a 2-pulse generator. The mA meter since it records average current will register half the value for the same filament temperature. In practice this effect is not seen as the filament temperature is increased to give the stated value of current whatever the generator type. When 1-pulse unit is self-rectified as is almost always the case today, the loading must be very restricted to ensure that the tube anode will never reach a heat at which electrons will be freed by thermionic emission and so able to pass current in the reverse direction across the tube, an action which would severly damage the tube.

During the reverse, unused $\frac{1}{2}$-cycle, there is no load on the HT transformer for no current is flowing during this period. Therefore there will be no voltage drop during this $\frac{1}{2}$-cycle and so provision must be made for the resultant increase in voltage (voltage without the drop) when the manufacturers calculate insulation requirements (Fig. 5.9).

2-pulse

A 2-pulse (full-wave rectified) generator uses both halves of the AC output from the HT transformer, doubling the X-ray output of the 1-pulse generator. The reverse $\frac{1}{2}$-cycle, which was unused in the 1-pulse unit, is re-routed by the use of two pairs of rectifiers so that there is a positive potential on the anode of the X-ray tube during both half cycles, providing unidirectional current across the tube during the whole cycle (see Fig. 5.10). The tube voltage has a 100% ripple, therefore in each cycle two pulses of X-radiation is generated, hence the name '2-pulse'; the alternative name, 'full-wave rectified', describes its waveform.

This type of generator is used for mobile units and many fixed units. It is comparatively inexpensive and although only medium

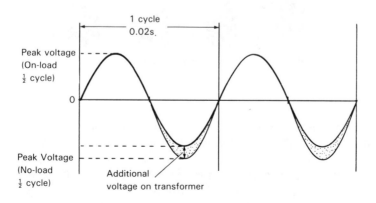

Fig. 5.9 'No-load' voltage on the HT transformer of a 1-pulse X-ray generator (extra voltage shown as dotted area).

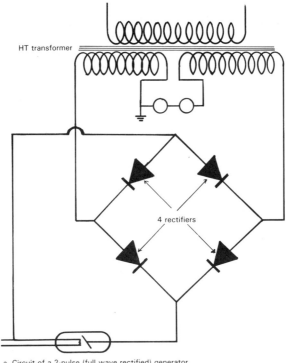

HT transformer

4 rectifiers

a. Circuit of a 2-pulse (full wave rectified) generator

b. Transformer waveform

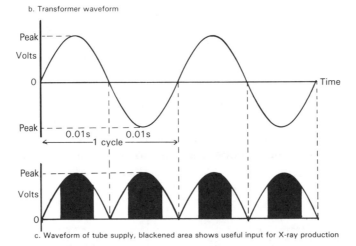

Peak

Volts

0 — Time

Peak

0.01s   0.01s
←————1 cycle————→

Peak

Volts

0

c. Waveform of tube supply, blackened area shows useful input for X-ray production

Fig. 5.10   2-pulse generator.

powered is adequate for most general work but its pulsed waveform prevents the use of very short exposure times.

The rectifiers are aligned in the circuit so that one pair conducts during one half cycle and the second pair during the other half cycle. Should a rectifier fail to conduct, which is an uncommon occurrence with solid-state rectifiers, one radiation pulse in each cycle is eliminated. The unit is said to be 'half-waving' with the output cut by half. Radiographically the film density is cut by half. The mA and mAs meters will show only half of their expected value.

Constant potential

The 2-pulse generator has two important disadvantages, resulting from its pulsating waveform. These are inefficient radiation production due to the intervals when the voltage across the tube is not great enough for X-ray production (occurring as a result of the 100% ripple on the tube voltage) and the inability to allow for the selection of very short exposure times. These disadvantages are overcome by the introduction of two capacitors to smooth the pulsating waveform to a constant potential for the whole time the tube is conducting.

The circuit shown in Figure 5.11 operates by interposing two large capacitors across the

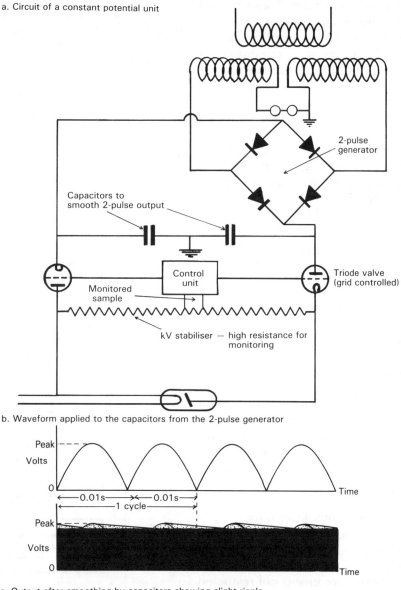

a. Circuit of a constant potential unit

b. Waveform applied to the capacitors from the 2-pulse generator

c. Output after smoothing by capacitors showing slight ripple
Blackened area shows smoothed useful output for X-ray production

Fig. 5.11 Circuit of a constant potential unit.

output from the four rectifiers of a 2-pulse unit before it is applied to the X-ray tube. The pulsating waveform is used to charge the capacitors and provided the capacitors are adequate, a constant potential can be applied to the tube. The waveform shown in Figure 5.11c illustrates the output from the capacitors. There may be a very slight ripple which is eliminated by HT triode valves in the circuit between the capacitors and the X-ray tube. These triodes trim off the highest voltage to give a constant potential. The introduction of triode valves in the secondary circuit has other advantages. It allows the tube voltage to be stabilised to the exact voltage selected and provides secondary switching.

The smoothing and stabilising are obtained by varying the resistance across the triode valve which changes the voltage drop across them, so adjusting the voltage across the X-ray tube. Resistance across the triode can be varied by altering the bias on the valve grid. The value of the bias required can be determined by fitting an electronic unit which responds by comparing the actual voltage across the tube against an accurately set reference voltage. The monitoring of the tube voltage is by means of a very high resistance potential divider connected in parallel to the tube. A small section of the divider provides a sample of the actual tube voltage. Once the actual tube voltage has been monitored it is corrected to the required value by the electronic unit which injects the correct bias on to the grid. Continuous small adjustments can be made to the bias ensuring the continuous delivery of constant potential at the exact voltage required even when there are mains voltage variations.

Advantages
1. Very high X-ray output per mAs.
2. A more homogeneous X-ray beam, the result of all electrons being accelerated by the same kilovoltage.
3. Choice of exposure time is not restricted.
4. The triode valves can provide very efficient rapid switching for cine techniques.

Medium-frequency (high-pulse) generator

A medium-frequency generator produces an almost ripple-free output from a single-phase mains supply, an output very similar to the constant potential generator already described or to the three-phase 12-pulse unit which will be described later. The very small, insignificant, ripple is obtained by the use of an invertor which generates a frequency of 5000 Hz; a waveform of 200-pulses is produced after rectification and when this is smoothed by capacitors the supply to the tube is virtually ripple-free.

Figure 5.12 is a block diagram to show the layout of the components. The invertor receives its supply from a rectified and smoothed single-phase mains. Once the in-

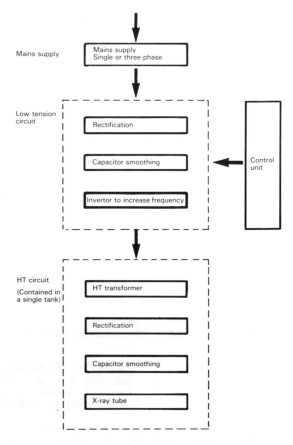

Fig. 5.12 Medium frequency (high pulse) generator.

vertor has generated the frequency of 5000 Hz this is connected to the HT transformer. The voltage is stepped-up in the usual way but more efficiently than with the conventional 50 Hz transformer because of the high frequency input. The high voltage is rectified and then smoothed by capacitors before being applied to the tube.

The advantages of this unit are in its very high output from a single-phase mains delivered by a very compact generator which may be housed in a single tank. The HT transformer, rectifiers, capacitor and the tube may be in the tank. This is possible because the transformer, as a result of its efficiency, can be smaller. The single-tank eliminates the cumbersome high tension cables and eliminates the generator tank. If required the unit can be connected to a three-phase mains supply.

Power storage generators (mains independent units)

Power storage generators provide a very high rate of radiation output from a poor mains supply which could not produce such an output by conventional means. There are two types: (i) capacitor discharge; (ii) battery storage.

Capacitor discharge — power is gradually stored from the mains supply in a large capacitor in the secondary circuit of the X-ray unit's HT transformer. Once this capacitor is fully charged it can be discharged through the X-ray tube as soon as the grid-controlled X-ray tube allows conduction. The rate of discharge is very much greater than the rate of storage allowing the required exposure to be delivered in a very short time by the use of a high mA which would not have been possible by a conventional unit connected to a poor supply.

The potential difference across the X-ray tube is controlled by the kV across the capacitor. The potential difference across the capacitor is controlled by the potential difference across the secondary winding of the HT transformer. Therefore if a different kV is required it can be obtained by selecting a different voltage on the primary winding through adjust-

ment of the kV selector on the autotransformer. The layout of the unit's components (Fig. 5.13) also illustrates the operating principle of the system.

The exposure commences when the grid-controlled X-ray tube allows conduction to take place. Once the required exposure time has passed the bias on the grid is re-applied preventing any further passage of current across the tube. A grid-tube is essential to ensure no uncontrolled generation of X-rays is possible from the residual charge on the capacitor and to provide the very accurate short exposures, measured in milliseconds, which are required when using these units with their high tube current, some units being rated as high as 500 mA. Once the immediate work is over, the capacitor is fully discharged to ensure that there can be no accidental X-ray exposure. Additional radiation protection is provided in some units by a heavy lead filter which is automatically brought across in front of the tube port when the unit is not in use. This filter is removed as soon as the unit enters the 'prepare' stage prior to an X-ray exposure.

This type of unit is very suitable for mobile use, especially where there is only a poor mains supply, or a battery-operated power supply or where no electrical supply is immediately available and power stored in a capacitor is the only method of generating X-rays. These units have advantages and disadvantages when compared with other methods of generating X-radiation in sites remote from the X-ray department.

Disadvantages

1. Problems resulting from the discharge characteristics of capacitors; for as the capacitor discharges during the exposure, the kilovoltage across the tube and the radiation output rate is continuously dropping (see Fig. 5.14). In practice, it is usual to determine exposure factors empirically and always initiate the exposure with a fully charged capacitor, or if this is not possible to determine the

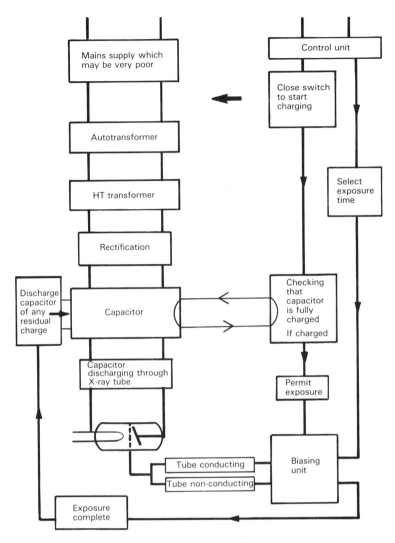

Fig. 5.13 Principles of a capacitor discharge generator

kV and mAs still available in the capacitor by reference to manufacturer's charts and graphs

2. Comparatively low output (30–50 mAs).

Advantages

1. Small size and weight.

2. Availability when mains supply is not available or very unstable.

3. High mA available allowing very short exposure times which will reduce unsharpness due to patient movement.

4. May avoid the necessity for expensive mains supply outlets in locations like premature baby units.

5. Eliminates trailing mains supply cable.

Battery storage — battery storage generators are designed to produce high power output without the need for continuous connection to the mains supply. The quantity of stored power is considerable and allows a number of exposures to be made without reconnection to the mains supply. This makes the unit ideally suited to mobile work.

The power is stored in large capacity, nickel

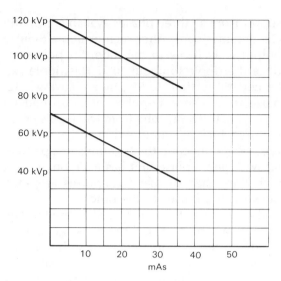

Fig. 5.14A Falling-off of kilovoltage during exposure.

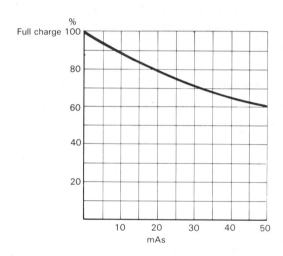

Fig. 5.14B Falling-off in radiation generated during exposure.

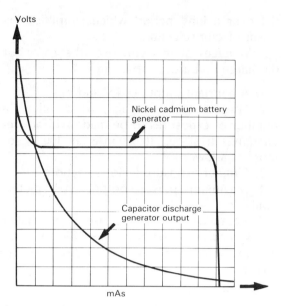

Fig. 5.15 Output of nickel cadmium batteries compared with the output from a capacitor.

X-ray tube (see Fig. 5.16). 500 Hz when rectified gives 1000 pulses per second generating a waveform which has virtually no ripple and can be equated to a constant potential or 12-pulse unit. Unlike the capacitor discharge storage unit, the output has a constant poten-

cadmium, rechargeable batteries. Nickel cadmium batteries are chosen for their resistance to corrosion and the character of their discharge curve (see Fig. 5.15). The output from the batteries is fed into a DC inverter which interrupts the DC voltage many times a second, generally 500 times. This produces a 500 Hz alternating supply.

The high frequency output is supplied to the primary winding of the high tension transformer. The output from the secondary winding is rectified before being applied to the

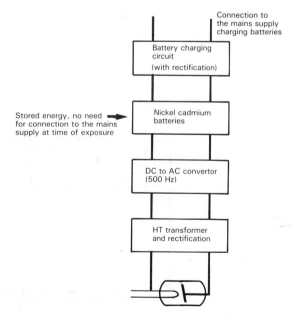

Fig. 5.16 Layout of components found in a battery storage generator.

tial over a long period which simplifies exposure factor selection.

Advantages of this unit over the capacitor discharge unit are:

1. A constant output of kV and mA.
2. Greater storage capacity which allows a number of exposures to be made without recharging. It stores 10 000 mAs at 100 kV or more at a lower kV.
3. Simpler exposure factor selection.
4. Maximum power output immediately available.
5. Reputed to allow the use of a smaller focus because of the units very efficient X-ray output which reduces the loading on the target.

Disadvantages

1. Heavy.
2. More expensive.
3. Requires regular battery maintenance.
4. Regular charging is necessary which takes up to 12 hours for a full charge.

THREE-PHASE GENERATORS

Another method of overcoming the 100% ripple produced by a 2-pulse unit is to use the supply from all three phases available from the Generating Board. After rectification a 6-pulse output is available to the tube. Six pulses reduce the ripple to about 10%. This ripple can be cut still further, to 5%, by employing a 12-pulse unit. These 12-pulses are obtained by supplying the X-ray tube from two 6-pulse generators which are mounted in series with the tube. By connecting the two units in a particular way, one 6-pulse unit has a 30° phase shift with the other so that its 6-pulses are sited between the pulses of the other.

The layout of the circuit is illustrated in Figure 5.17 where the two three-phase generators are described in more detail. If a truly constant potential is required this can be easily provided by including triode valves in the secondary circuit which can be made to trim off the ripple. In practice this is rarely necessary as the 5% ripple gives no observable radiographic effect.

6-pulse generator

To utilise the three phases, triple auto and HT transformers are used. Each autotransformer supplies its own HT transformer. The primary and secondary coils of the three HT transformers are mounted on a single core with three limbs; each set of coils is mounted on

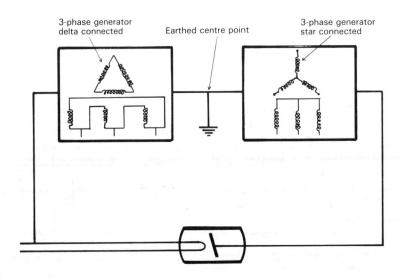

Fig. 5.17 Two HT transformers connected in series: one a delta-connected, the other star-connected.

one limb as shown in Figure 5.18. The output from the three secondary windings is connected through six rectifiers to provide the 6-pulse waveform across the X-ray tube (Fig. 5.19). Figure 5.20 illustrates the principles in a simple

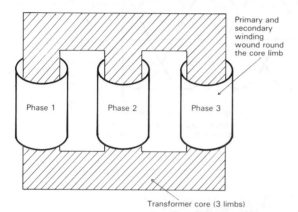

Fig. 5.18 Three-phase transformer showing how the windings are distributed on the limbs.

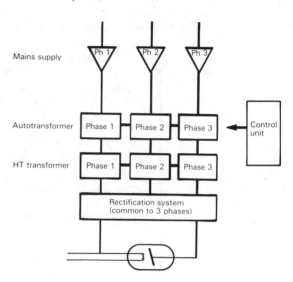

Fig. 5.20 Layout of a three-phase generator (6-pulse).

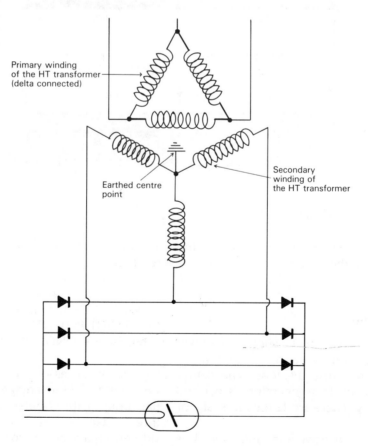

Fig. 5.19 Circuit of a three-phase 6-pulse generator (secondary winding — star connection).

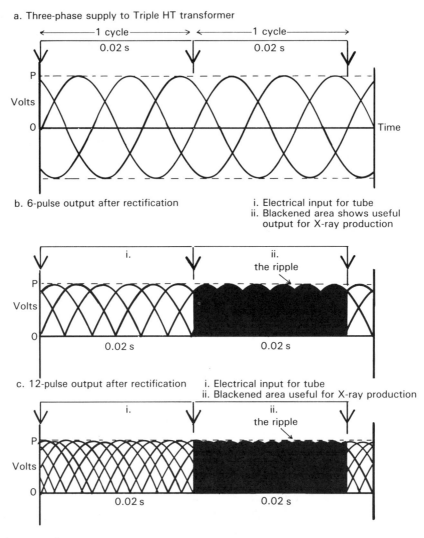

Fig. 5.21   Three-phase waveform.

block diagram while Figure 5.21 shows the waveform across the tube.

12-pulse generator

Examination of Figure 5.22 shows how two generators are connected to provide a 12-pulse waveform across the tube. The centre point between the two generators is earthed giving symmetry. There are 12 rectifiers, six for each generator.

This is a very expensive and bulky unit. It is only used where its very high output is necess-ary and rapid repetitive short exposures are required.

ADVANTAGES AND DISADVANTAGES OF CONSTANT POTENTIAL COMPARED WITH THOSE OF A SINGLE-PHASE PULSED UNIT

For the purposes of a comparison of the advantages and disadvantages of constant potential units with 2-pulse single-phase units, three-phase 6- and 12-pulse units are considered equivalent to constant potential units because of their very low percentage ripple.

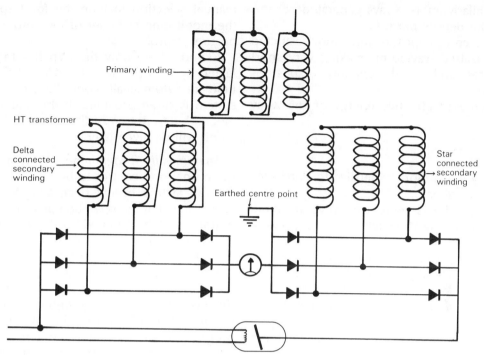

Fig. 5.22 Circuit of a 12-pulse three-phase generator.

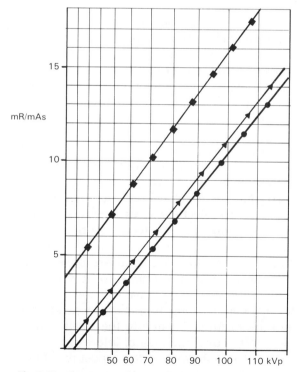

● Output from a 2-pulse generator

▲ Output from a 6-pulse generator

■ Output from a 12-pulse generator

Fig. 5.23 Comparision of the X-ray output from a 2-pulse, 6-pulse and 12-pulse X-ray generator.

Advantages of a constant potential unit

1. More efficient conversion of electrical power to X-ray energy, therefore better use of available power.

2. More X-rays generated per mAs because the kinetic energy acquired by the cathode electrons does not fall below 90% of peak value making all electrons capable of conversion to X-rays. Figure 5.23 compares the output of mR/mAs for a 2-pulse single-phase generator, a 6 and 12-pulse three-phase generator.

3. With more X-rays produced per mA, the exposure time can be shorter with less risk of unsharpness due to movement.

4. Similarly, more X-rays generated per mA more film density per mA.

5. Choice of exposure times not restricted by the pulsed waveform, making very short exposures and rapid repetitive exposures possible.

6. Increased effective energy of the X-ray beam.

Disadvantages

1. Very much more expensive to purchase, instal and maintain.

2. X-ray tube is more expensive to allow very high loading to match the output power of the generator.

3. Loading over 0.5 s is less than for a 2-pulse unit, although in practice this is not a real disadvantage as the exposure times needed to produce the required density are less anyway.

4. More homogeneous X-ray beam reduces image contrast.

5. X-ray tube target deteriorates more rapidly as a result of the greater loading.

6. The generator is much larger because of the triple transformers.

OTHER X-RAY GENERATORS

The high tension circuits described up to now in this section are basic circuits. Their output can be modified by the addition of control systems to make them more suitable for the nature of the work they are to undertake or to simplify their use.

The types of control system available today can be divided into groups based on the way the exposure factors are selected. These are:

3-knobs for kVp, mA and exposure time. All of the knobs must be set manually together with factors like the focal spot. This 3-knob unit is the common conventional form of control and is much cheaper than any of the others listed.

2-knobs for kVp and mA are selected manually, while the exposure time is controlled automatically. Other factors which also need manual selection include the focal spot and the monitoring chamber of the automatic exposure control.

1-knob where only the kVp has to be selected by the operator, the mA and exposure time are automatically controlled. This control system is often provided in the 'falling load' mode. A description of the operation of such a unit will be given later.

Anatomically programmed generators require only one control to be operated manually, all factors having been programmed in such a way that the operation of a single push-button switch labelled with a particular technique introduces a set of factors, which provide a suitable exposure. Alternatively, selection may be made by tapping a code into a micro-processor which performs the same function as the array of push-buttons but with the advantage of allowing the operator to re-programme the system when circumstances change with much less trouble than with push-button selection.

The falling-load generator

A falling-load generator will correctly expose a radiograph in the shortest possible time. The shortest possible exposure time is obtained by using a high speed tube and by the unit automatically selecting the highest mA available for as long as the rating permits and then moving to the next highest mA for as long as this is permitted and then the next highest mA and so on until the exposure is terminated by the automatic timing device.

To operate a falling-load generator, it is necessary to select the focus if this is possible, for often only the large focus can be selected in the falling-load mode, and to choose the kVp which will provide adequate penetration and allow the image contrast to be set at the required level. The automatic exposure monitoring chamber must be accurately positioned and the beam collimated to the smallest field needed to cover the area of interest.

Figure 5.24 shows how the exposure is fitted in within the rating of the particular tube focus.

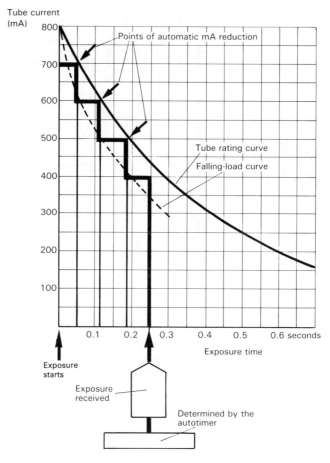

Fig. 5.24 Relationship of mA and the tube rating chart in a falling-load generator.

Figure 5.25 is a block diagram to show the system by which the unit operates. To provide the reducing mA it is necessary to introduce additional resistance progressively into the filament circuit. The extra resistance reduces the supply to the filament and so cuts the tube current, the mA. A control circuit varies the resistance as the rating limit for the mA is approached. In order to maintain a stable kVp as the mA reduces, a resistance is placed in the primary of the high tension circuit which is adjusted by linkage with the variable resistance in the filament circuit. As the mA decreases, the resistance in the primary of the HT circuit is increased.

The advantage of this form of generator is the very short exposure time, shorter than

could be obtained by conventional means.

The disadvantages are the very heavy loading applied to the tube, which always operates close to the limit of its rating. It can only be used with automatic exposure control. There is no advantage when exposure with low mAs is required for these will almost always be possible within the rating limit of the highest mA particularly if the kVp is relatively low as in chest radiography. The sophisticated control system needed to provide this facility is very costly.

The disadvantages of the system clearly indicate why a conventional 3-knob system must also be provided by the unit if all techniques are to be possible.

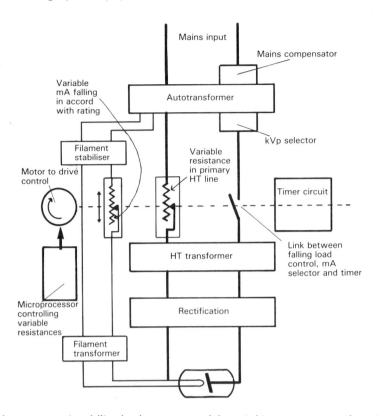

Fig. 5.25 Layout of components in a falling-load generator and the mA drive motor to vary the mA delivered.

The cost of generators

Generators increase in price as their facilities and sophistication increase. Therefore the elaborate units should only be selected when the techniques they are to perform justify the extra cost, not only because of the advantage the special generator has over the simpler unit but by the frequency of demand for these special features.

The cost of generators may also be reduced by other means such as shared generators where one generator serves a number of tubes in different rooms. Each room has a separate control unit equipped with all the radiographic controls. There is a master control ensuring that there is no simultaneous exposure from the different rooms and that the loading on the generator is within the rating limit of the generator.

The disadvantage of the system is that should the generator or the master control fail all the satellite units are out of use.

Modular design enables the purchaser to select only the features required for the work the unit is required to perform, for instance falling-load control or the angiographic facility may not be required and so the unit can be purchased without these facilities in the knowledge that they can be added at a later date should they become necessary.

Detailed information on all forms of generators is available from the manufacturers' data sheets and these should always be carefully considered when selecting equipment. Chapter 21 gives information on equipment selection.

THE RATING OF GENERATORS

Manufacturers of X-ray equipment indicate the rating of their generators by quoting:

a. kW — determined at 100 kV

b. maximum kVp under no-load conditions

c. maximum current allowed on continuous running

d. maximum current for a short time, not exceeding one second.

Also specified will be the maximum mA at various kV settings, for example:

32 kW 2-pulse generator
    500 mA at 90 kVp
    300 mA at 125 kVp
    250 mA at 150 kVp
100 kW 12-pulse generator
    1250 mA at 80 kVp
     500 mA at 150 kVp

Other generators are available with ratings of up to 200 kW.

THE SELECTION OF X-RAY GENERATORS

Before selection of a generator a detailed specification should be drawn up listing the:

available power supply (240 or 415 V, single or three-phase)

size of the cable supplying the unit and its effect on impedance

size of the room into which the unit must be installed

available funds.

The nature and volume of work to be performed including information on:

number of tubes to be energised

typical exposures

single exposures only or single and rapid sequences

kVp — maximum and minimum and number of increments

mA — maximum and minimum and intermediate values

time — maximum and minimum and number of intermediate values

type of timing control required

any specific radiographic requirements or techniques

radiography only or radiography and fluoroscopy

generator waveform

maintenance arrangements

pre-installation requirements

installation and commissioning time.

With this information the data sheets of the generators available can be compared with the specification and the best match selected.

THE CONNECTION OF MORE THAN ONE TUBE TO THE GENERATOR OUTPUT

The X-ray generator may supply more than one X-ray tube, often two: one in the overcouch position and one for the undercouch position; sometimes three with the third tube for a specialised unit such as skull or mammography unit. Occasionally four or even six tubes may be supplied from one generator, but this will necessitate the introduction of a selector unit which will energise the appropriate tube. With bi-plane work, a programming unit can be linked to the generator so that connections can be made to energise the particular tube required by the programme.

To energise an X-ray tube, it is necessary to connect the tube with the high tension and the filament supply. Both connections are made in the high tension circuit and so for safety must be operated remotely with the actual switch in the HT generator tank. The connection between the HT tank and the tube is made through a HT cable, whose design is considered at the end of Chapter 6 on the X-ray tube.

The actual connection is through a high potential cable termination plug and a receptacle socket assembly. Two sockets are provided for each tube in the top of the HT generator tank, one socket for the cathode cable and the other for the anode cable. The terminations at each end of the cable are exactly alike so that the cables are interchangeable and can be plugged into the receiving sockets of the gen-

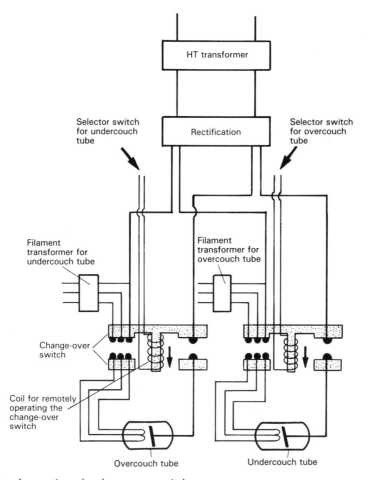

Fig. 5.26 Layout and operation of a change-over switch.

erator tank or the X-ray tube. If the tube is grid-controlled a special four conductor cable is required for the cathode and the cable ends and socket fittings will be different for the cathode and anode connection. Figure 5.26 shows the method of connecting two tubes from a generator and the arrangement for the remotely operated change-over switch to supply the X-ray tube selected.

6

X-ray tube and its electrical connections

X-RAY TUBE

The X-ray tube is central to the X-ray unit being responsible for the generation of a beam of X-rays. The basic requirements of an X-ray tube are that it shall provide a beam of radiation:

1. generated from as near a point source as possible, without damage from the accompanying heat, to produce a radiographic image with the maximum image detail.

2. which can be accurately controlled to provide the quantity and quality of radiation needed to penetrate the part being radiographed and in the quantity needed to produce the required image density in as short a time as possible so that the patient's movement is 'frozen' and that the same quantity and quality of radiation shall be generated on each occasion the same exposure factors are selected.

3. a housing for the source of the X-rays which

   a. allows the radiation only to emerge through an opening in its shielding. It must be possible to vary the size of the opening to restrict the area covered by the beam to that of the area under examination.

   b. is compact and shaped to allow it to be securely supported but still capable of easy movement into any position that may be required and once positioned remain in that position

   c. by design allows easy maintenance and cleaning

   d. is electrically safe.

By describing the design and construction of a fixed (stationary) anode tube assembly, it can be shown how these basic requirements are fulfilled and later in the text how adaption of this simple design can provide for the needs of the radiographic examinations undertaken today.

Design of a fixed anode X-ray tube assembly

The fixed anode X-ray tube assembly has two parts, the X-ray tube or insert and the housing or tube shield which contains the insert. The layout of the tube assembly is shown in Figure 6.5 (p. 70).

X-ray tube insert

The X-ray tube insert (Fig. 6.1) is basically a specialised diode valve and will be described in its three parts: the cathode and anode assemblies and the highly evacuated vessel that contains them.

The cathode assembly has a dual function; it must act as the negative electrode of the valve and as the controlled source of the beam of electrons, which after acquiring extra energy by acceleration interacts with the anode target to generate X-radiation.

The electrons are produced by heating a tungsten wire, known as the filament, to a pre-

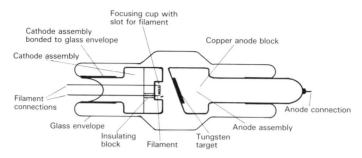

Fig. 6.1 Fixed (stationary) anode tube insert with single focus.

selected temperature. It is the temperature of the wire which controls the quantity of electrons freed by thermionic emission. The temperature of the filament is raised or lowered by varying the current passing through it. The control on the X-ray unit to vary this current is the mA selector. The mA, the tube current, depends upon the number of electrons passing from cathode to anode which of course depends upon the number released from the filament.

The temperature required for electron release is very high and will cause evaporation of tungsten from the filament — the higher the mA selected, the greater the rate of evaporation. It is important to reduce the rate of evaporation as quickly as possible to extend the life of the tube, therefore as soon as an X-ray examination is over, the unit should be turned off and when an exposure is going to be made the filament should only be raised to its required temperature for the shortest time possible. When a unit is switched on, the filament is held at a low temperature where evaporation is minimal; it is not until the 'prepare' position is reached that the unit controls cause the filament temperature to be raised to its correct value. Reference to the filament circuit details described in Chapter 4 will show how filament temperature is stabilised at the exact temperature necessary to release the desired number of electrons to provide the selected mA.

Electron source — the cathode head — the head is made of pure nickel and the filament supported by it from fine tungsten wire. It is designed to act as:

1. the negative electrode of the X-ray tube
2. the source of electrons and the means of controlling the dimensions of the electron beam as it crosses to the anode.

On the face of the head of a dual focus tube are two slot-like grooves, in one the filament helix for the large (broad) focus is fitted and in the other the filament for the small (fine) focus. A single focus tube has a single central groove. The position of the filament helix in the groove is critical for the margins of the slot provide electrostatic focusing to shape the electron stream.

The high loading capacity of the tube and accurate focal spot sizes results from:

1. accuracy in the siting of the machined grooves and the size of the slot
2. positioning of the filament within the groove
3. the size, length and diameter of the filament helix
4. sharp edges of the groove which increase the electrostatic charge operating on the electron stream as it leaves the slot.

The dual focus tube's filament grooves may be sited one above the other or more commonly side by side (see Fig. 6.2). When they are positioned side by side, they are angled so that the electron stream they produce will fall on the same point on the anode. This arrangement ensures that the X-radiation is generated from a focal spot on the target of the anode which is in the same position for both foci. When they are positioned one above the other, the electron streams they produce are

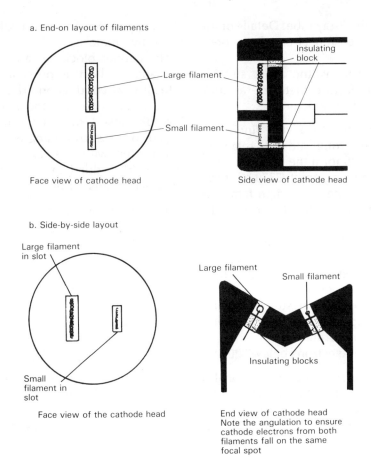

a. End-on layout of filaments

Large filament

Small filament

Face view of cathode head

Insulating block

Side view of cathode head

b. Side-by-side layout

Large filament in slot

Small filament in slot

Face view of the cathode head

Large filament

Small filament

Insulating blocks

End view of cathode head
Note the angulation to ensure cathode electrons from both filaments fall on the same focal spot

Fig. 6.2 Cathode head of a dual focus tube.

directed to two different target positions on the anode. This results in X-ray beams generated from two focal spot sites. There are times when this arrangement is useful but they do not arise in the work for which a fixed anode tube is likely to be chosen. In view of this details of the advantages and disadvantages of this filament arrangement will be considered when the rotating anode tube is described (p. 90).

The advantages of a dual focus tube are that it allows selection of a wider range of exposure factors and techniques than is possible with a single focus tube. The choice can be made between a small focal spot producing less penumbra giving less geometric unsharpness in the radiographic image or the relatively greater unsharpness of the larger focus offset

by the freezing of patient movement by the shorter exposure time permitted by the greater heat tolerance of the larger focal spot.

The filament helix is made of fine tungsten wire drawn into a very precise diameter and wound into a helix of precise size. The dimensions of this helix along with other factors determine the 'large' or 'small' focal spot size. By insulating one end of the filament winding from the cathode head assembly it is possible to apply a potential difference across the filament helix which will generate the required amount of heat in the filament to release the number of electrons needed to provide the selected tube current. When a different tube current is required, the potential difference across the filament helix is varied whilst still retaining the same potential between the cathode and anode of the X-ray tube. Details of the filament and high tension circuit have been described.

Tungsten is chosen as the most suitable metal for the manufacture of the X-ray tube filament because of its characteristics:

1. It can be drawn into a very fine wire, which is still quite strong and will retain its shape when twisted to form the filament helix.

2. It has a high melting point (3370 °C) making it possible to operate at the high temperatures necessary to release the electrons at the required rate.

3. It has a relatively low rate of vaporisation.

4. It has a fairly low work function compared with other metals which might have been selected.

5. It has good mechanical strength which allows it to stand up to the tube movements which must be made during use.

6. It ceases to emit electrons below 2200 °C.

These features combine to give a reasonably long life and a consistant output which will not cause any appreciable change in the size of the focal spot or X-ray generation throughout the working life of the tube provided it is handed with care and not held in 'prepare' for very long periods.

The anode assembly has two main functions. It is the positive electrode of the valve and it acts as the target of the beam of electrons travelling across from the cathode. In addition, it is designed to remove as quickly as possible the heat produced by the interaction of the electron beam, the input load, with the target so that a reasonably large input of energy can be safely applied to the target without risk of damage from overheating.

A fixed anode X-ray tube for general use has a tungsten and rhenium target button implanted in the surface of a solid copper block. The target button is very firmly bonded into the bed of copper by silver solder to ensure that the heat created in the target area is removed by conduction as efficiently as possible across the tungsten/copper boundary and that there are no problems resulting from the different coefficients of expansion of tungsten

and copper. Silver has a coefficient between those two metals.

The copper block has a large diameter and is made as short as possible to increase the rate of heat conduction. The end of the copper block extends into the oil which surrounds the tube insert so that the heat can be conveyed to the surrounding oil.

Tungsten with a small percentage of rhenium (10%) added to it is used as the target material because it has:

1. high melting point
2. high atomic number
3. high density
4. reasonable absorption of heat
5. fairly high thermal conductivity
6. good mechanical strength
7. reduced risk of surface crazing — the result of the added rhenium.

The face of the anode is angled to provide a larger actual target area to receive the bombardment of electrons but still provide an apparently smaller effective source of X-rays when viewed through the tube port. This arrangement is described as the 'line focus principle' (Fig. 6.3). In a fixed anode tube the angle of the target face is generally about 16 ° to the central ray of the X-ray beam. By this means a greater input load can be applied to the target whilst still maintaining a small focal spot to reduce the level of geometric unsharpness in the radiograph.

The size of the effective focal spot is controlled by:

1. The area of the target receiving bombardment by the electron beam from the cathode. The beam dimensions are determined by the:

   a. size of the filament and the degree of electrostatic control applied by the slot containing the filament
   b. distance between the cathode and anode
   c. potential difference between the cathode and anode.

2. The angle of the target face.

The size of the actual target area determines the amount of input load that can be applied

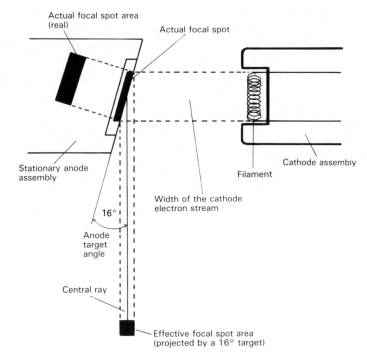

Fig. 6.3 Line focus principle.

to the tube by a single exposure. Therefore by the use of an angled target face, a greater X-ray output can be delivered from a small effective focal spot which is actually considerably larger in area because of the geometry of the line focus.

Bonding of the metal electrodes to the glass vessel — metal to glass bonds are required at either end of the vessel. These bonds are difficult to achieve with the different coefficients of expansion for metal and glass. With technical skill the difficulty can be overcome by joining the glass of the vessel to a different type of glass with a slightly greater expansion coefficient, and then to continue adding further rings, until after three additional rings of glass of progressively increasing expansion coefficient, the final ring is a very near match to the metal. This allows a solid and permanent bond which will withstand the heat changes which arise during use. The strength of the bond will allow the vessel to be pumped free of gas during manufacture giving it the vitally important high vacuum essential to precise electron control. A further glass to metal bond has to be made where the electrical con-

ductors supplying the cathode pass through the glass into the vessel. Glass is heated to mould it into a very efficient seal around each conductor and then bonded to the insert so preserving the vacuum and providing insulation between the conductors.

The glass vessel (envelope). The cathode and anode assemblies of the X-ray tube are sealed within a highly evacuated hollow glass vessel. Examination of a glass vessel will locate the remnants of the connection point for the evacuation pump used during manufacture.

The position of the cathode and the anode and their relation to each other is critical. Even a slight malalignment of either will cause the focus to be incorrectly sited and may cause the actual focal spot size to vary. The width of the gap between cathode and anode is carefully calculated to ensure that there will be no arcing across the gap at the tube's maximum kVp, therefore this gap must be correct; to be too narrow will run the risk of severe damage at high kVs and to be too wide will reduce the control of the electron beam's dimension and so allow the focus to become larger than intended. Therefore in manufacture each electrode is very securely bonded to the glass vessel in its exact location. The type of glass for the actual vessel is chosen for its low coefficient of expansion so avoiding change in size resulting from the very wide range of temperature the tube is subjected to during its working life and its high dielectric properties. Borosilicate glass has these properties, and is marketed under various trade-names with 'Pyrex' perhaps the most common.

The shape of the vessel, expanded in its central third to increase the insulation between the electrode face and the glass vessel by increasing the distance between them, is another feature of the X-ray tube insert.

The wall of the glass vessel attenuates the beam as it leaves the tube and forms part of the inherant filtration of the tube. In low energy tubes this may be reduced by grinding down the glass over the area transmitting the useful beam. This is not required in modern tubes used for general radiography. The code of Practice (Para. 3.10.2) requires a total filtration equivalent to 2 mm of aluminium for voltages above 70 kV and up to and including 100 kV, and 2.5 mm of aluminium equivalent at voltages above 100 kV. Therefore the aluminium equivalent of the glass can be allowed for in the calculation of the filtration which must be added to reach the required total.

The cylindrical shape of the outer thirds of the glass vessel, fitting quite closely around the electrode assemblies, is an important feature since it aids the dissipation of generated heat from the electrodes to the surrounding oil.

Therefore the functions of the glass vessel are:

1. to contain the electrodes
2. to provide a gas-free container
3. to secure the electrodes relation to each other very precisely and in particular to site the focal spot very accurately
4. to insulate electrically the electrodes from each other and isolate them from the tube housing
5. to aid the dissipation of heat from the anode and the cathode filaments

6. to allow electrical connections to be made with the electrodes
7. to provide a carefully regulated filtration of the beam by forming part of the inherant filtration of the X-ray tube.

This list of functions applies to a fixed anode tube. In a rotating anode tube there is an additional function the transmission of the magnetic field to cause the rotation of the anode which will be considered later.

Here the X-ray tube insert described has a glass envelope. Until recently there was not an alternative material suitable for this purpose but now some tubes have metal and other ceramic envelopes. These will be considered on page 95.

Drawing of a fixed anode tube insert. Figure 6.4 illustrates a method of drawing a fixed anode tube insert ensuring that the relationships and shape are correct.

X-ray tube housing
The X-ray tube housing is a cylindrical thick-walled aluminium alloy casting which is the container of the X-ray tube insert and its surrounding oil. Aluminium is used as it provides rigidity and strength and can be welded so allowing the addition of cable socket receptacles. To provide the necessary radiation barrier, it is lined, where necessary, with lead sheet ensuring that the leakage radiation does not exceed the maximum permitted level. The lead is very carefully arranged so that there is overlap where the sheets meet. To keep the weight of the tube to a minimum the heavy lead sheet is only laid down where it is needed and its thickness governed by the intensity of the radiation falling upon it. For instance the heavy anode block is more than adequate to protect the anode end of the shield.

The cylinder ends are closed by removable caps which allow access to the contents. The joints between cylinder and caps are carefully sealed to prevent any loss of oil. If oil is lost the level of electrical insulation is reduced. The operator must regularly check that there is no leak by wiping round the joint with a tissue for evidence of oil.

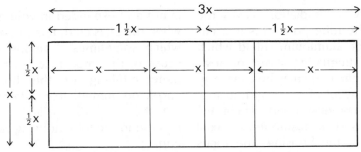

a. In pencil draw a rectangle 3 times longer than its height
   Divide it in half in both axes
   Divide the length into thirds

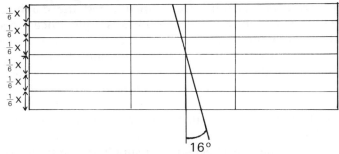

b. Divide the height into 6—3 in each half as shown
   Draw a line at 20° to the vertical through the mid-point

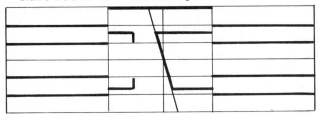

c. Outline in heavy pencil the basic lines of the tube as shown

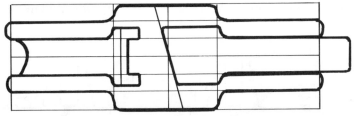

d. Join up the lines as shown remembering to round off all the angles apart from
   the corners of what will be the focusing cup of the cathode assembly. Examine
   the shape of the tube insert and other details; modify if necessary.

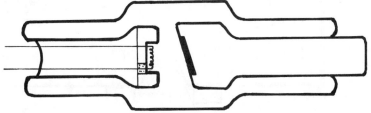

e. Ink in the tube insert shape and the other details; rub out the pencil

Fig. 6.4 Method of drawing a stationary anode tube.

The useful beam of X-radiation leaves the housing through the tube port. This is a circular opening in the aluminium shield which is covered by low attenuating plastic or nowadays a thin aluminium plate may be used. Figure 6.5 shows the layout of a typical housing.

Positioning of X-ray tube insert within the shield. The tube insert is positioned co-axial with the cylinder of the housing, the focus lying precisely on the axis of the tube port. It is held in this position by highly insulating plastic supports which are about a centimetre thick having a central opening which closely fits the glass insert at either end; the circumference fits inside the housing, with provision made for circulation of the oil through them. These fittings are very important as they ensure the correct alignment of the focus within the shield and its relation to the tube port. The position of the focus is essential for accurate collimation and should be checked from time to time and certainly when a replacement tube is fitted even though the manufacturer will undertake tests before delivery.

Provision for changes in oil volume with changing temperature. At the cathode end of the housing the oil is contained by a flexible diaphragm allowing no oil to leak round it. By its flexibility it can alter its shape to accommodate the volume of oil in the housing, bulging out towards the housing end when the oil is hot and expanded in volume, and drawn in when the oil is cold. It is this plastic diaphragm which sometimes develops a leak, and because of the importance of maintaining complete oilfilling of the housing must be corrected immediately if damage to the insert is to be avoided. The leak will be evident by oil around the tube housing cap at the cathode end.

As the X-ray tube insert heats up with use, the heat is transferred to the oil causing it to expand, and the diaphragm to move slowly outwards. This process continues without any significant increase in pressure within the housing until the diaphragm reaches the limit of its permitted movement. At this point the diaphragm exerts pressure on a microswitch. This microswitch is in an interlock circuit which when operated will prevent any further generation of X-rays by cutting off the electrical supply to the tube, so protecting the tube from damage due to excessive heat. It must be remembered that this safety device only operates when the oil becomes very hot which will take a comparatively long time and so will not prevent overheating resulting from a single or a few radiographic exposures. Further information on heat input, its dissipation and the overload protective devices will be given on pages 136–144.

X-ray tube window (tube port). The X-rays radi-

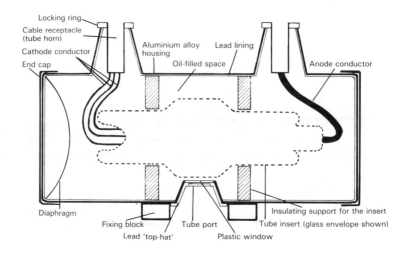

Fig. 6.5 Essential features of stationary (fixed) anode X-ray tube.

ated from the focus travel in all directions. The useful beam is simply those X-rays forming the cone of radiation which is directed through the tube port. The remaining X-rays radiating in all other directions are attenuated by the tube housing. The tube port is an area where the attenuation of the housing is deliberately kept low. The material used to form the tube port is either plastic or thin aluminium. It is shaped like a 'top hat' and projects into the cylinder, thus reducing the depth of oil between the insert and the port to reduce the attenuation of the beam and allow better elimination of off-target, extra-focal, radiation from leaving the tube. The 'top hat' has its sides lined with lead and the top partially covered with lead, leaving a central area clear of lead allowing an X-ray beam to emerge of the exact dimension required to cover the maximum field area that has to be exposed. Care must be taken to check the inherent filtration of the tube when it is first installed or replaced so that the correct amount of additional aluminium can be added to meet the requirements of the Code of Practice.

The window plate forms an accurate base for the attachment of the colliminating devices.

Details of the tube port are shown in Figure 6.5.

Provision for mounting. The housing is strengthened around its centre to allow for the clamp fittings which are used to attach the tube to its support. This fitting usually incorporates friction locks and scales to allow the tube to be angled precisely in both axes.

Tube housing high tension cable receptacle socket assemblies. The tube housing has two lead lined alloy 'horns' attached to its basic cylindrical shape. The 'horn-like' receptacles are designed to accept the HT cable plug and socket and provide for connection of their conductors to the tube insert within the housing. A choice of cable receptacle positions in relation to the X-ray beam is available although the range of choice is limited for fixed anode tubes, since their use is limited. The different positions for the horns are necessary to avoid restriction in tube movement. The two most commonly used types are those with cable re-

ceptacles 90° from the axis of the X-ray beam and at right-angles to the long axis of the cylindrical tube housing and at 90° from the axis of the X-ray beam in the direction of the cylindrical housing (see Fig. 6.15).

The design of the cable socket assembly (Fig. 6.6). A highly insulting plastic receptacle socket is fitted into each horn: one for the reception of the cathode cable plug and the other for the anode cable plug. The dimensions of both sockets are alike, making them interchangeable; each socket has three pin-like sockets in its base which receives the pin termination of each cable conductor. Inside the housing the cathode socket has three connections for the cathode filaments. The anode socket has all three terminations joined together to provide one conductor for connection to the tube anode.

The socket is very carefully made so that it exactly matches in shape and size the cable plug. There is a slot in the side wall of the socket and a ridge on the surface of the plug so that the plug must enter the socket correctly orientated with the socket to ensure correct connections are made. It is very important that the plug and socket fit very tightly so that all air is excluded. Air is a poor insulator and if air is present tracking can occur between the

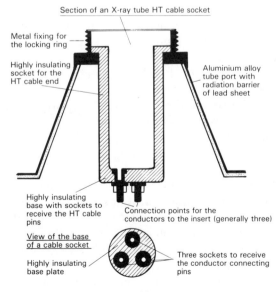

Fig. 6.6 Cable socket assembly.

highly charged internal parts of the socket and the earthed tube housing or earthed outer covering of the cable. The cable plug is secured in the socket by a threaded locking ring so ensuring no accidental extraction of the plug or poor connection between the cable conductor pins and their sockets.

Cables should only be removed by qualified X-ray engineers when the unit is totally isolated from the mains supply, and once removed must be immediately earthed to discharge any residual charge on the conductors. Poor connection within the socket will increase the resistance across the connection and result in reduced filament current and consequent reduction in X-ray output.

Functions of the tube housing

1. To act as an effective barrier against the radiating X-ray beam generated by the anode target, only allowing the emission of the useful X-ray beam from the very carefully controlled tube port.

2. To protect the fragile glass insert from mechanical damage.

3. To provide a means of securing the insert within itself in a very precise location.

4. To provide electrical safety for the patient and the operator by providing very effective earthing.

5. To contain the oil which surrounds the insert. The oil acts as an electrical insulator, as a means of removing heat produced by the insert and to a limited extent prevents tube overloading.

6. To provide highly insulated sockets for high tension cables.

7. To secure the tube to its support so that the X-ray beam can be aligned in the required direction.

8. To provide a mounting for the collimator.

The functions listed above are those for a fixed anode tube; with the rotating anode tube (p. 78) there is a stator motor within the housing and this will add to the function of the housing.

Whilst making provision for all these functions the tube housing must be kept as small as possible to allow a wide range of movement in a restricted space and to limit as far as possible the weight.

Uses of fixed anode X-ray tubes

Fixed anode X-ray tubes have few applications in today's X-ray service because they are so severely limited by their inability to tolerate anything more than a very small exposure load. They may be used for the following:

Dental units where a small, light manoeuvrable X-ray tube is needed and the poor loading characteristics are not a problem with the low exposure factor necessary and the short focus-to-film distance.

Portable units where the unit is required to have minimal weight allowing use without elaborate counterweight so that it is possible to manhandle the unit. These units can be operated from low powered electrical mains supply and with the very fast film/screen combinations can be used for a wider range of work than was previously possible.

Other low-powered units which may use fixed anode tubes include: mobile image intensifier units, mammographic units and orthodontic units. Details of these specialised units will be considered later.

Rotating anode tube assembly

To increase X-ray output whilst still retaining a small effective focal spot, the fixed anode tube has been replaced by the rotating anode tube for almost all applications as illustrated by the very short list of uses given earlier.

The essential difference between the two is that the electron stream from the cathode falls upon a rotating anode target instead of a stationary one. By rotating the target the generated heat is spread over a much greater area so allowing many times the maximum input load of a fixed anode tube to be applied to the target area before it reaches the limit of its heat tolerance. The rotation of the target does not exclude the use of the line focus principle to give a small effective focus. Therefore the rotating anode tube provides a high rate of X-ray generation whilst still retaining a fine focus giving a low level of geometric unsharpness and by shorter exposure times freezes patient movement.

In this section the design of the components of the basic rotating anode X-ray tube assembly are considered where their design varies from that found in the fixed anode tube previously described. Modifications to this basic design will be considered on pages 87–96.

X-ray tube insert

Figure 6.7 shows the layout of the cathode and anode and its surrounding glass vessel. It also shows the method of drawing the rotating anode insert.

Cathode assembly. The shape of the nickel cathode focusing cup and the layout of the tungsten filaments are identical in design to those of the fixed anode tube but their position within the tube is different. The focusing cup is mounted on a nickel support off-centre to the central axis of the tube, so that the electron stream is directed to the border of the target disc. The actual location of the cup is governed by the diameter of the target disc.

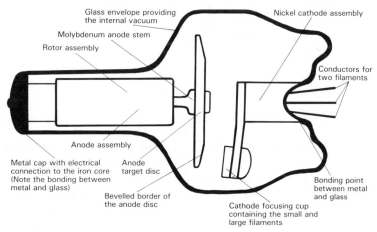

Fig. 6.7A Rotating anode tube insert.

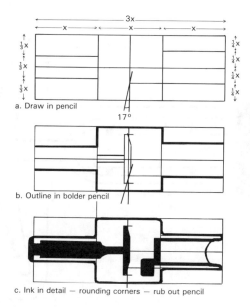

Fig. 6.7B Method of drawing a rotating anode insert.

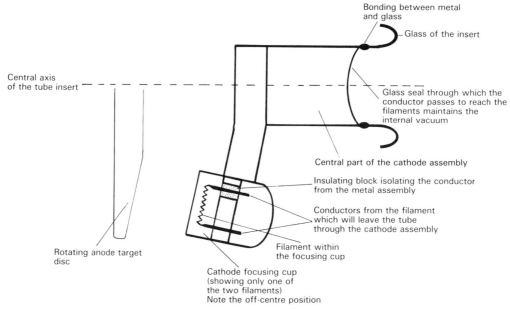

Fig. 6.8 Rotating anode cathode assembly.

Figure 6.8 shows the detail of the cathode assembly.

Anode assembly. The design of the anode assembly is shown in Figure 6.9. The disc-shaped target rotates freely on a central stem.

Figure 6.10 shows the relation of the disc to the cathode focusing cup. When the electron stream is directed to the border of a rotating disc the area bombarded is an annular track around the disc allowing very much more heat

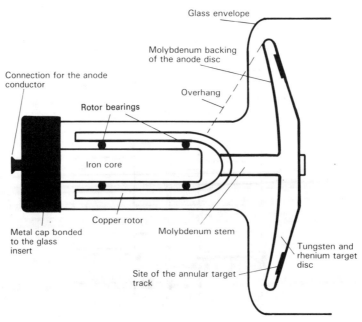

Fig. 6.9 Rotating anode tube anode assembly.

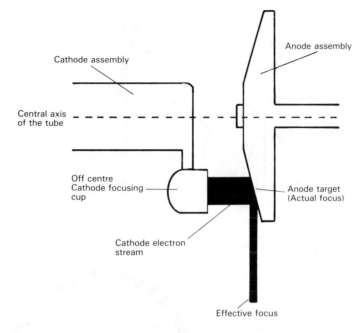

Fig. 6.10 Relationship of the rotating anode target disc to the cathode focusing cup.

input to be tolerated than on the small target area of the fixed anode tube, and by bevelling the edge of the disc the line focus principle is maintained affording a larger actual focal spot than effective focal spot. Thus a rotating anode tube can provide small focal spots whilst still accepting a vastly increased electrical input load. Figure 6.11 illustrates the target area and the calculation set out below shows just how great the difference in area is between a typical fixed anode and a rotating anode tube having the same effective focal spot size.

Details of the target areas for comparison

Effective focus   2 mm × 2 mm
Target angle   17 °
Rotating anode target disc   100 mm diameter
See Figure 6.12.

1. By line focus principle

$$= \frac{\text{effective focus}}{\sin 17°}\text{mm}$$
$$= \frac{2}{0.2924}\text{mm}$$
$$= 6.8 \text{ mm}$$

2. Target area of:
  (i) Fixed anode
     'a'   = 6.8 mm
     'b'   = 2 mm   (note there is no enhancement of this dimension)

    Therefore area   = 'a' × 'b' sq.mm
                     = 6.8 × 2 sq. mm
                     = 13.6 sq. mm

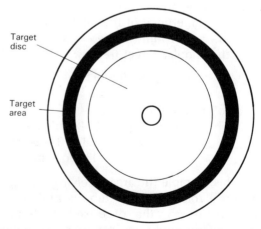

Fig. 6.11 Rotating anode target disc showing the target area.

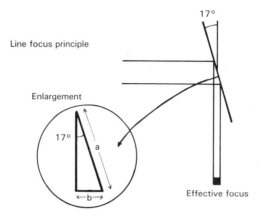

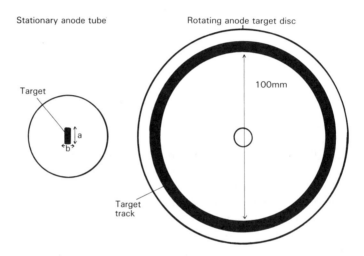

Fig. 6.12 Comparison of the target area of a rotating anode tube and a fixed anode tube.

(ii) Rotating anode
Circumference of the target area 'b'
'b' = 2π r mm (where r is the radius of the annular target track)

$$'b' = 2 \times \frac{22}{7} \times 50 \text{ mm}$$

'b' = 314 mm
Therefore the area = 'a' × 'b' sq.mm
= 6.8 × 314 sq.mm
= 2135 sq.mm

So in this example the area receiving the input load on a rotating anode tube is 2135 = 157 times greater than that of a fixed anode tube — one of the great advantages of a rotating anode compared with a fixed anode tube.

The anode assembly is formed of a target disc, rotor and bearing assembly.

The target disc is generally formed of a surface and backing layer:

front surface — also the target surface; made of tungsten with 10% rhenium added to improve its thermal capacity, so allowing increased loading over longer periods and to reduce the cracking and pitting of the surface which shortens the tube's useful life;

backing of molybdenum, which by its low thermal conductivity prevents some of the heat produced on the surface travelling through the disc to the bearing assembly. Molybdenum is a light metal which allows the disc to be expanded into a bi-convex disc to increase its mechanical strength. Note bi-convexity is a design feature of a modern rotating anode disc.

Manufacturers make X-ray tubes with target discs of different diameters ranging from 80 mm–150 mm, allowing selection to match the demands of the work that the unit is required to undertake; a larger diameter will increase the maximum tube loading that can be safely applied. Also there are different target angles available, from 6 °–17 ° and this too must be considered when selecting a tube for it has an effect on tube loading and also on effective focal spot and X-ray field size. The speed of rotation of the disc alters the single load rating of the tube. Examination of Figure 6.13 shows the length of track bombarded during a short exposure with the anode rotating

at the standard speed (3000 revolutions per minute) and the much longer track bombarded by the same short exposure time when high speed rotation (9000 revolutions per minute) is used. The illustration indicates that if the exposure time exceeds that of a single revolution, bombardment is applied again over the same track. From this it is easy to understand that when serial exposures are made in rapid succession there is no loading advantage to be obtained.

The target disc is attached to the rotor by a molybdenum stem. The stem is made as thin and long as possible to restrict the conduction of heat generated on the target disc from reaching the bearing assembly. The limitation on the length and diameter of the stem is determined by the need to provide the stability and mechanical strength necessary where a heavy disc is rotated at high speed.

The rotor. The rotor in which the foot of the molybdenum is firmly embedded is made of copper and forms a sleeve-like cover over the bearing assembly. Copper having high thermal capacity and being a good conductor prevents some of the generated heat from reaching the bearing and with the outer surface blackened and roughened improves the heat loss by radiation off the rotor.

Induction currents are produced within the copper rotor by the magnetic field produced by the windings of the stator motor and these cause the rotor with its attached target disc to rotate.

The bearing assembly consists of a steel spindle, the core. At each end of the core there is a race filled with steel ball bearings, allowing very free rotation of the copper rotor with its attached anode disc around the central core. The steel bearings are lubricated by a thin film of soft metal, silver or lead. It is essential that the bearings are protected from overheating if the free and easy rotation is to be maintained so that the tube will have a long useful life.

Securing of the anode assembly. The central steel core is secured to a cup-shaped steel cap which is securely bonded to the glass insert by a series of rings of different grades of

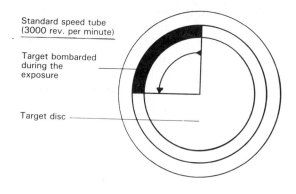

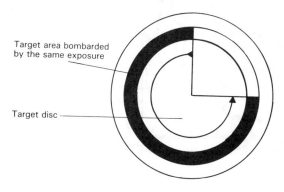

Fig. 6.13 Comparison of the target bombarded by an exposure on a standard and a high speed tube.

glass allowing the attachment of the metal cap to the main body of the glass insert.

The secure fixing of the central core to the glass provides the firm support for the anode, ensuring the vibration free rotation and accurate location of the anode target so that the focal spot is precisely sited. The electrical connection to the anode is made through the central core and the bearings on to the rotor which is continuous through the stem to the target disc. The conductor is fixed to the end of the core. In some tubes connection through the bearings is not considered adequate and an additional connecting switch is fitted between the end of the core and the undersurface of the rotor sleeve close to its bonding with the anode stem.

The glass vessel (insert casing or envelope). The vessel containing the two electrodes of a rotating anode is similar to the fixed anode vessel. It is normally made of borosilicate glass although metal (p. 93) is being used occasionally as an alternative to glass.

The vessel has an expanded central third to accommodate the anode disc and the offset cathode assembly, and a narrowed anode end around the rotor assembly. The narrowing here is important to ensure that there is the smallest gap possible between the stator motor windings sited outside the glass insert and the rotor inside the glass. The actual dimensions of the vessel are precisely calculated to provide adequate electrical insulation.

X-ray tube housing (shield)
Figure 6.14 shows the design of the rotating anode housing and its contents. The functions of the housings are as follows, including all of those for the stationary anode plus some additional requirements resulting from rotation of the anode:

1. to surround the tube insert with a conducting sheath which will provide an efficient connection to earth
2. to enclose the insert in an effective radiation barrier apart from the site of the tube port so that the intensity of radiation transmitted by the barrier is very low even under the most adverse conditions and at no time exceeding the maximum specified in the International Recommendations of Radiation Protection
3. to provide highly insulated high tension cable receptacle socket assemblies allowing the high tension and filament supplies to be connected to the insert electrodes

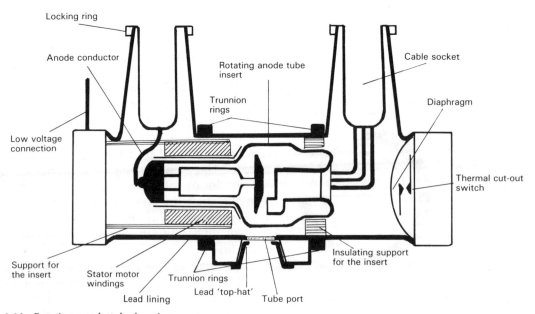

Fig. 6.14 Rotating anode tube housing.

4. to contain oil which will provide electrical insulation and cooling and allow for thermal expansion and contraction

5. to provide support for the insert ensuring that the focus is precisely positioned within the tube, the location of the focus must be clearly indicated on the outside of the housing

6. to carry a trunnion mounting ring allowing secure fixing of the tube to its support and a mounting block for the beam collimator to be fitted around the X-ray beam as it leaves the tube through the tube port

7. to provide housing and a firm support for the stator motor windings which cause the anode to rotate.

Whilst providing for all these functions the housing must be as small and as low in weight as possible to allow a wide range of movement in a restricted space and as light as possible to minimise counter-balancing difficulties.

General description of the housing. *The outer shell* is made from light aluminium alloy having sufficient thickness to give it adequate strength and rigidity to fulfil its function. Alumium alone cannot provide the radiation barrier so the housing is lined with lead sheet to reduce the leakage radiation to well below the minimum permitted level over its total surface. The lead is carefully arranged with overlaps at all joints with its thickness adjusted to suit protection requirements and cut the overall weight as much as possible.

The ends of the shield are removable to allow access to the insert, but they are carefully sealed to prevent leakage of the contained oil. The seal may break down with use so the operator must be alert for any evidence of this and deal with the situation at once as loss of oil reduces the level of electrical safety provided.

Positioning of the tube insert within the housing. The tube insert is co-axial with the main cylinder of the housing, the focus lying precisely on the axis of the tube port.

The end-casting of the housing, as well as closing the anode end of the housing, supports the insulator which fixes the anode end of the insert securely in position and also

holds the windings of the stator motor in their correct position. The other end of the tube insert is held in a highly insulating plastic support which is securely fixed within the shield. It is most important that the insert is held in position when the tube is turned into different positions and subjected to rotational stress. If the anode moves even a slight amount, malalignment of the X-ray beam will occur.

The plastic or rubber diaphragm (bellows) and thermal limit switch. The cathode end of the housing is closed by a plastic diaphragm fitted inside the end cap. The diaphragm is flexible and allows the change in oil volume which arises with changes in its temperature to be accommodated. As the temperature of the oil rises with the heat transferred to it from the insert, the oil volume expands causing the diaphragm to bulge outwards. This process can continue without any significant rise in pressure within the housing until further diaphragm movement is prevented by a stop-plate. At this point a micro switch is operated by the diaphragm which prevents further radiography or fluoroscopy by operating an interlock circuit. It is important to remember that the thermal limit switch is very slow in its operation and therefore cannot prevent radiographic tube overload.

X-ray tube port (window). X-rays radiate in all directions from the target area, the useful beam being the cone of radiation which is allowed to leave the tube housing through the tube port (window). The port is merely an area of low attenuation made of aluminium or plastic and formed into a cup-shape which is sealed into the housing. The walls of the cup are lined with lead and the base of the cup, which is directed into the housing, is fitted with lead into which is cut an opening with its dimensions carefully calculated to restrict the beam area to the maximum field size that the beam is required to cover. The cup-shape allows the beam limitation to be made as close as possible to the radiation source. This position restricts the exit of extra-focal (off-focus) radiation effectively and reduces the attenuation effect of the contained oil. The reduced attenuation by the oil is insignificant in general radiography, where a 2.5 mm Al, e.g. filtration, must be provided but will be significant in mammography where very low energy radiation is required and filtration has to be limited severely.

The face-plate of the cup is secured to the housing mounting block so that the collimation is accurately positioned.

Tube trunnion mounting ring. The housing is strengthened around its centre to enable the whole unit to be very firmly and safely attached to the mounting block on the tube support. This fitting generally incorporates friction locks and scales which allow the tube to be angled precisely in both axes or in a combination of both. The location of the focal spot must be indicated on the outside of the tube housing.

The housing cable receptacles for a rotating anode tube are similar in design to those described for the stationary tube (see p. 71). There are a number of housing types available the variation being in the location of the cable receptacle 'horns' in relation to the X-ray beam axis. The type of housing selected is governed by the location of the tube, for the tube 'horn' must not be the cause of limited tube movement. There are three main types available (see Fig. 6.15):

1. both cable receptacles at 90 ° from the axis of the X-ray beam and at right-angles to the long axis of the cylindrical tube housing
2. both cable receptacles at 135 ° from the axis of the X-ray beam and at right-angles to the long axis of the cylindrical tube housing
3. cable receptacles 90 ° from the X-ray

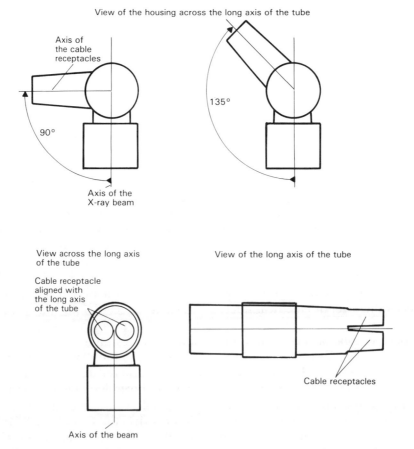

Fig. 6.15 Three types of tube housing showing the different positions of the cable receptacles.

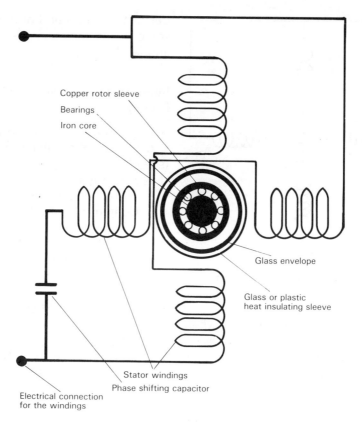

Copper rotor sleeve

Bearings

Iron core

Glass envelope

Glass or plastic
heat insulating sleeve

Stator windings

Phase shifting capacitor

Electrical connection
for the windings

Fig. 6.16 Cross-section of anode end of a rotating anode X-ray tube to show the location of the stator motor windings.

beam axis in the direction of the cylindrical housing with both cables leaving at the same end.

Stator motor windings. The anode is rotated by an induction motor located within the tube housing with the rotor inside the glass insert and the windings arranged around the rotor outside the glass insert. Figure 6.16 shows the relation of the various parts around and within the anode end of the glass vessel.

The externally placed stator windings and the anode rotor form the induction motor. The stator winding consists of two pairs of coils positioned so that the axis of one pair in at 90° to the other pair and directed through the centre of the rotor. The coils are supplied from an AC supply either single or three-phase depending on whether the anode is to rotate at 3000 revs per minute or whether it may be required to reach a rotation speed of

9000 revs per minute. The coils of each pair are connected in series and the pairs in parallel.

A capacitor is introduced into the circuit of one pair as shown in Figure 6.17 which causes the magnetic field of one pair to reach maximum when the field generated by the other is at zero. This makes for maximum rotational efficiency when one pair of coils is set at 90° to the other. Thus the copper rotor is subjected to a rotating magnetic field which induces eddy currents in the rotor, since the rotor is of conducting material and is being cut by the lines of force from the coils.

These eddy currents set up their own magnetic fields which react with those from the coils to cause the rotor to rotate. When high speed rotation, 9000 revs per second, is used it takes longer to reach full speed, requiring a longer 'prepare' delay. As a result of the ad-

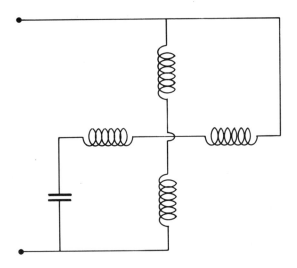

Fig. 6.17 The electrical supply of the stator windings showing the position of the phase shifting capacitor.

ditional stress and strain on the rotor when high speed is used, it is usual to find provision for dynamic braking to reduce the speed as quickly as possible once the exposure is over to reduce the wear and tear on the unit.

The high speed rotation is often obtained from a tripling transformer. This is a three-phase tranformer with its coils wound on a heavily saturated core. The output windings from the three-phases are connected in series so that a single-phase output is produced at three times the input frequency. Much heat is generated by this transformer but it can be reduced to some extent by careful selection of components to produce resonant frequencies which give high efficiency with a comparatively low heat production.

It must also be remembered that the heat input from the stator windings especially when they are generating high speed rotation is very considerable and must be taken into account when assessing the heat input into the X-ray tube from a rapid series of exposures.

Some manufacturers place a plastic or lead glass cylinder with a funnel-shaped end between the insert and the stator windings to protect the rotor bearings from some of the heat generated by the stator windings; the expanded end which lies behind the outer bor-

der of the anode end of the insert attenuates some of the radiation passing back from the anode.

Information found on the outside of the tube housing

1. The position of the focal spot.
2. On a label attached to the housing (shield)
    Shield type
    Shield serial number
    Content of the tube shield
      Tube type
      Insert serial number
      Focus, e.g. 0.6/1.2
      Maximum tube voltage, e.g. 150 kVp 4 or 6 pulse
      Maximum voltage to earth, e.g. 75 kVp
      Maximum continuous rating, e.g. 100 W on target
      Target drive 50–60 Hz
        50 Hz acceleration time, e.g. 1 sec
        150 Hz acceleration time, e.g. 30 sec
      Inherant filtration e.g. 0.7 mm A1 e.q.
Manufacturer.

Factors which will extend the useful life of an X-ray tube

When an X-ray tube is in use it is subjected to considerable strain. This strain causes wear which in time leads to a total tube failure or a gradual deterioration in X-ray output and an increase in image unsharpness which progresses until the deterioration reaches an unacceptable level and the tube must be replaced.

The tube manufacturers, the equipment suppliers and the radiographers can extend the useful working life of a tube by:

1. attention to design
2. care in manufacture
3. selection of a tube suitable for the work it is to perform
4. correct installation and adjustment
5. careful handling

6. knowledge of its operation and its limitations
7. good radiographic practice.

Tube selection

It is important that the tube selected is rated highly enough to withstand the demands put upon it. It must have a very large anode heat capacity if the work to be undertaken necessitates a very high loading so that it will not need to be operated near its maximum loading. In practice most units are set so that the tube loading is restricted to about 90% of maximum. Frequent loading over those limits shortens the life of the tube.

Good radiographic practice

Prevention of damage to the tube anode from the generation of excessive heat by:

a. avoiding unnecessarily high tube current or use of fine focus when the radiographic examination does not require it. This will result in exposure loading approaching the maximum permissible loading particularly if exposures are repeated without adequate cooling time between them.

b. using a 'run-up' procedure before a very large injection of heat is applied to a cold anode. Failure to do this may result in cracking of the target disc through differential expansion, the result of a sudden application of great heat on the surface of a cold anode disc. Four exposures of 70 kVp 200 mA 2 s with 1 minute intervals using the large focal spot if there has been no exposure for more than 30 minutes is suitable before a very heavy exposure is to be made with high output machines.

Extension of tube filament life by:

a. using a low mA when possible; conscientious use of immobilising devices will often allow a longer exposure time to be used without risk of motional unsharpness.

b. holding the unit in 'prepare' for the minimum of time. When the unit is in 'prepare', the filament is supplied with the higher boosted current which will evaporate the tungsten from the filament more rapidly than at the lower temperature produced by the standby current.

c. minimising careless handling of the tube which may cause mechanical damage to the filament.

Reduction of wear on the bearing of the rotating anode by keeping their running time at top speed to a minimum. The anode of the selected tube starts to rotate as soon as the exposure sequence commences and is running at its correct speed by the time the prepare period is over and remains running at this speed until the exposure is over. To reduce the running time the unit should not be held in prepare for any longer than necessary. If high speed rotation is available, this should only be selected when it is essential and not routinely. The high speed unit is fitted with a braking system which rapidly slows the speed down so limiting the wear.

Reduction in the rate of tungsten deposition on the internal surface of the glass envelope will delay tube failure through puncture of the glass or reduction in the insulation provided by the glass. Tungsten is deposited on the tube walls by condensation of tungsten vapour freed from the filament or the target by the very high operating temperatures. Limitation of the generated heat will reduce the amount of vapour available for deposition. The metal or ceramic tube envelopes will repel the deposition of tungsten.

Use of rating charts and full understanding of the protective devices incorporated in the unit will ensure the optimum use of the equipment and extend its useful life.

Checking of the tube shield for evidence of oil leak will allow replacement of oil before too much is lost and the insert subjected to undue strain.

Faults in X-ray tubes

With use the X-ray tube gradually deteriorates until the point when its output is unacceptable or a fault occurs. Faults can be classified into those which involve the glass envelope and its contents and those which arise in the housing or the stator winding within the housing.

Faults affecting the tube insert

Glass envelope. This is required to act as an insulator ensuring electrical isolation between the cathode and anode, but if tungsten is deposited on the internal surface of the glass there is reduction in insulation, and the wall has less negative charge. The loss of negative charge allows more electrons to bombard the wall because they are no longer repelled by the charge. As more and more tungsten is deposited the situation deteriorates until a point is reached when the glass is under constant heavy electron bombardment throughout the exposure.

When the rate of gas released from the glass by the bombardment exceeds a certain level, the gas released into the envelope in the narrow space between the shoulder of the rotor and the envelope becomes ionised, leading to a massive increase in the bombardment of the glass, and the production of copious gas leading to tube breakdown. If the gas in the tube does not actually cause perforation of the glass and total failure of the tube through entry of surrounding oil into the tube, the gas in the tube will cause the tube current, the mA, to increase uncontrollably and the kV to fall in response producing a radiograph which is grossly under-exposed and under-penetrated. The tube is described as gassy. This is a serious fault and no further exposures should be attempted as damage to other parts of the unit may occur as a result of the excessive current flow. A punctured tube can be diagnosed by a radiographer as the oil sucked into the insert will slop when the tube is turned and this can easily be heard.

The tungsten film will add extra filtration to the total filtration of the tube. This will harden the beam although in practice it will not be apparent as the deposition is gradual. Checks using a penetrameter or other technique to measure filtration should be undertaken occasionally.

The glass envelope may be broken by careless handling and sometimes stress fractures may occur especially as it has to carry the weight of the heavy anode assembly being rapidly rotated.

Anode. Every exposure heats the anode. The heat is applied to the surface of the disc causing it to be much hotter than the deeper layers. This leads to differential expansion and results in surface crazing. Crazing causes reduction in radiation output, increased anode heel effect and an increase in image unsharpness. If the anode does not start to rotate or ceases to rotate during the exposure all the heat is applied to a small area which will melt and release gas.

The anode disc may split through the sudden injection of great heat. The run-up procedure already described will reduce the risk of this occurring and some tube manufacturers have redesigned the anode disc to a discus shape which strengthens up the region under stress.

Rotor and its bearings. Deterioration of the bearings is indicated by increased noise whilst running and by a shorter slowing down period after the exposure is complete. Occasionally the bearings may seize, with an exposure on a stationary anode which will result in total tube failure. There is no method of servicing the bearings once they are installed in the insert. They must rely on the silver coating to act as the lubricant for their whole life. The amount of wear can be reduced by only rotating the anode for the minimum time necessary and by providing braking to reduce speed as soon as an exposure requiring high speed is over. Interlock circuits in the stator circuit prevent exposure or terminate exposures if the anode is not rotating in the generally forlorn hope of preserving the insert.

Filament. A break in the filament may occur as the filament thins with age through evaporation or by mechanical damage. The rate of thinning of the filament depends upon the rate of evaporation which is governed by the temperature of the filament and the time it is held at the temperature. The life of the filament can be extended by only boosting the filament to the high temperature for the shortest time possible and avoiding a high mA unless necessary. The filament as it thins will increase its resistance and this will reduce the mA. To ensure standardisation of exposure the mA values must be set up regularly by the X-ray engineer who adjusts the mA selector resistance until the mA is seen to be correct by examining the mA meter. A broken filament will mean no electrons to carry the tube current therefore no X-ray production. Identification of this fault may be made by trying the other focus of a dual focus tube; if this is functioning correctly the fault must lie with the filament supply or most commonly the filament itself. If the fault is intermittent it is generally a fault in the filament circuit rather than the filament, for instance a loose connection or break in the HT cable or in the HT socket may present an intermittent or persistant loss of mA.

Tube housing and the stator windings

Tube housing. The gasket sealing the oil within the tube housing may fail allowing oil to escape from the housing. This must be repaired at once before the loss is enough to reduce the insulation level of the tube. A radiographer should watch for evidence of leak, noticing the presence of oil on the outside of the housing, or sometimes a spot of oil on the floor under the tube after it has been left for the night.

Stator windings. A break in the windings or in the supply cable will result in no rotation or intermittent rotation of the anode—both are harmful to the target. The safety circuit provided in the unit will terminate the exposure as quickly as possible but even with fast operating relays this is rarely fast enough to prevent damage occurring. The most common fault is a break in the supply cable which is subjected to considerable strain through frequent changes in the position of the tube. The radiographer may reduce the strain on the cable by ensuring that it is not twisted or trapped by the tube support.

Notes on materials found in X-ray tubes

Glass

The tube envelope is made of borosilicate glass (Pyrex) which has a low coefficient of expansion.

Coefficient of Pyrex is $10^6 \times 3$ per metre per °C

Ordinary glass $\qquad 10^6 \times 9$ per metre per °C

Therefore Pyrex has a high resistance to thermal stress.

In order to bond the Pyrex type glass to the metal parts of the tube, it is necessary to have two or three intermediate glasses to increase gradually the expansion of the glass to match the expansion of the steel ring which links the electrodes to the insert.

Nickel

The cathode is made of nickel because it is a metal which is light and capable of being made to a very precise shape and retaining this shape even when heated. It is strong and can be used as a thin sheet.

Tungsten

As a filament material tungsten can be drawn into a very fine wire which can be shaped into a very small helix and retain this shape even when heated to incandescence. It has a reasonable work function, i.e. it does not require high energy to remove electrons from the highest filled energy level of the atom. It does not free electrons in any number until it is raised to a temperature in excess of 2200°C when it releases copious numbers. It has a low rate of vaporisation, boiling at 5400°C so protecting the internal vacuum of the tube.

As a target material it has a high atomic number, can be shaped precisely and has a high melting point. It has a high thermal capacity despite its poor specific heat coefficient because it is a very dense material. Thermal capacity is equal to the product of mass and specific heat. It can be worked to a smooth surface but is a rather brittle material so is not suitable for the stem of a rotating anode disc.

Rhenium

This metal has very similar properties to tungsten but as it is a very expensive material, 10% is added to tungsten to form an alloy which is more resistant to crazing than pure tungsten. By reducing crazing the tube has a longer useful life, the X-ray output does not fall off so quickly, anode heel effect is lessened and the definition of the image is maintained at an acceptable level for longer.

Molybdenum

Molybdenum is a strong material which will stand up to stress and can be machined to a precise shape, so it is suitable for the stem of a rotating anode target disc. It is a light material with half the density of tungsten and a poor conductor of heat, which makes it ideally suited as a backing for the tungsten target disc where it is useful to reduce the weight to be rotated and to prevent the heat produced on the target face passing back to heat up the bearings. Molybdenum can be used as a target material for low energy use. Mammography tubes have molybdenum targets, since the low kV is needed to improve image contrast and with molybdenum characteristic radiation produced at about 29 kV the X-ray output is greater for the same input power. Precise machining makes molybdenum a substitute for nickel in the cathode assembly.

Copper

In the stationary anode tube copper is used as the anode block into which the tungsten target button is embedded; it is valuable here as its high thermal conductivity removes the heat quickly away from the target. In the rotating anode tube it acts as the rotor sleeve helping to protect the bearings from the generated heat and because it is a good conductor eddy currents are developed in it which cause the anode to rotate. Copper is used elsewhere as electrical conductors for connecting the electrical supply to the electrodes within the insert. It is also used as the material forming the windings of the stator motor.

Graphite

Graphite is used in some modern tubes where high loading is required and where the weight of the target disc is unacceptably heavy for high speed rotation. The use of graphite as the support for an annular track of tungsten has been used and here the use of graphite greatly reduces off-focus radiation.

Stainless steel

This is used for the inner spindle of the rotor and for the bearings. The steel spindle concentrates the magnetic field from the stator windings.

Lead/silver

Lead/silver is used as the lubricant for the bearings. Silver is used to fix the tungsten target button into the copper anode block of the stationary anode tube.

Aluminium alloy

The X-ray tube housing is generally made of this material.

Lead

Lead lines the tube housing so that the leakage radiation is reduced to permitted levels.

Plastic

In the tube port the low attenuation of plastic allows the useful beam of radiation to leave the tube. Plastic is strong and can withstand the pressure of the contained oil. Highly insulating plastic is used for the HT cable sockets and as the support for the insert within the tube, maintaining it in an exact position. A flexible plastic sheet is used to form the diaphragm placed across the end of the tube housing so that the increased volume of heated oil can be accommodated.

Oil

Oil surrounds all parts within the tube housing acting as an insulator and as a means of removing heat from the insert.

Titanium and zirconium

These are sometimes used in very small quantities to strengthen the molybdenum back of the rotating anode tube target disc.

Different types of X-ray tube

The basic design of a rotating anode X-ray tube is modified to make it perform specific functions more efficiently. The modifications may allow the safe application of very high input loads or may meet the particular needs of a specialised radiographic technique.

Tubes designed to give a better performance for general radiographic techniques

High speed rotating anode tubes. These tubes have a similar stator windings to the basic tube but have the windings supplied with a three-phase electrical supply instead of the more usual single-phase. At normal speed the anode rotates with 3000 revolutions per minute, whereas the high speed tube with a three-phase supply rotates at 9000 revolutions. As an alternative to the three-phase the same or a greater rotational speed can be obtained with a frequency convertor. The high speed tube allows a very much increased input load, some 75% more than the same tube operated at the normal speed. However, this gain only applies to very short exposure times.

Figure 6.18 contrasts the loading of a stan-

dard rotational speed and a high speed tube. From this it can be seen that the high speed tube allows a much higher mA to be used for short exposure times but after about 1 second there is very little to choose between them. The restriction is now dependent upon the rate of cooling of the target block which is similar for both.

Figure 6.19 illustrates the distribution of the input load of a very short exposure time on the target track of a rotating anode tube operating at the standard speed of 3000 revs per minute and at the higher speed of 9000 revs per minute. From the diagram it is easy to understand why the rating of a high-speed tube is greater for short exposure times and how the advantage of high speed rotation falls off with longer times. With short exposures, the

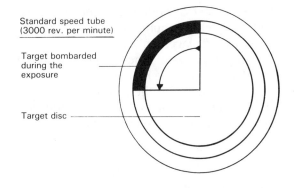

Standard speed tube (3000 rev. per minute)

Target bombarded during the exposure

Target disc

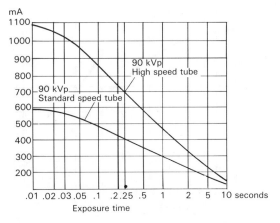

Fig. 6.18 Loading of a standard and high speed tube at 90 kVp.

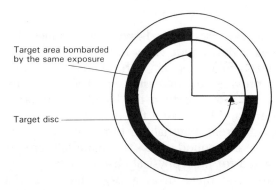

High speed tube (9000 rev. per minute)

Target area bombarded by the same exposure

Target disc

Fig. 6.19 Comparison of the target bombarded by an exposure on a standard and a high speed tube.

heat input is spread over a longer track as the anode rotates more quickly in front of the stream of cathode electrons. For longer times the input load is put time and time again on the same target track as the anode rotates a number of full revolutions before the exposure is completed.

The advantages of the high speed tube are:

1. Increased short-time loading, allowing the use of high mA and consequent shortened exposure time so reducing the risk of motional unsharpness.
2. Possible use of smaller focal spots, because of the increased input loading permitted. A micro-focus can be used enabling macro-radiography to be performed with a reasonably short exposure time.

The disadvantages are:

1. Initial cost of equipment, more sophisticated equipment required to operate the unit. Costly tube replacement.
2. Longer 'prepare' time because more time is needed to reach the higher rotational speed.
3. Greater wear on the bearings.
4. Greater heat injection from the high speed rotor windings. (Heat in excess of 9 kW can be produced by the stator windings of a high speed anode tube).
5. More stress on the anode stem, the result of high speed rotation. Therefore anode 'overhang' has to be reduced. This reduces the protection afforded to the bearings by the comparatively long thin anode stem.
6. Need for a braking system to rapidly reduce the rotation speed.

X-ray tubes with heavy duty anodes. The heavy duty anode X-ray tube has a very large heat storage capacity. The increased loading is provided by increasing the diameter of the target disc to extend the length of the target track and by making the disc from a number of different materials to form what is known as a compound disc. The materials are selected for their physical characteristics. Tungsten and rhenium as a target face material, molybdenum with a small amount of titanium and zirconium as the centre block, and graph-

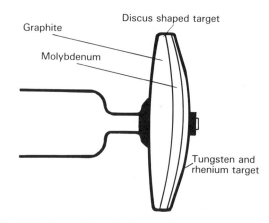

Fig. 6.20 Heavy duty rotating anode target.

ite as a back plate. Sometimes a thin skin of tungsten is applied to the back of the disc to give it added strength. It is shaped like a discus to provide greater strength than the older saucer-shaped disc.

Figure 6.20 is a cross-section of a heavy duty anode and shows the distribution of the various materials. Graphite and molybdenum are light materials and make it possible to increase

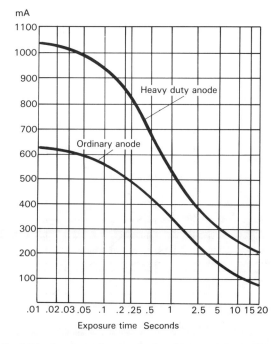

Fig. 6.21 Loading of a standard and heavy duty anode at 90 kVp.

the diameter and thicken the disc without producing weight which cannot be safely rotated at high speed. The anode disc forms a considerable block which has a large heat storage capacity.

Comparison of the rating chart of standard and a heavy duty tube is shown in Figure 6.21.

Steep angle target tubes
Manufacturers produce rotating anode tubes with different target angles. The conventional angle of 17° is suitable for general radiography

for it will provide an X-ray beam to cover a 43 cm field at 100 cm. However, if the maximum field is less than 43 cm, as in a skull unit, a steeper angle of 10° which will cover 30 cm may be selected. The geometry of a steep angle tube gives a smaller effective focal spot at the same loading or the same effective focal spot at an increased loading since the actual focal spot is larger and so able to accept a greater loading. Figure 6.22 illustrates the geometry of a conventional 17° target and the smaller effective focal spot or increased actual focus provided by a 10° target. It also indicates

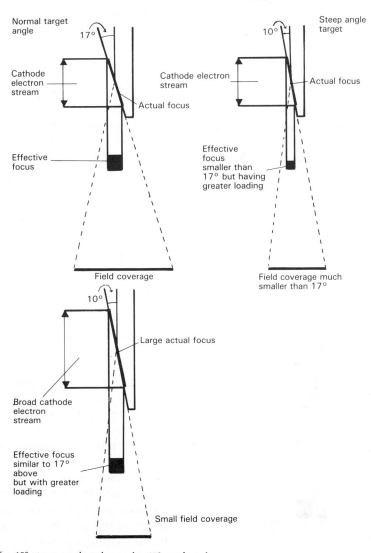

Fig. 6.22 Geometry of a 10° steep angle tube and a 17° angle tube.

the reduced field size covered by the beam of the steeper angle target.

The radiographic techniques to be performed by the tube must be specified before the tube is ordered as the geometry of the beam cannot be adapted after manufacture.

Bi-angular X-ray tubes. Such tubes have the target face bevelled to provide two different angles. The cathode electrons from one filament are directed to one angle and the electrons from the other filament to the other angle. Figure 6.23 shows the cross-section of such a tube. The advantage of the tube is that it provides a choice of high loading with an average focal spot size or a lower loading on a smaller effective focal spot. Therefore with a dual focus tube it is possible to select an arrangement to suit the needs of the radiographic examinations being undertaken on the unit.

Figure 6.23 illustrates the actual and the effective focus of the option with a steep angle, 10° and an average 17° angle tube. It must be remembered when considering a bi-angular tube that a steep angle target face can only be used where the field to be covered is small and that as the filaments must be arranged one above the other that the two focal spots will not be in the same position within the tube making it impossible to accurately align the collimator to coincide with the radiation field from both foci.

Very great care must be taken when selecting these tubes. Rating charts and other data must be examined to ensure that their output, focus and field coverage will satify the demands of the range of radiographic techniques that may be undertaken with the tube.

Grid tubes

Grid tubes can perform two functions. They can switch the X-ray output or less commonly control the focusing of the cathode electron stream to produce a micro-focus.

The grid in these tubes is rarely an actual wire grid sited in front of the cathode but is the cathode focusing cup supplied with an additional biasing voltage so that it can operate as a grid. The action of the biasing voltage is to increase the electrostatic force developed around the slot containing the filament. The space charge generated may cause the electron stream to be unable to leave the cathode so acting as a switch or it may not be great enough to stop the flow but will compress the electron stream so that it interacts with a much smaller actual target area giving a micro-focus. Once the additional biasing is removed, the tube returns to its normal focus size. The additional biasing is only provided for one focus of a dual focus tube.

Figure 6.24 illustrates the variable focus principle and Figure 6.25 the grid switching function. It can be seen from the illustrations that an additional conductor is required to connect the unit providing the additional biasing voltage to the cathode focusing cup.

A grid tube for switching purposes is used for pulsed cine work where rapid switching is essential and where the current to be switched is less than 1000 mA. It is also a useful tube for techniques where the exposures are extremely short as in paediatric work. Further detail of the switching method is given under the section on exposure switching on page 105. Ca-

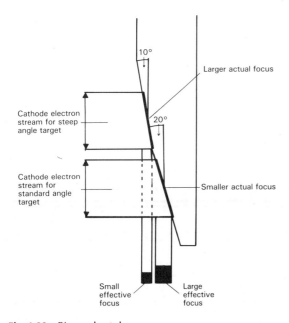

Fig. 6.23 Bi-angular tube.

a. Normal focusing cup

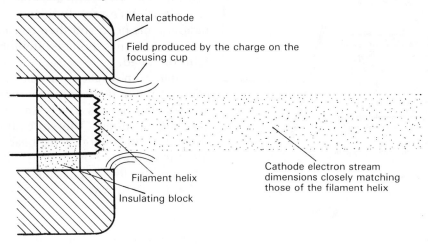

Metal cathode

Field produced by the charge on the focusing cup

Filament helix

Insulating block

Cathode electron stream dimensions closely matching those of the filament helix

b. Focusing cup with biasing applied

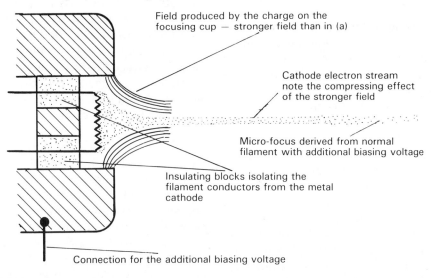

Field produced by the charge on the focusing cup — stronger field than in (a)

Cathode electron stream note the compressing effect of the stronger field

Micro-focus derived from normal filament with additional biasing voltage

Insulating blocks isolating the filament conductors from the metal cathode

Connection for the additional biasing voltage

Fig. 6.24 Variable focus.

pacitor discharge units are generally fitted with grid tubes so that X-rays cannot be produced when the capacitor has discharged to a point where its energy has fallen below the level when it can play no further part in image formation but merely increase the patient dose. This action is discussed on page 267.

Some dental tubes are grid tubes. They are used because it enables the manufacturer to prevent the passage of low energy electrons across the tube. The spectrum from these tubes is more homogeneous and with higher average energy. This eliminates X-radiation produced by electrons whose energy can play no part in image formation.

A grid tube providing a variable focus. These tubes allow macro-radiography to be performed when needed but without restricting the normal use of a dual focus tube. Foci as small as 0.1 mm^2 can be provided by this

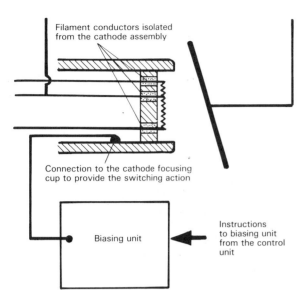

Filament conductors isolated
from the cathode assembly

Connection to the cathode focusing
cup to provide the switching action

Biasing unit

Instructions
to biasing unit
from the control
unit

Fig. 6.25   Grid switched X-ray tube.

method. The great advantage is that for most of the time the tube can accept a useful loading which cannot be provided by a dual focus tube with one focus devoted to macro-radiography as the micro focus can only have a very limited use. Some manufacturers have increased the loading of these tubes on all foci, micro included, by water cooling the tube.

The disadvantage of grid tubes is the cost; not only is the tube more expensive but the biasing unit needed to operate it is also an expensive item. The modified focusing cup method of providing the grid facility is more economical than the true grid tube. In the tube with an actual grid, if the grid fails the facility is lost; with the modified cathode focusing cup the tube can continue to be used and anyway the likelihood of failure in this form of tube is no greater than the normal tube. There are no delicate parts to fail.

Tubes designed for special purposes
Some radiographic techniques are better performed by the use of an X-ray tube specially designed to suit the particular needs of the examination.

These tubes will be considered by examination of how the basic design is modified to provide for the particular need. For each tube it is necessary to identify the special radiographic need and then consider how the manufacturer has modified the tube design to fulfil the need.

Mammography tubes. For maximum visualisation of the soft tissue of the breast it is essential that there is a very sharp image with very high contrast. Therefore the tube must produce a low energy X-ray beam from a fine focus in a short exposure time with the patient dose kept as low as possible.

The modifications necessary are:

(i) The anode target is of molybdenum, not tungsten. Molybdenum characteristic radiation is produced at 29 kV and so when using a low kV between 20 and 40 for increased contrast, X-ray production is greater because of the added characteristic photons, which would not be present with a tungsten target until the kV used exceeded 69.

(ii) The target angle of the mammography tube is reduced (steep) as the field under examination is small. This gives a fine focus with a reasonable loading. A fine focus is essential for the demonstration of micro-calcification which is a useful diagnostic feature.

(iii) The cathode and anode are brought much closer together, less than a centimetre apart, to ensure close control of the dimensions of the electron beam to give a fine focus. The small gap between cathode and anode is permitted because of the restricted kV.

(iv) Because the glass insert would cause considerable attenuation of the useful beam, a beryllium window is fitted in place of glass and the shield designed to reduce the amount of oil within the shield that must be traversed to a minimum. This modification is also possible because of the low operating voltage.

(v) The spectrum of the beam is further modified to provide maximum useful photons at as low an energy as possible for increased contrast, and at the same time eliminating photons which have too low energy to take part in the image formation and only add to the patient dose. This alteration in the spectrum is made by means of a molybdenum filter. No aluminium filter is present as it would attenuate the useful low energy beam excessively.

(vi) The layout of the contents and the shape of tube housing are adapted to allow easy positioning of the patient.

These tubes are supplied by an ordinary X-ray generator which will most probably supply one or two other tubes being used for general work. The mammography tube supply will be fitted with limiting devices to ensure that this tube cannot be supplied with a kV in excess of 40 kV and cannot exceed the safe loading of this low output tube.

Dedicated mammography units are available which use stationary anode tubes with their anode hooded to eliminate extra focal radiation and in order to provide an adequate loading the anode is water cooled. Further details of mammography units are given on page 260.

Stereography tubes. Stereography can be performed satisfactorily by displacement of the central ray of an ordinary tube, but with the advance of photofluorography displacement of the tube presents logistic problems as well as difficulty in exposing two films in rapid succession.

Specialised stereoscopic tubes can overcome these problems. There are two methods:

The X-ray tube has one of its dual filaments dupletised. The two parts of this filament are set side by side of the normal filament position. The electron beam from each is directed to a different target area so that the X-ray beam generated from one of the filaments produces an image with displacement towards one side and the other an image with the displacement to the other side. When these two images are viewed through 3-D glasses or a stereo-mirror system, a stereoscopic view of the image is perceived (see Fig. 6.26). The disadvantage of this system is that there is only one filament remaining for normal radiography.

The X-ray tube insert is fitted into the tube housing so that it can be electrically turned through a few degrees within the housing in response to an electrical signal from the control unit. In this way the filament can be pos-

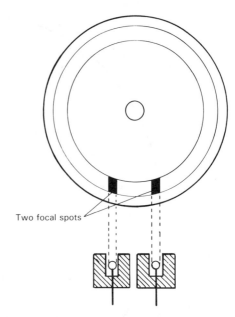

Fig. 6.26 Dedicated stereoscopic X-ray tube having two focal spots with no facility for normal radiography.

itioned 15° off-centre in one direction and the collimator automatically adjusted to suit the beam for one of the stereo-pair of films and then turned 15° the other way with further adjustment of the collimator for the second film of the pair. The pair of films when viewed with 3-D glasses gives a stereoscopic image. The effective focal spot size is very small. The filament's normal position being central allows normal use of the filament, extending the range of options available (see Fig. 6.27).

Stereoradiography provided in this way permits:

(i) use with photofluorographic systems

(ii) immediately available stereoscopic pairs at up to two films a second useful in vascular radiography

(iii) enlargement techniques because of the small focus

(iv) digital image enhancement and subtraction techniques of stereoscopic images

(v) normal use of one focus in the first option and both in the second.

Metal/ceramic tubes. These have been designed to provide very compact units able to accept extremely high loading. This makes

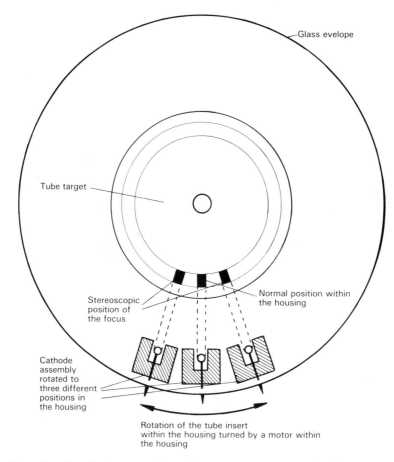

Fig. 6.27 Stereoradiography tube allowing normal use when stereoscopy not required.

them ideally suited for techniques requiring long runs of rapid repetitive exposures.

The shape and features of one type of these new style tubes (see Fig. 6.28) are:

1. A metal insert envelope instead of traditional glass.

2. Ceramic (aluminium oxide) for electrical insulation around the conductors.

3. A large diameter anode disc mounted on an axle with bearings at either end to provide greater stability and reduced stress on the shaft.

4. An extended tube life through elimination of the risk of a punctured envelope and the effect of a tungsten film on the inside of the insert.

Earthing of the metal envelope ensures that the electrical fields developed within the tube are stable and do not change as tungsten vapour is deposited on the inside of the insert.

5. Extra-focal radiation is reduced by removal of stray electrons through the earthed metal envelope.

6. The HT cables enter the insert at one end.

Examination of Figure 6.28 shows how the components and their layout can be arranged as a very compact unit; the use of ceramic insulation and the earthing of the envelope ensuring electrical safety despite its small size. The design of the tube insert gives great thermal capacity. Unless forced cooling of the oil is provided the tube rating may be limited not by the insert but by the rate at which oil can

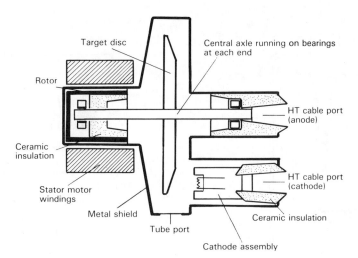

Fig. 6.28 Metal/ceramic X-ray tube.

dissipate the generated heat. The metal shield improves the rate of conduction of heat from the insert components to the oil.

The advantages of this type of tube are:

1. Higher rating.
2. Improved image quality through elimination of much of the extra focal radiation and the possibility of using smaller focal spots because of the improved rating.
3. Compactness.

Disadvantages are:

1. Cost.
2. Tube insert and housing are not interchangeable with conventional units.

Tubes for computed tomography. Computed tomography requires longer exposure times than those needed for general radiography. The stationary tubes used for radiotherapy units have been used but these are being superseded by heavy duty rotating anode tubes with very high thermal capacity. Some of the tubes are grid-controlled to reduce patient dose by pulsing the radiation.

Extra focal radiation degrades the reconstructed image so it must be reduced to the absolute minimum by very close beam collimation, possibly the use of an earthed metal tube insert envelope and in stationary anodes

by the use of hooded-anodes to absorb any stray electrons.

The stationary anode tubes have their cathode filaments turned through 90° to normal to provide the fan beam but in rotating anode tubes the cathode filament is in normal alignment and the fan beam provided by a slit diaphragm.

Tubes with forced cooling
Forced cooling is used to allow higher loads to be safely applied to the tube and to extend the life of the tube by enabling it to be operated well within its maximum loading. Detailed information on tube loading is dealt with in later chapters. The principal means of providing forced cooling are by:

An external fan. An external fan improves the air circulation around the tube housing. It is commonly attached to the housing of undercouch tubes to move forcibly the air within the metal covers surrounding the tilting table. The fan is switched on as soon as the tube is energised. The rate of cooling can be doubled by the use of a fan.

A heat exchanger. Heat exchangers (Fig. 6.29) are used where the X-ray techniques require very high load sequential exposures — cine-angiography is a good example of a technique which can be extended by the use of a heat

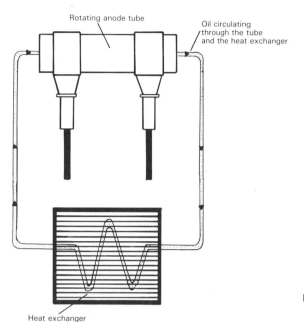

Fig. 6.29 X-ray tube fitted with a heat exchanger to cool the oil from the tube housing.

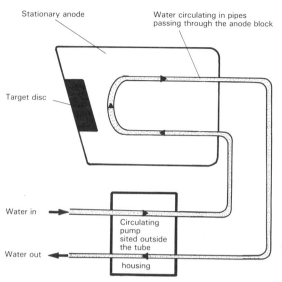

Fig. 6.30 Water-cooled stationary anode tube.

exchanger. The tube insert is designed to accept very high input loads using very high mA within its anode maximum thermal storage capacity but the surrounding oil cannot dissipate the heat conveyed to it rapidly enough. This would prevent the full use of the tube's potential so the oil is pumped through long flexible hoses to an externally sited heat exchanger; here the oil is passed through a radiator where the oil is cooled before being returned to the tube. A heat exchanger can remove about 100 000 HU per minute.

Water-cooled stationary anode tubes. Water cooling for the anode is provided by pumping cold water through fine pipes up behind the target face (see Fig. 6.30). It is used where the heat generated at the target cannot be removed rapidly enough by conduction through the copper stem of the anode. Some dedicated mammography units use this method of cooling. An interlock system is provided to prevent operation of the tube should the water circulation not be taking place.

THE ELECTRICAL CONNECTIONS TO THE X-RAY TUBE

The X-ray tube requires electrical connection with the HT generator and with the low voltage control circuit supplying the thermal cut-out switch, and in the rotating anode tube a supply for the stator motor.

High voltage connection

The X-ray tube cathode and anode are connected to the output of the HT generator by high tension cables specially designed to ensure electrical safety despite the high voltage supply they carry. HT cables are always fitted unless the generator and the X-ray tube are contained within a single tank. The cables are terminated in plugs which fit into the sockets in the tube housing or the HT generator tank top. The cables are reversible and interchangeable so that they can be used as cathode or anode cables. To reduce the insulation required in the tube and generator connection and in the cable itself, X-ray tubes are energised symmetrically about earth so that each cable and its connectors carry only half of the potential across the tube. This safety feature has been described in the section on the HT transformer (p. 40). It will be recalled that the centre point of the secondary winding is earthed so that the cathode operates at negative potential in respect to earth and the anode at positive potential to earth. By this means thinner and more flexible cables can be used to provide the required level of electrical safety.

Construction of a high tension cable

The cable (Fig. 6.31) has a central core of three or occasionally four separate conductors surrounded by a thick layer of insulating material. The thickness of this layer is determined by the maximum kilovoltage to be applied to the conductors and the insulation coefficient of the material used. Modern cables use insulating plastic rather than rubber. Outside the insulation is a sheath of flexible aluminium or copper foil. This mesh is bonded to the metal covering of the cable ends, providing a continuous path to earth extending from the tube housing and all along the cable to the generator tank; this earth pathway also

provides earthing for the tube support. The outer covering of the cable is smooth plastic allowing easy cleaning and protection for the aluminium or copper mesh from mechanical damage.

The central core contains the three conductors, or four if the cable is to supply the cathode of a grid tube. Each conductor is covered by a thin plastic sleeve to insulate it from the other conductors. There is no need for thick insulation since the potential difference between each conductor is only about 12 V (the filament voltage). The thick outer insulation encompassing all the conductors is needed as the potential difference between the conductors and earth is half the maximum kVp across the X-ray tube; in diagnostic tubes with a maximum voltage of 150 kVp this will be 75 kVp.

The cathode cable in a dual focus tube has its three conductors connected thus: one to an end of the small focus filament, one to an end of the large focus filament and the third as a common lead for both. The common conductor is also used to connect the cathode to the negative HT supply. In the case of a grid tube the fourth conductor carries the biasing voltage to be applied to the cathode focusing cup. The anode cable being similar in construction to the cathode cable has three conductors but as only one supply is required by the anode the ends of the conductors are joined together so they act as one.

The cable ends

The cable terminates in special plugs which fit into the cable receptacles (sockets) of the X-ray tube and the generator tank. The plug has an outer case of highly insulating plastic, and the conductors pass down through the centre of this plastic sleeve which is filled with bitumen or araldite, highly insulating materials that ensure electrical isolation of the conductors as they pass into the tube or generator tank. Figure 6.32 shows the layout and shape of the cable end. The conductors emerge through the base as metal pins which plug into the bottom of the sockets.

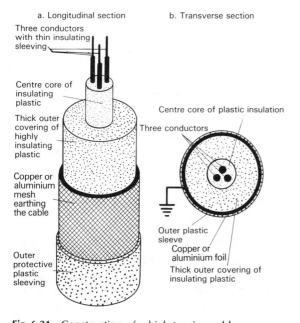

a. Longitudinal section   b. Transverse section

Three conductors with thin insulating sleeving

Centre core of insulating plastic

Thick outer covering of highly insulating plastic

Copper or aluminium mesh earthing the cable

Outer protective plastic sleeving

Centre core of plastic insulation

Three conductors

Outer plastic sleeve

Copper or aluminium foil

Thick outer covering of insulating plastic

Fig. 6.31   Construction of a high tension cable.

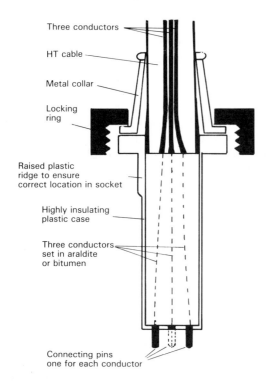

Three conductors

HT cable

Metal collar

Locking ring

Raised plastic ridge to ensure correct location in socket

Highly insulating plastic case

Three conductors set in araldite or bitumen

Connecting pins one for each conductor

Fig. 6.32 High tension cable end.

The cable plug is securely fixed into the socket. To reduce the stress exerted by movement of the cable close to the tube a metal collar is fitted over the cable and under the locking ring so that the first centimetres of the cable are supported. The fit between cable plug and socket must be extremely close as an airtight seal is required to prevent arcing; a silicon lubricant is sometimes used to ensure that all air is excluded.

Care in handling HT cables
HT cables should be supported and carried to the X-ray tube in a way which will avoid any strain on them, through pulling or acutely bending them. This could ultimately break one of the conductors. The radiographer must take care not to cause strain by twisting the cables around the tube support as the tube is positioned or by trapping them between parts of the equipment. If the conductor is broken the cable must be replaced or if the break is very

close to one end it may be possible to shorten the cable and refit the end plug. This is a skilled job and cannot be done on site.

Evidence of a cable fault may be apparent by a zero reading on the mA meter or inconsistency of mA if the break is not total. It is difficult to isolate the fault to the cable as a tube fault may present the same symptoms, shown radiographically or on the meter. Occasionally, when a short circuit of a cable occurs there is a smell of burning insulation material, which will not occur with a tube fault.

If the locking ring fixing the plug into the socket works loose, which may happen with constant movement of the tube as in tomography, the connections in the base may not be good and the resistance created will effect the tube output and can be a cause of variable results.

Removal of the HT cables
Removal of the HT cables must only be undertaken by an X-ray engineer who will take great care to isolate the unit first by switching off the mains supply. He must also discharge the charge built up in the cables before they are handled. The length of the cable acts as a capacitor, having the conductor as one electrode and the earthed metal sheath as the other electrode and the insulating layer the dielectric. This effect is useful in practice as it does provide some smoothing of a pulsed supply. However, if the cables are very long and the mA very small there may be a noticeable effect on the output from the tube when compared with a similar unit with short cables.

Other connections to the X-ray tube

Stator motor connection
The cable bringing the supply to the windings of the stator motor enters the tube housing through the anode end cap passing into the oil-filled cylinder through a rubber encircled opening which provides an oil sealed entrance for the cable.

Thermal cut-out switch supply

The circuit containing the thermal cut-out switch reaches the switch inside the end cap of the tube with the cable supplying the stator windings, but it does not enter the oil-filled cavity as the switch is placed outside the plastic diaphragm forming the end wall of the cavity.

Tube load monitoring devices

The cable connecting these modern monitoring devices also enters the end cap with the other cables and through a rubber seal to reach the sensor device sited behind the anode.

None of these cables carry a voltage in excess of the normal domestic voltage of 240 V and so require no additional safety features. The cables having left the tube are carried back to their control units beside the high tension cables tied to the cables for protection against mechanical damage. Figure 6.33 shows the position of the HT cables and the other cable exits from the tube.

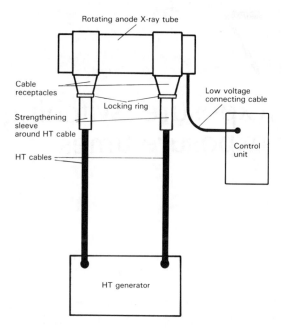

Fig. 6.33 Position of the HT and tube voltage cables connected to the X-ray tube.

7

Exposure switching and the control of exposure times

X-rays are produced when electrons are released by the X-ray tube filament and when the high tension is applied to the tube electrodes. This occurs when the exposure contactor is closed and continues until it is reopened. The interval between the closing and reopening of the contactor is the exposure time. This interval is controlled by the exposure timer circuit which operates remotely on the exposure contactor.

Therefore for accurate control of exposure time three operations must be working efficiently:

1. The circuit supplying the high tension to the tube must close so that current may flow through the X-ray tube.

2. The length of time during which the current will flow must be accurately measured.

3. The circuit must cease to pass current immediately the measured time interval has elapsed.

Therefore to understand the control of exposure time appreciation of the operation of exposure switching and of exposure timing is necessary. Accuracy and consistency of exposure time cannot be obtained if one or both parts of the system are inadequate or defective. In practice the degree of accuracy necessary is governed by the length of the exposure time; an error of a few milliseconds is insignificant on most occasions. The accuracy of the system is determined by the sophistication of the circuit and the quality of the components used in it. These factors are reflected in the cost of the unit.

EXPOSURE SWITCHING

Exposure initiation and termination is the function of the exposure switch. Switching may take place in the primary circuit of the high tension transformer where it is necessary to switch high currents at a low voltage or in the secondary circuit where a low current must be switched at a high voltage. Both systems require that the time taken to perform this function is short and unchanging. In most general units the switching occurs in the primary circuit and is termed primary switching. Secondary circuit switching is found where rapid repetitive exposures are made as in cine radiography or where extremely short exposure times are required as in paediatric work.

Primary switching

There are two types in use today: the solid state switch and the electro-mechanical contactor. The mechanical contactor is gradually being phased out but as it can cause loss of X-ray output it will be considered. Figure 7.1 shows the location of these switches in the X-ray circuit. Often two switches in series are provided, one operating to close the circuit and allow the exposure to start, the other to open the circuit and end the exposure.

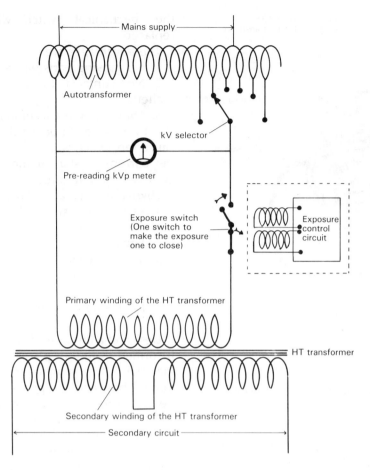

Fig. 7.1 Location of the exposure switch in the primary circuit.

The electro-mechanical contactor

The electro-mechanical contactor (Fig. 7.2) consists of a solenoid whose coil is wound around an iron core which supports two copper contact pieces. The contacts are specially designed to ensure their rapid response to magnetic attraction, closing them without bounce. There is however unavoidable inertia in this form of mechanical switch.

The contacts must be able to withstand the high temperature produced at their point of contact and so are faced with silver or tungsten alloy; the rest of the contact is made of copper to reduce the resistance of the unit.

There may be a single contactor in the circuit making and breaking the exposure although two positioned in series are more efficient, one making and the other breaking the exposure. Each operates more positively in response to a magnetic attraction than is possible with a spring operated release. It is important that the switching action takes place when the alternating voltage is at zero potential; if it is not at zero; arcing will take place as the contacts come together causing a high temperature to be developed which will distort the contact surfaces. Any distortion of the surface will result in poor contact and a progressively increasing level of resistance arising in the switch. There will be evidence of this radiographically, as the output of the unit will progressively fall off. Therefore regular servicing is essential to ensure the phasing of the switching, to keep the contact surfaces smooth and to check that there is no bounce when the contacts close. Bounce will

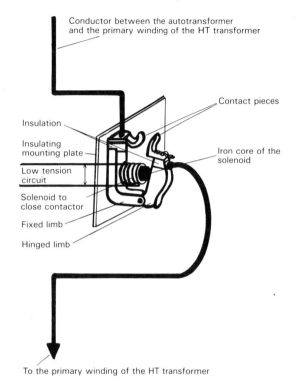

Conductor between the autotransformer
and the primary winding of the HT transformer

Contact pieces

Insulation

Insulating
mounting plate

Iron core of the
solenoid

Low tension
circuit

Solenoid to
close contactor

Fixed limb

Hinged limb

To the primary winding of the HT transformer

Fig. 7.2 Principal parts of an electro-mechanical exposure contactor.

lead to overheating. The radiographer will recognise this form of switching by the distinctive sound as the contacts close and should suspect the presence of high resistance in the switch if the exposure factors have to be progressively increased to overcome a falling X-ray output.

Disadvantages of an electro-mechanical contactor are:

1. The need for frequent servicing to maintain the contacts in good condition.

2. Regular replacement of expensive contacts.

3. Inertia of the moving parts making the unit unsuitable for short exposures.

Solid state switching

Solid state switching is provided by a pair of thyristors. This form of switching is very efficient and is found in most modern units. The thyristor has replaced the gas-filled triode valve. The thyristor and the older equivalent the gas-filled triode valve are much better than

the mechanical switch which they have replaced.

The advantages are:

1. No moving parts, so less inertia.

2. No contacts to become distorted or melted.

3. They operate accurately, allowing very short exposures to be made with accuracy because the switch will only allow conduction of the current to start at the zero point of the cycle and end at zero.

Thyristors have additional advantages:

4. Almost indestructible and do not vary during their life.

5. Small.

6. Voltage drop across them is very small and does not vary.

7. Action is very rapid.

8. No filament to heat.

Design of a thyristor. The solid-state thyristor is formed from four plates of semi-conducting material. Three junctions: N-P, P-N, N-P, are formed between the plates. Current can pass freely across the N-P junctions but cannot cross the P-N junction until a positive pulse is introduced into the P-type to overcome the barrier. The positive pulse is introduced through a conductor, known as the gate, which is welded to P-type material.

Operation of a thyristor as a switch. A thyristor when used as a switch in an electrical circuit provides a means of starting a current flow which will continue until the potential across it falls to zero. In an alternating circuit this will occur at the end of each half cycle. Therefore the thyristor will be either fully conducting or non-conducting. They will only conduct when their polarity is correct. This will mean that a pair of thyristors must be provided aligned so that one will conduct in one half cycle and the other in the second half cycle when the polarity is reversed. If a pulsing or triggering unit keeps applying a signal (a pulse of short duration) to the gate of the thyristors at the beginning of each half cycle, then the current will continuously. The flow will continue until the pulsing signal ceases causing the current to cease the very next time the zero point of the

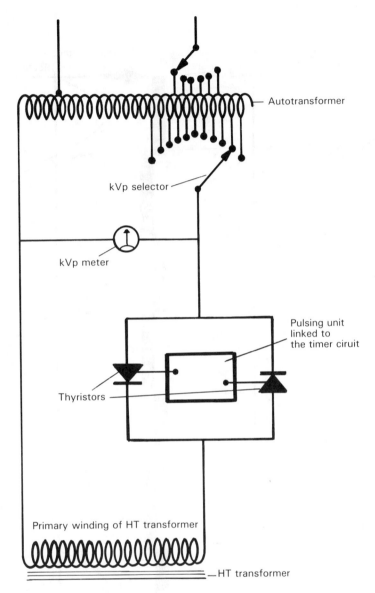

Autotransformer

kVp selector

kVp meter

Pulsing unit
linked to
the timer ciruit

Thyristors

Primary winding of HT transformer

HT transformer

Fig. 7.3 Solid state exposure contactor.

supply waveform is reached. Figure 7.3 shows the arrangement of the thyristors and the pulsing unit in a primary circuit switching unit. The pulsing unit forms part of the timing circuit and because a very low voltage is required to make the unit conduct it provides a means of switching high current with safety. Figure 7.4 is intended to illustrate how the trigger pulse operates first on one thyristor and then on the other as the polarity of the alternating supply changes.

Thyristor switching is only possible in the low voltage primary circuit where it will provide a very accurate switch for times which are greater than 0.01 s, the time of one half cycle of the supply. Three-phase generators provide high output and so may need exposures in milliseconds. These very short times can be controlled by modifying the supply to the thyristor switch so that it is not restricted by the low frequency of the supply. Figure 7.5 shows the modification. The thyristor controls the

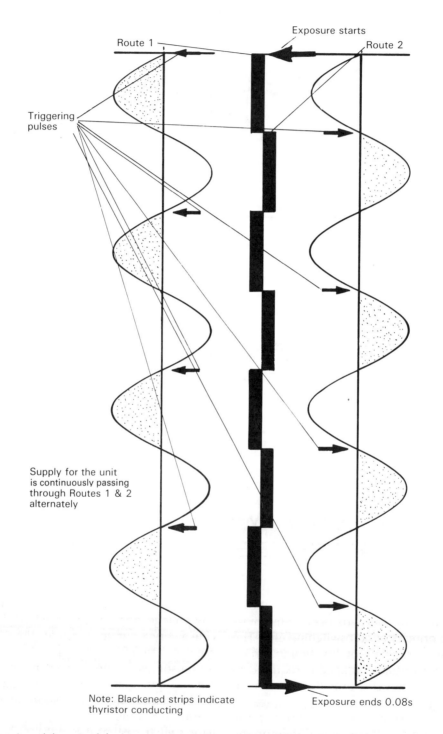

Exposure starts

Route 1

Route 2

Triggering
pulses

Supply for the unit
is continuously passing
through Routes 1 & 2
alternately

Note: Blackened strips indicate
thyristor conducting

Exposure ends 0.08s

Fig. 7.4 Triggering of the pair of thyristors.

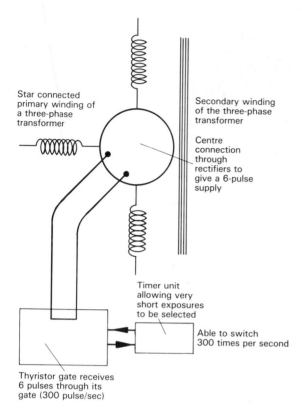

Star connected
primary winding of
a three-phase
transformer

Secondary winding
of the three-phase
transformer

Centre
connection
through
rectifiers to
give a 6-pulse
supply

Timer unit
allowing very
short exposures
to be selected

Able to switch
300 times per second

Thyristor gate receives
6 pulses through its
gate (300 pulse/sec)

Fig. 7.5 Principles of the solid state thyristor switch designed for rapid switching of very short exposures.

supply to the primary windings of the three HT transformers by connection into the earthed centre point of the 'Y'-connected primary windings. A rectifier bridge is provided making it possible for a single thyristor to switch the supply 300 times a second, each time one of the rectified phases drops to zero. Such accuracy will call for electronic circuits which reduce the time taken for initiating and terminating the exposure.

Secondary switching

Switching of the supply to the X-ray tube may take place in the secondary circuit of the HT transformer either by means of triode valves or by use of a grid controlled tube. Both systems are very satisfactory although more expensive to provide than the primary switching previously described.

Triode valve switching
Special triode valves are used which are designed to operate up to 150 kVp. They act as an electronic switch making and breaking the tube current. They can also be used to stabilise the kV and trim off the ripple from a waveform to provide a constant potential.

The advantages of triode valve secondary switching over primary switching are:

1. Extremely short exposure times can be used.
2. No moving parts are involved as in mechanical switching.
3. A stabilised constant potential can be delivered to the X-ray tube.

The circuit of a typical triode valve secondary switch is shown in Figure 7.6. When a negative bias is applied to the grid, which is in excess of the cathode negative potential, the passage of current across the valve is totally blocked. Therefore the valve is acting as a switch for once the bias is removed current can pass and can be stopped again by reintroduction of the bias. The bias is applied by a control unit which is directed by the timer.

Grid controlled tube
When a grid controlled X-ray tube is used it acts as a switch as well as performing its primary function of producing X-rays. The tube acts as a triode instead of a diode valve. There is no actual grid within the tube, the cathode focusing cup operating as a grid. If an additional bias of 2–3 kV is applied to the focusing cup it will produce a space charge effect great enough to prevent any passage of electrons through the tube. Therefore a biasing unit is provided which keeps a bias on the cup until instructed by the timer or other control unit to remove it. Once removed electrons flow and X-rays are produced, the reintroduction of the bias on instruction from the controlling unit will immediately block further electron flow. The system of switching can be extremely fast allowing filming rates of up to 500

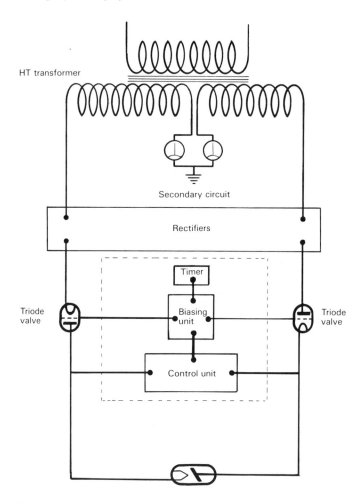

Fig. 7.6 Secondary switching.

frames per second in cine radiography. It is important to know that this relatively simple inexpensive method of secondary switching is only satisfactory where the mA does not exceed 500. Higher mA values require the passage of so many electrons across the tube that the biasing focusing cup cannot effectively block them all. A triode valve system is necessary for switching these high mA values.

To provide the biasing voltage an additional conductor is brought through the cathode high tension cable to the cathode focusing cup, making four conductors in the HT cable. The modification to the cathode is very simple. It is only necessary to insulate all the conductors supplying the filaments from the as-

sembly. The HT supply remains connected to the common filament conductor. The biasing voltage is then quite separate from the other cathode connections (see Fig. 6.25).

The uses of grid controlled tube switching are:

1. where very short exposure times are required, for example in paediatric work.
2. when a rapid repetition of short exposures is required in cine techniques.
3. where pulsed exposures are required to cut unnecessary radiation.
4. to ensure that there can be no accidental exposure from a residual charge on the capacitor or battery of an energy storage mobile unit.

THE CONTROL OF EXPOSURE TIME

The interval between the closing and reopening of the exposure switch is the exposure time. The interval is controlled by the exposure timer circuit, which operates the exposure switch.

The timing circuit starts to conduct at the same time as the exposure switch closes and continues until a preselected time has elapsed. At the end of this time, the timing circuit terminates the exposure by causing the exposure switch to break the supply. The timing circuit must operate effectively every time and be consistent in its operation. It must always be matched with a suitable type of exposure switch, for however accurate the exposure timer may be, variation in the actual exposure time will occur if the exposure switch does not take the same time to operate on each occasion.

Selection of a timing system

There are many types of timing control available and the selection of the most suitable is dictated by the type of unit it is required to control. A low-powered unit requiring a relatively long exposure time to expose adequately the radiograph because of its low rate of X-ray generation will not require the accuracy of a high-powered unit producing X-rays at a high rate. For example an error of 0.01 s in an exposure of 0.5 s will not be noticeable radiographically and this unit may well have fluctuations of tube current through its simple circuit. On the other hand the same error of 0.01 s certainly would be apparent in an exposure of 0.04 s and an error of much less than this would be unacceptable in a very high powered unit. Therefore as the X-ray output rate increases so the degree of accuracy provided by the timer circuit must increase. From this, it can be seen that a variety of timing methods will be found in X-ray units ranging from the simple cheap units to the highly sophisticated very expensive units. In addition to timing the exposure time they are generally designed to operate the exposure switch in

the primary circuit of the HT transformer or more rarely in the secondary circuit of the HT transformer

Types of timers found in X-ray equipment

Electro-mechanical — found only in very old low-powered equipment:

   (i) spring operated clockwork timers
   (ii) synchronous motor driven timers.

Electronic — the most common type:

   (i) simple electronic timer
   (ii) mAs impulse time
   (iii) auto-timers.

Pulse counting timers:

   (i) pulse counting circuits
   (ii) logic circuits using quartz crystal oscillation.

Description of the operation of the various types

In the text emphasis will be placed on the operation of the most commonly used forms of timer circuit — the electronic timers. Electro-mechanical timers will be described as they may still be found in departments. Pulse counting circuits will be described briefly.

Electro-mechanical timers
Spring operated clockwork timers. These timers are only suitable for low-powered self-rectified units such as dental units and truly portable units. They are found measuring time for other purposes such as the control of delineator lamps and some fluoroscopy timers. The system is very inaccurate, but can be adequate in some circumstances provided it is consistent in the intervals measured and the exposure time to be measured is sufficiently long so that small inaccuracies will not be apparent radiographically.

Operation. This simple timer operates by manually rotating a ratchet wheel from one position to another where it is held in position by a catch against the pull of a spring stretched by the rotation until it is under considerable tension. When the exposure switch is operated the X-ray exposure commences and the catch released to allow the ratchet wheel to return to the start position. Once this position is reached, a pair of contacts are broken causing the exposure to cease. The speed of the ratchet wheel's return is calibrated and when a dial is attached to the wheel the settings for different time intervals can be displayed, so that the timer can be set to take the time predicted to return to the start position where the X-ray exposure will end.

Synchronous motor timers. Synchronous motor timers (Fig. 7.7) are found on old mobile units and some small fixed units. Although similar in operation to the spring operated clockwork motor timers they are more accurate. Time is controlled by an electric motor which has its rotational speed linked to the mains frequency. The motor rotates a central shaft at a constant speed. The shaft is connected through a series of reducing gears to a disc which takes about 10 s for a full rotation. The rotating disc faces a second disc which has an arm attached to its border. The second disc is scribed with divisions which indicate the proportion of the time of a full rotation.

The exposure time is set by turning the second disc to the selected exposure time. When the exposure is set the arm on the disc moves away from a pair of contacts causing them to open. The timer is now ready for use. When the exposure switch is operated the mains contactor is closed, the exposure starts and simultaneously the arm bearing disc of the timer is drawn by a magnetic field into contact with the rotating dic. The two discs now move together taking the arm back through the preset angle until it closes the contacts. Once the contacts are closed a solenoid is energised to open the exposure contactor and terminate the exposure.

This type of timer is not satisfactory for short exposures and cannot be used for repetitive

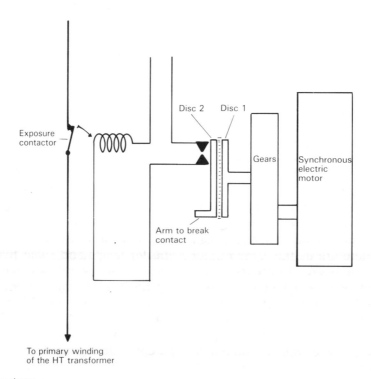

Fig. 7.7 Synchronous timer.

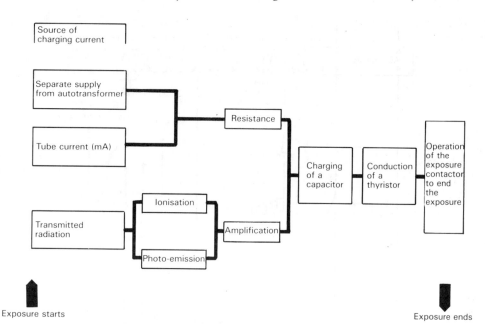

Fig. 7.8 Operation of three types of electronic timers.

exposures as it must be reset between each exposure. It is however quite useful for other purposes like fluoroscopy timers and the motor can be used to rotate a spinning top.

Electronic timers
Almost all timing methods for X-ray exposures other than the electro-mechanical methods described previously and the counting of pulses just being developed for routine use, use the charging of a capacitor as the basis of measuring exposure time.

The differences between the various types available lie mainly in the way the capacitor is charged and to some extent the location of the exposure switching, i.e. in the primary or secondary circuit of the high-tension transformer.

The block diagram shown in Figure 7.8 indicates the operating principles of the three main types of electronic timers: the simple electronic, the mAs impulse timer and the auto-timer. Consideration of the simple electronic timer will aid the understanding of the other types.

Simple electronic timer. Figure 7.9 is a circuit of this type of timer which is best described in three sections:

1. the circuit which determines the length of the exposure.
2. the circuit which on receiving instructions from the timing circuit will energise a relay and so cause the exposure switch to open and terminate the exposure.
3. the exposure contactor itself and its operating method. Details of the exposure switch were considered on pages 100–107.

The circuit determining the length of the exposure. The time of an exposure is governed by the time taken to charge a capacitor to 63% of full charge. 63% of full charge is termed the critical voltage as this is the voltage which will initiate the sequence of events which will terminate the exposure. The supply voltage and the capacitor value are chosen to provide the critical voltage at 63% of full charge. Examination of the charging curve of a capacitor shown in Figure 7.10 will clearly indicate that the time taken to reach 63% is very definite whereas 100% is difficult to determine with any accuracy.

Three factors control the time taken to reach the critical value, these are:

a. the value of the supply voltage

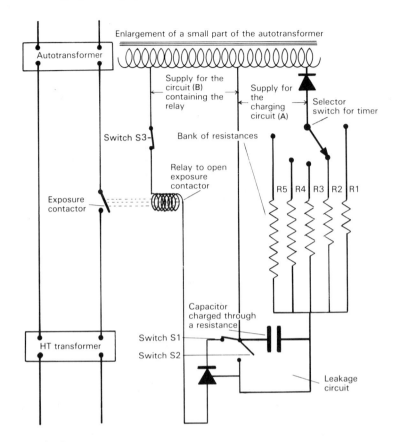

Fig. 7.9 Electronic timer circuit.

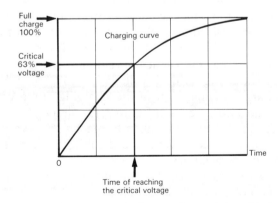

Fig. 7.10 Charging curve of a capacitor and the critical voltage.

b. the value of the capacitor
c. the resistance in series with the capacitor.

Once the first two values are fixed as described the only variable is the resistance. In Figure 7.11, the graphs show the charging curve for five different values of resistance. The five curves show the different times taken before the critical voltage is reached. The provision of a range of different resistances provides the range of exposure times.

It is important if accurate time is to be measured that there is no residual charge on the capacitor. This is assured in timing circuits by providing a short-circuit to leak away any residual charge before timing starts. This short-circuit must be broken before charging commences. Figure 7.9 shows a typical charging circuit found in many X-ray units. The supply voltage is taken from the autotransformer. This will be an alternating supply which must

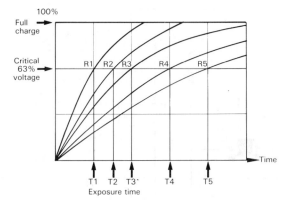

Fig. 7.11 Five charging curves indicating how the time of reaching the critical voltage varies with different resistance values.

be rectified before it can be used to charge a capacitor. The charging process is started by closing a switch. Figure 7.9 shows the rectifier; the switch S1 which must be closed before the charging of the capacitor can begin and five resistances of different values. Selection of a particular resistance by a rotary switch places it in series with the capacitor and causes the capacitor to take a particular time to charge. In modern units there will be many different resistances so that there is a wide range of time intervals available to the operator. The circuit shown in Figure 7.9 is in the charging mode, with the switch S2 in the leakage path open.

The circuit containing the relay which operates the exposure switch. At the same time as the timing circuit (A) starts to charge the capacitor, another circuit receives a supply from the autotransformer. This circuit (B) contains a relay which will, when energised, open the exposure switch and terminate the exposure. Initially this circuit (B) cannot conduct as the thyristor in its circuit is not able to conduct until the blocking bias on its gate is removed. The thyristor gate is connected to the timing circuit (A) so that when the critical voltage developed on the capacitor is applied to it, the bias on the gate is removed. The thyristor is then able to conduct allowing current to pass through the relay coil, energising it to terminate the exposure. Once the exposure switch is opened, switch S3 is broken and switch S2 closed so

that any residual charge can leak from the capacitor. The timer circuit (A) is then ready for another timing sequence as soon as S1 and S3 are closed and S2 opened.

The exposure time is varied by selection of a suitable resistance. This is the only variation that can be made by the operator, as all other component values are preset by the manufacturer. The bank of resistances are either mounted around a rotary switch so that a particular one can be connected into the circuit by turning the knob or through one of a bank of resistances each having its own push-switch which when operated will connect the resistance behind it into the circuit. The timing circuit operates at a low voltage and so can be safely mounted on the control panel.

mAs impulse timer. This form of electronic timer takes its voltage supply from the secondary circuit of the high tension transformer. The exposure switch which it operates remains in the primary circuit.

The timing circuit is similar in layout to the simple electronic timer just described, except for its source of charging current. In this type of unit the capacitor is charged by the actual X-ray tube current. The timer circuit is connected into the centre of the secondary winding of the high tension transformer, where the voltage is very low (near the earthed point) but passing the same current as that passing through the X-ray tube. The great advantage of this system compared with the simple unit is that the capacitor receives a charging current which suffers any change that the tube may receive and will automatically make an adjustment to the exposure time to compensate for it. Therefore the mAs values will always be accurate even if the mA is not quite correct since the time will be increased or decreased accordingly as the capacitor will receive a higher or lower current causing a shorter or longer charging time.

Operation. Before exposure the connection to the primary of the high tension transformer is broken by the switch S2 (see Fig. 7.12). Switch S3 is closed and will only open when the exposure is to be terminated. The capacitor in the timing circuit is short-circuited by

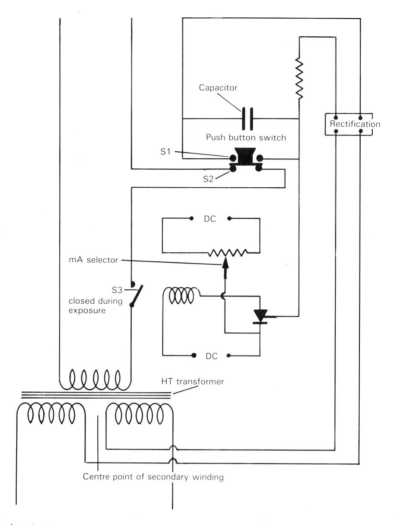

Fig. 7.12   mAs impulse timer.

switch S1 to ensure that there is no residual charge on the capacitor.

On pressing the exposure button the capacitor charging can begin; this action will break the short-circuit at S1. Simultaneously, the circuit to the primary winding of the high tension transformer is completed by closing S2.

The exposure is terminated when the bias on the thyristor in the timing circuit is overcome and conduction can take place across it. As in the simple electronic unit once the thyristor conducts, the exposure switch S3 is opened by the relay in the circuit.

Note. In modern units the exposure switch will not be a mechanical switch but a solid-state switch. The result of operating either switch is the same and because it makes appreciation of the operation of the timing circuit easier to understand the older mechanical switch is shown in the circuit diagrams.

The charging current is obtained from the centre point of the secondary winding of the high tension transformer. This will of course be an alternating current and must be rectified before it is applied to the capacitor of the timing circuit. The current once rectified is passed through a resistor. This will modify the voltage which is to charge the capacitor to the value necessary to overcome the bias on the gate of the thyristor. Should the tube current vary from its selected value the charging time will vary to compensate for the error.

The selection of mAs is obtained by varying the time taken for the thyristor to conduct. In this type of unit the charging current is at a fixed value, the selected mA, so the negative potential on the collector (cathode) of the thyristor must be manipulated instead. The degree by which the collector of the thyristor is made more or less negative depends upon the value of the resistance in the circuit applying the extra negative potential to the collector. Note that the collector potential is the combined potential of the fixed supply and the variable. The variable resistance is the mAs selector and is calibrated in mAs.

Auto-timers

The timers described previously require operators to select exposure factors which they think will provide a satisfactorily exposed radiograph. The selection of factors is based on the skill and experience of the operators and their knowledge of a similar examination on a patient of the same build and similar medical condition. This empirical approach is not infrequently the cause of re-examination giving the patient an unjustifiable increase in radiation dose and making the examination more costly.

Auto-timers have been designed to ensure that the exposure factors used for a radiograph will almost always provide an acceptable result for diagnostic purposes. It is however generally agreed that the result may not be aesthetically as good as the best operator selected technique, but will be a marked improvement on the poorer work. The quality of the radiograph produced with the aid of an auto-timer can be improved to match more nearly the ideal by the operator who fully understands the principle by which the auto-timer operates, carefully uses its controls and recognises the limitations of the system. Once correctly set up, the unit will continue to produce radiographs of a similar density indefinitely.

Operating principles of an auto-timer. To determine exposure factors for any radiographic or fluoroscopic examination, it is necessary to select a kilovoltage which will penetrate the most dense part of the area under examination and provide the image contrast necessary to allow the range of subject densities to be displayed on the radiograph. Once this kilovoltage has been selected, it is only necessary to determine when the number of X-ray photons has fallen on the film to give the required density. The number of photons needed for the satisfactory exposure of a radiograph for diagnostic purposes will vary with the speed of the X-ray film, the type of intensifying screen used, the type of cassette front and to a limited extent the density level required for different techniques.

To avoid frequent re-programming to allow for the factors listed above, it is usual to standardise the cassette type and choose a film/screen combination which is suitable for the majority of the work to be undertaken and then use it for all examinations using the auto-timer. This will allow the controls to be set up when the unit is installed and only changed when different materials are put into use. The remaining control is the one which allows a slight change in film density to be produced when required and even this is not often changed in practice.

Once the controls are set, the auto-timer will determine when the film will be satisfactorily exposed and will continue to do so for all the work undertaken with the unit so ensuring standardisation of results. The unit operates by monitoring the number of X-ray photons passing through a specific area either by their ionisation or photo-electric effect. The monitored area is sited so that it receives a fixed proportion of the radiation which will fall upon the film and thus when the monitored area has received a specified amount of radiation it will be an indication of the amount received by the film. By careful selection of components the manufacturer uses the ionisation or photo-electric current to terminate the exposure when the film will have been correctly exposed. The ionisation or photo-electric current after amplification is used to charge a capacitor as in the electronic timer units.

There are two types of auto-timer unit. The ionisation unit and the photo-electric unit. Both types will be described more fully later.

The time taken for the required number of photons to pass through the auto-timer monitoring area will depend upon the rate at which the X-rays are generated by the tube, the focus to monitored area distance, and the absorption taking place in the patient and in any other intervening structures such as a grid or filter. The mA selection is made by the radiographer after consideration of the tube loading capability and the degree of image unsharpness both geometric and motional that can be tolerated. By monitoring the transmitted radiation leaving the patient, varying absorption within the part being examined will be automatically allowed for by the unit. This is one of the advantages of auto-timing, but it does require careful positioning and selection of the monitoring site to ensure that the monitoring of the transmitted beam is taken over the correct area. Another advantage is that auto-timing will automatically compensate for any variation in the tube current, mA, by extending or reducing the exposure time to obtain the correct number of X-ray photons.

Guard timers in auto-timer circuits. In all auto-timer circuits there is a guard timer which will operate if the auto-timer fails to terminate the exposure. This is essential for the patient's protection against excessive radiation exposure and as an added protection for the tube against overload damage. One of the occasions when the guard timer might operate would be when the monitoring field is overshadowed by a large amount of opaque contrast agent which attenuates the majority of the photons expected to reach the unit.

Location of the monitoring areas (the chambers). The manufacturers call the monitored area, the chamber. These chambers are positioned strategically over the areas most suitable for determining the exposure of a wide range of examinations. An example of their distribution is shown in Figure 7.13.

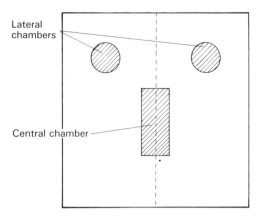

Fig. 7.13 Location of the monitoring areas (the chambers).

They may be found in the bucky of a table, on the explorator and in the chest stand and anywhere else where a chamber can be satisfactorily located.

The auto-timer control unit allows the operator to choose the most suitably positioned chamber or chambers for the particular examination to be undertaken (see Fig. 7.13). For example:
— for spinal radiography — a centrally sited chamber
— for chest and abdominal radiography — laterally placed chambers
— for contrast examination of the alimentary tract using large format film — all chambers
— for small format film examinations — a chamber in the centre of the explorator.

Factors affecting the efficiency of auto-timers. In addition to the factors already considered it is important to remember that the chamber(s) will only assess the number of photons falling on the whole monitored area and not a part of the area and that the area monitored is only a proportion of the whole area radiographed. These limitations do not generally present problems with film density if the user is aware of their effect and is careful with the positioning of the patient over the chamber. However, areas of high absorption in the patient resulting perhaps from a collection of dense barium sulphate overlying the chamber will extend the exposure time as the auto-timer takes longer than it should to collect the required number of photons. The result will be a radiograph with above average density. On the other hand there are occasions when part of the chamber is overshadowed by a very low attenuating part or even free of any overshadowing by the patient, as in the oblique view of the abdomen of a very thin patient. This will cause the exposure to be terminated too early with the resultant film underexposed.

Satisfactory results will depend on very careful beam collimation for if this is not arranged the amount of scatter produced will vary because of the increased or decreased volume irradiated, or if part of the chamber is excluded from the field by collimation the film will be overexposed.

Problems may also occur if the number of photons required by the film is very low, as with some very fast 'rare' earth intensifying screens. The small auto-timer current will require such an amount of amplification before it can be used to charge the capacitor that it may introduce error unless a very sophisticated amplification system is provided. In addition a very low current can be influenced by external interference. This difficulty with interference may well preclude the use of auto-timing in paediatric work, adding to the problems of poor exposure control resulting from the use of monitoring chambers which will on general units be too large for the size of the child.

Photo-electric timers. Photo-electric timers are most commonly found controlling exposure in photofluorographic units, although some X-ray equipment manufacturers use them for general work. The unit uses the ability of X-rays to cause certain materials to fluoresce.

Operation

1. With closure of the exposure switch, X-rays are generated. The X-rays which pass through the patient and the anti-scatter grid when used, interact with a fluorescent screen before reaching the film.

2. The fluorescent screen produces light which is collected from a selected area(s) by means of a lens or mirror system and directs it on to the photocathode of a photomultiplier tube, where the light is converted to an electric current and amplified to a useful value by the photomultiplier tube. The photomultiplier tube will be described later.

3. The amplified current is then used to charge the capacitor in the timer circuit to its critical value. The time taken for this value to be reached will depend upon the magnitude of the current derived from the light produced by the fluorescent screen.

4. When the capacitor reaches its critical value, the thyristor in the timing circuit will conduct causing the exposure to be terminated.

Figure 7.14 shows by block diagrams the operation of this system. There are technique modifying controls which can be adjusted to allow for differences of film/screen combination, different techniques and different chamber sites so that the resultant density on the film will be correct. The value of a resistance in the capacitor charging circuit is altered when the controls are adjusted so increasing or decreasing the time taken for the thyristor gate bias to be overcome allowing the thyristor to conduct and terminate the exposure.

In common with all automatic exposure timing systems there is another timer, the guard timer, in parallel with the automatic system which is ready to operate if there is long delayed or nonfunction of the automatic unit. The functioning of the guard timer is most important as it ensures that excessive exposure cannot be given to the patient through failure or malfunction of an automatic unit. It operation must be regularly checked.

The photomultiplier tube. The photons of light directed on to the photocathode of the photomultiplier tube cause electrons to be released by the photo-emissive layer on the first electrode, normally described as the first dynode. These electrons are accelerated by a positive potential to interact with the photo-emissive layer on a second dynode behind the first giving rise to an increased number of electrons. These electrons are then accelerated by the third dynode at a greater potential than the last to increase their energy so that when they interact with the photo-emissive

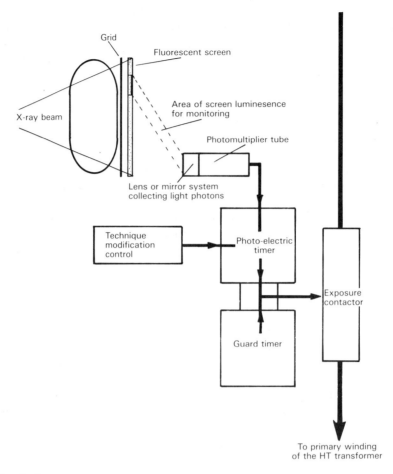

Fig. 7.14 Photo-electric timer.

layer on the third dynode there will be many more electrons released. If the photomultiplier tube has 10 dynodes with 150 V potential difference between each, and each electron causes three to be produced when it collides with the photo-emissive layer, it can be seen that the number of electrons developed at the exit of the tube will be 3^{10} more than initially. Therefore the photomultiplier tube has increased the current by 3^{10} times. Figure 7.15 shows the arrangement of a photomultiplier tube and the enlarged diagram illustrates the amplification in the number of electrons produced. The figure shows the 'venetian' blind-like arrangement of the dynode. The gaps between the angled strips of metal with their coating allow the electrons to pass back from

one dynode to the next without obstruction.

The photocathode and the dynodes are contained in an evacuated glass tube which has a flat optical glass input face at the photocathode end and a series of connecting pins emerging at the other end. These pins allow the potential differences to be applied between each dynode and the amplified current to be applied to the capacitor. As the number of electrons produced at the photocathode depends upon the number of light photons collected from the fluorescent screen which depends upon the number of X-ray photons transmitted by the part being monitored, it can be seen that if the output number of X-rays is fixed by controls based on the particular recording mediums need, the input (exposure)

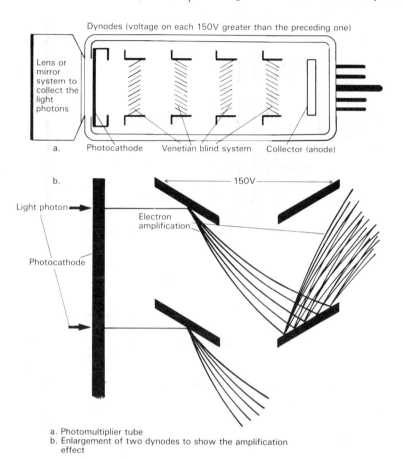

a. Photomultiplier tube
b. Enlargement of two dynodes to show the amplification
effect

Fig. 7.15 Photomultiplier tube.

will continue until this value is reached, because the amplified current will cause the exposure to terminate when the number of transmitted photons reaches the desired level.

Ionisation timer. Ionisation timers are used for controlling exposure time in many types of radiographic and photofluorographic techniques undertaken in the X-ray department.

Operation. The system is similar to the photo-electric system, except that it is the ionising property of the X-radiation which is used to control the exposure and not the ability to cause fluorescence. Figure 7.16 shows the essential features of the system.

A thin parallel plate ionisation chamber is placed between the patient and the cassette under the grid. The chamber has an even and very low attenuation factor. The central elec-

trode is charged in the area selected for determining the film density to a potential of 300 V above earth.

The radiation transmitted by the patient and the grid passes through the chamber to reach the film. In its passage across the chamber, ionisation of the air within the chamber occurs, and the ions produced are attracted by the potential to the chamber plates causing a current to flow. The current generated depends on the rate of X-ray photons passing through the chamber. This current is very small indeed and so before it can be applied to the capacitor charging circuit it must be amplified.

As in the photo-electric system, adjustment for different techniques must be provided. A variable resistance is used to modify the time taken for the ionisation chamber output to charge the capacitor.

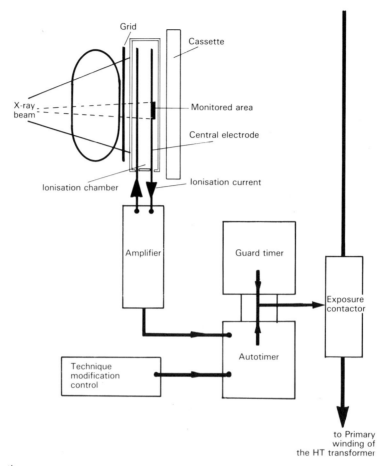

Fig. 7.16 Ionisation timer.

The most suitable area for controlling the exposure is chosen by selecting the most appropriate chamber location.

Electronic amplification. In an ionisation timing system there is need for amplification to increase the input voltage derived from ionisation of the air in the chamber to a value that can charge the timer capacitor. To achieve the output required, it is necessary to use a number of amplifiers arranged in series, known as a cascade, so that their combined effect will give the required amplification; one amplifier output providing the input for the next (see Fig. 7.17a).

In a simple amplifier circuit the input voltage is applied to the base of a transistor where it controls the current flowing through the transistor (emittor to collector). The small base voltage (input voltage) causes a large current to flow and since the amplification factor of a transistor is a constant, the value of the input voltage is reflected by the output current. The output current by flowing through a high resistance produces a potential difference across the resistance. It is the voltage across this resistance which provides the amplifier's output voltage (see Fig. 7.17b).

Pulse counting timers

Once an exposure time falls to less than 0.01 s (the time taken for one half cycle of the mains supply) or greater accuracy is required, the capacitor charging method of measuring exposure time is not adequate. Therefore in order to take full advantage of the more powerful generators available today it must be

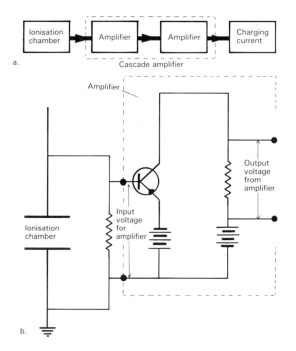

Fig. 7.17 Electronic amplification.

possible to measure very short exposure times in milliseconds or even nanoseconds.

The method of measuring accurately very short exposure time is by use of a pulse generator with a very high oscillating frequency. Such a unit will produce pulses lasting for only a short time. If the time per pulse is known and the pulses counted electronically, exposure times can be accurately measured.

There are two ways of providing the high rate of pulse generation: the electronic generation of high frequency and piezo-electricity. These underlie the two types of pulse counting timers.

Pulse counting circuits. Pulse counting circuits are contained within a printed circuit board. The mains frequency of 50 Hz is increased by an invertor to 500 Hz which when rectified gives 1000 pulses. This timer will measure milliseconds but can by circuit modification measure even shorter exposure times. A binary counter is used to determine when the preselected number of pulses has been generated and when this point is reached the circuit causes the exposure to cease.

Quartz crystal oscillation. A quartz crystal produces oscillations due to the strain of the crystal lattice when an electrical potential difference is applied to opposite faces of the crystal and conversely, if the crystal lattice is strained by pressure a potential difference is produced between the opposite faces of the crystal. The phenomona is known as piezo-electricity. The frequency of oscillation, i.e. the number of pulses, depends upon the crystal material, the area of the opposing faces and the distance between the faces. In the case of quartz, the pulse frequency is in megahertz (MHz). The rate of pulse generation is constant unless the crystal is changed.

The MHz pulse frequency can be arithmetically reduced by logic circuits to a rate suitable for the length of exposure timers required. These pulses are then counted and when the required number has been reached a further linked circuit operates to terminate the exposure.

These very short exposure times must be matched by exceedingly rapid acting exposure switching.

8

The nature of the X-ray beam

The X-ray photons generated at the focus radiate in all directions. The photons directed onto the target are attenuated by the tungsten. Only a narrow beam of those remaining emerges through the radiolucent tube port. The rest are absorbed by the lead lining of the tube housing and the other metal parts within the tube (see Figs 6.5 & 6.14).

X-RAY ENERGY DISTRIBUTION

The cone of useful radiation is formed by X-ray photons of all energies up to a maximum which is governed by the applied kVp. They arise as a result of the Bremsstrahlung process and characteristic radiation occurring at the focus.

X-RAY INTENSITY DISTRIBUTION

The intensity distribution falling on a plane at right-angles to the central axis of the useful beam is not uniform. Examination of Figure 8.1, which is an illustration of the typical distribution of X-ray photons from a 20° target angle stationary anode tube, reveals that the number of photons arriving at the anode end of the field is only 31% of the number at the centre of the field. This reduction is spoken of as the 'anode-heel' effect. In normal practice, this effect has little radiographic significance as the tube designers carefully choose the target angle and the dimensions of the tube port

to ensure that only the central part of the radiation cone where the variation in intensity is not very marked is used to form the image. This is indicated in Figure 8.1.

However, an understanding of the anode-heel effect is essential for as the X-ray tube ages, the target surface becomes progressively rougher. This leads to a marked anode-heel effect, which arises because some electrons interact in a hollow and the X-ray photon produced is attenuated by the surrounding target material. Radiographically this will be noticeable as uneven exposure of the radiograph with less blackening beneath the anode end of the tube. Accelerated electrons can pass into the target for a finite distance so X-rays are produced within the target itself, and their path within the target may be in any direction. The target material is a barrier to most of these X-rays and in steep angle tube there is less possibility of escape for the X-ray photon because of the angle of the target. Therefore these tubes are more subject to anode-heel effect and they will more rapidly present uneven density across the field which is unacceptable radiographically. A regular check should be kept on the progress of anode-heel effect.

EXTRA-FOCAL (OFF-FOCUS) RADIATION

When considering the nature of the X-ray beam it was assumed that all the X-ray photons

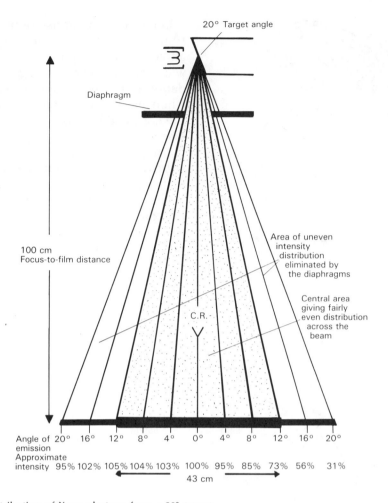

Fig. 8.1 Typical distribution of X-ray photons from a 20° target.

forming the beam of radiation originated from the focus. If this were so it would be ideal since it is only radiation from the focus that provides useful image information. However, unfortunately X-rays are also produced outside the focal spot and may contribute up to 20% of the total. This radiation is known as extra-focal or off-focus radiation. The X-ray photons generated off focus should be eliminated as far as possible as they do not carry any image information and only degrade the image. Their effect is:

1. to degrade the image by adding to the image forming focal radiation a percentage of non-image forming radiation which is distributed at random over the image.

2. to make it impossible to produce a sharp cut-off of the irradiated field.

3. to increase the patient dose.

The chief source of extra-focal radiation arises from the interaction of cathode electrons which have escaped from the focusing effect of the cathode focusing cup and hit the anode outside the focal spot. They have approximately the same energy as the focal radiation. They are more numerous in the rotating anode tube as there is more tungsten in the anode than in the stationary anode. In the stationary anode tube electrons which are not focused are likely to interact with copper and the radiation produced will be of low energy and readily absorbed within the tube structure.

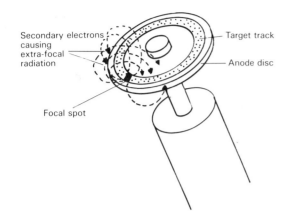

Fig. 8.2 Rotating anode tube target disc showing the source of some extra-focal radiation.

Other X-ray photons are produced by electrons back-scattered by the target and then re-attracted to the anode. The X-rays produced will have a lower average energy. Molybdenum characteristic radiation may be produced when electrons fall on the molybdenum on the edge and back of the rotating anode target disc.

The generated X-rays may interact with any structure they pass through and give rise to scattering, the scattered photon being deviated from the direction of the incident photon.

Consideration of the sources of off-focus radiation will show that although it may form

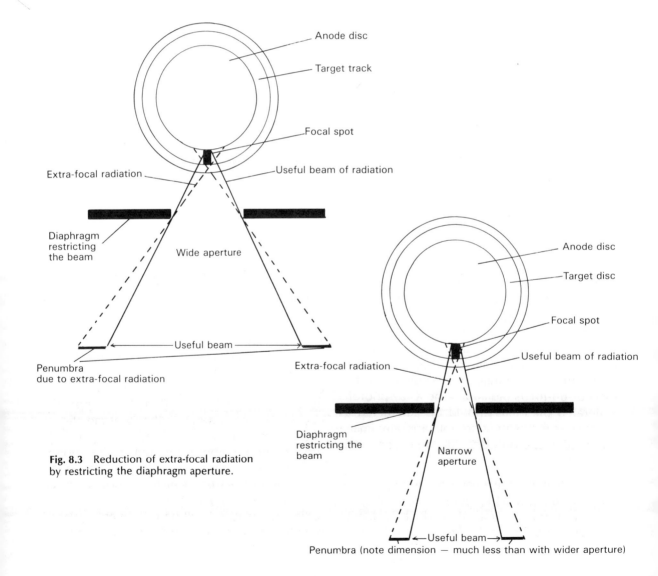

Fig. 8.3 Reduction of extra-focal radiation by restricting the diaphragm aperture.

some 20% of the radiation many of the photons will have low energy and will not influence the image but they will increase the dose to the patient. Therefore it is essential to eliminate them as far as possible. Figure 8.2. illustrates the back-scattering of electrons.

Reduction of extra-focal radiation can be provided by:

1. Close collimation of the beam as near as possible to the source of the radiation (Fig. 8.3). Figure 14.1 shows a 'top-hat'-shaped lead diaphragm for fitting in the tube port. The top of the hat has an aperture cut to the smallest size which will permit the radiation field to cover just the maximum area that will be required in the particular tube location and collimate the beam very close to its source.

2. Collimating the beam as close to the film as practical. This will attenuate some of the photons directed away from the main beam (see Fig. 8.4). The use of multileaved diaphragms and an additional localising cone attached to the delineator face will eliminate very effectively extra-focal radiation particularly if a lead 'top-hat' diaphragm is fitted into the tube port.

3. Filters fitted close to the tube port will if carefully selected remove much of the low energy radiation both focal and extra-focal produced but because of the lower average energy of extra-focal radiation more of this unwanted radiation will be eliminated.

4. Anode disc design has attempted to reduce extra-focal radiation by eliminating radiation produced off-focus. The target of tungsten has been made into an annular strip which is set in graphite, but to date the bonding of the tungsten to the graphite has not

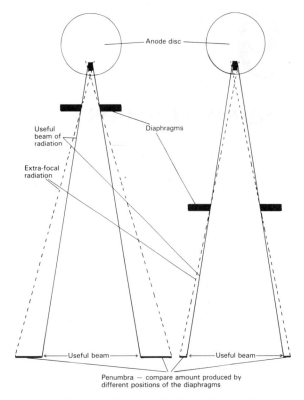

Fig. 8.4 Effect of collimating the beam close to the object — causes reduction in extra-focal radiation.

been very successful. Tungsten set in molybdenum has been used with more success. In the case of graphite, no X-rays will be generated when subjected to bombardment of high energy electrons and with molybdenum only low energy X-rays are produced.

5. Metal tube inserts remove unfocused electrons so reducing extra-focal radiation production. The metal walls of these tube will attenuate low energy photons more effectively than the usual glass.

9

Safety devices

The manufacturers of X-ray equipment fit many safety devices to their units which automatically protect patients, operators and the equipment from damage through malfunction of a component or poor performance through operating under less than optimum conditions. They can be divided into five groups for descriptive purposes based on the hazard they are designed to prevent, namely:

1. electrical hazard
2. mechanical defect
3. avoidable ionising radiation
4. burning or over-heating
5. equipment operation below acceptable standards.

All safety devices must be regularly checked to make sure that they will operate efficiently to overcome the hazard should the occasion arise. Regular maintenance and a quality assurance programme should include checklists to make certain that every safety device is checked and any malfunction recorded and corrected at the earliest possible moment. The engineer and/or the person performing quality assurance checks has a responsibility to report any defect and to make sure that no one can use the equipment again until the fault is cleared if there is any risk of accident or further damage. The operator should report any failure of a safety device to operate even when its failure has not resulted in accident or damage.

Examples from the five groups are set out below; they represent only a small proportion of the devices that can be provided. When new equipment is handed over by the manufacturer's representative the safety devices should be specified and their function and method of operation demonstrated and the information used to draw up checklists.

PROTECTION AGAINST ELECTRICAL HAZARDS

Switches, circuit breakers and fuses

(i) Sockets which have removable plugs are provided with a switch in their live line so that the supply can be switched off before the plug top is removed.

(ii) Major X-ray equipment has an isolator switch which completely severs the electrical connection to the unit.

(iii) Fuses prevent the drawing of excessive current by a circuit or part of a circuit provided that the fuse is the correct value for the circuit (see the section on fuses, p. 127).

(iv) Circuit breakers — an alternative to fuses.

Containment of components carrying current

(i) Covers are placed around electrical parts with the components mounted on insulating material and adequately separated from each other and the cover so that the surrounding air gap is wide enough to prevent arcing between components or between the equipment and the cover. The metal covers are connected to earth.

(ii) High tension equipment is enclosed in a metal cover but to avoid arcing and to keep the container as small as possible the unit is filled with oil. Oil has a much higher dielectric coefficient than air.

(iii) Covers require a tool to open them and in some sites a lock with a key is fitted to ensure the unit is only opened by an approved person and when the key is turned the electrical supply to the unit is immediately disconnected.

(iv) All conductors are covered with an insulating sleeve. The thickness of the insulating cover is determined by the supply voltage. In high voltage cables as used to supply the X-ray tube there is an earthed outer sheath to provide greater protection.

Isolation of high tension circuits

(i) High tension circuits are always operated remotely. A low tension circuit is provided which operates switches in the high tension circuits, ensuring that the operator does not switch on a high tension circuit directly.

(ii) Other controls are designed to operate at 240 V or below.

(iii) By winding the secondary coil of the HT transformer in two halves, the centre point can be earthed so that the HT cables only carry half the tube voltage.

(iv) All components have edges and points rounded off so that charge does not build up on these sites to cause arcing between components operating at very different potentials; if this was not done the separation between components would need to be greater.

(v) The high tension transformer and the filament transformer primary windings are isolated from their secondaries which are are at high potential, the filament secondary through its connection with the high tension transformer.

Earthing

All equipment is earthed; the fixed unit has a substantial earthing tape connected directly to earth. The earthing tape or conductor is a very low resistance pathway to earth and must have few connections in its path, as connections can become places where resistance develops reducing the effectiveness of the whole. The earth for each piece of equipment must be checked to see that its impedance does not exceed the mandatory value.

PROTECTION AGAINST MECHANICAL HAZARD

Switches which operate to stop a motor-driven movement when a collison would occur if the movement continued are commonly installed. Examples of their use are:

(i) on a tilting table to stop the tilt should the longitudinal movement be too great for clearance of the floor by the undercouch tube or image intensifier.

(ii) on the collimator of a ceiling suspended X-ray tube to prevent the continuing downward drive of the tube if it should touch an obstruction.

Slipping clutches are provided on some drive shafts to slow or stop them when the plate carried on the shaft meets an obstruction. This safety device is commonly found on power assisted explorators.

Covers around moving parts prevent injury by preventing access.

In older units damage by collison was prevented by limiting switches and carefully designed units but in modern units which provide very complex movements a purely mechanical form of protection is not satisfactory and is replaced by a minicomputer which can consider the effect of many movements, anticipate their result and take evasive action to avoid collison(s) occurring.

PROTECTION FROM UNNECCESSARY RADIATION

The examples listed below are some of the protective devices provided on or by the X-ray unit itself. There are many other ways of protecting patients, staff and others which are not related directly to the unit. These will not be listed here.

Shielding against primary radiation and limitation of the irradiated area

(i) Lead-lined X-ray tube shield.

(ii) Collimators to limit the size of the primary beam. Automatic devices are provided by some units to restrict the area of the primary beam to the area of the recording media. Manual controls are also provided to enable the operator to restrict the field still further.

(iii) Interlock circuits prevent the generation of X-radiation if the primary barrier afforded by an image intensifier and its support is not in place.

(iv) Mechanical linking is provided between the X-ray tube and the image intensifier to ensure that the beam of radiation is always directed to the centre of the recording field.

Restriction of the length of the X-ray exposure and the tube current

(i) Fluoroscopy time is measured by a timer which indicates audibly and then cuts off the radiation when a preselected time has been reached. The resetting of the timer draws the operators attention to the length of the screening time and allows a record to be kept of the factors used and the time for which they were used.

(ii) Fluoroscopic mA controls have restrictors fitted to prevent excessive mA selection, generally a 3 mA maximum.

(iii) Guard timers are fitted to cut an exposure not terminated by an automatic exposure control.

Restriction in the use of short focus-to-skin distance

(i) Mechanical blocks to prevent the tube coming down too close to the patient during fluoroscopy

(ii) Tilting table height selected to permit an acceptable focus-to-table top distance when the tube is sited beneath the table.

(iii) Face pieces fitted on X-ray tube to prevent source of radiation being placed too close to the patient, for example dental tube cones, mobile image intensifier and other tube collimators built so that their length prevents too short a distance being used.

(iv) Mechanical linking of tube and film support so that they can only be used at a fixed focus-to-film distance.

Indicators to reduce human error

(i) Indicator light on the tube to show which tube is being energised.

(ii) Indicator lights over entrance doors to show when X-rays are being generated

(iii) Indicator lamps to show which factors and accessories have been selected.

(iv) Interlock system to ensure the correct setting of a technique.

(v) Indicator lamp to show that an exposure by a particular tube has been selected.

PROTECTION AGAINST BURNING OR OVERHEATING

Protection of personnel

The use of a time switch on the light beam delineators ensures that the metal covers do not become excessively hot which will occur if the lamp within the housing is left on for long periods.

Protection of equipment

(i) Interlock circuits to prevent the tube becoming damaged by overheating through an input load in excess of the maximum permissible load.

(ii) Indicator systems which display the level of heat at the tube anode enabling units to be used within prescribed limits.

(iii) Provision of rating charts to enable safe exposure factors to be selected. The information from the charts may be stored within a computer so that it will control the unit automatically and when linked to technique programmes eliminate operator error.

(iv) Thermal cut-out switches are provided in various sites to ensure that parts are not allowed to become overheated, e.g. the X-ray tube thermal cut-out operates if the oil becomes excessively hot.

SAFETY DEVICES TO PREVENT THE USE OF EQUIPMENT WHICH HAS NOT REACHED ACCEPTABLE STANDARDS

Delay circuits provide sufficient time for tube filaments to rise from their standby value to operating value, the anode to reach its correct rotation speed and auxiliary equipment to reach operational standards.

Covers are provided over sensitive components to prevent accumulations of dust which could interfere with their operation.

Fuses and circuit breakers, interlock circuits and X-ray tube rating are now considered more fully. Other safety devices are explained in the text when they arise as part of the component being described.

FUSES, CIRCUIT BREAKERS AND INTERLOCKS

It is essential to protect a circuit and its components from damage resulting from the passage of a higher current than the design allows. All components have a maximum current which must not be exceeded, a current in excess of this maximum is known as an overload current. An overload current can be prevented by the use of:

Fuses

Fuses are short lengths of wire connected in series in a main or subsidiary circuit which are just capable of carrying the normal maximum current for the particular circuit and fail, breaking the continuity of the circuit, if an abnormally high current occurs. The passage of an excess current causes the temperature of the wire to increase to a point when it melts causing it to fail. The point at which the fuse fails is determined by:

(i) the temperature at which the material forming the fuse melts. Tin and tin/lead alloy are materials of choice. Tin melts at 232°C, tin/lead alloy 327°C.

(ii) the diameter of the wire.

In X-ray circuits different types of fuses are used:

1. rewireable fuses — not commonly found today.
2. cartridge fuses — these are in plug tops and must be very familiar to all radiographers. They are also used in complex circuits where they may be mounted in an array in a place easily accessible to the X-ray engineer. The normal type of fuse will fail within milliseconds of receiving an overload.

Other types allow some control over their speed of operation by preventing their failure for a short time. These fuses are known as anti-surge or time-delay fuses. They permit a very short-lived surge of current that the equipment can withstand to pass without causing the fuse to fail but will operate as the normal fuse if the overload current persists. One type of anti-surge fuse has the wire connected through a spring so that there is some 'give' in the fuse connection. Figure 9.1 illustrates the design of a normal and an anti-surge cartridge fuse.

Fuses must never be uprated (increased in value) they must always be the weakest part of the circuit to ensure that when there is a fault the fuse fails before serious harm can be done, protecting the equipment, preventing fire and

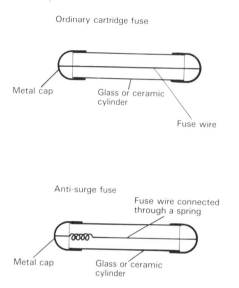

Fig. 9.1 Cartridge fuses.

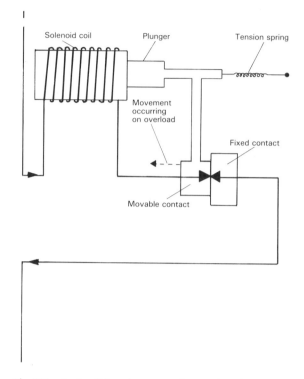

Fig. 9.2. A circuit breaker — used to replace fuses in some locations.

providing electrical safety for the operator. Equipment manufacturers will specify the correct value of the fuse in amps that must be used. If this is not given the wattage of the component and the circuit voltage can be used to calculate the correct value of fuse to be fitted.

Fuses have a serious disadvantage — they must be replaced once they fail before the unit can be used again. This has led to the introduction of circuit breakers which can be easily reset after operation. But like fuses it is essential to investigate the cause of failure before attempting to use the unit again. A higher rated fuse should never be fitted to prevent the operation of what is provided as a safety device.

Circuit breakers

A circuit breaker (Fig. 9.2) will break the continuity of a circuit when an overload current or short circuit occurs; when tripped it can be reset by simply pushing a lever or a button. These units are frequently used to protect a ring main.

The circuit breaker is placed in series with the circuit it is protecting. The current drawn by the circuit passes through a pair of con-

tacts, which are normally closed and a coil which forms part of the circuit breaker.

In normal conditions the magnetic field generated by the current passing through the coil is too weak to pull the plunger against the tension spring so leaving an unbroken circuit. Should a high current be drawn because of overload or short circuit the magnetic field will be greatly increased and by its strength will overcome the force of the spring and draw the plunger forward, and this will, through a series of levers, cause the movable contact to separate from the fixed contact causing the continuity of the circuit to be broken. Once the cause of the overload has been removed the plunger and the contact can be returned to their normal position by operating a lever or reset button.

It is possible to obtain a circuit breaker which will tolerate a short-lived surge by fitting a piston in place of the tension spring holding back the plunger. This piston is controlled by a silicone filled dashpot which delays the operation of the plunger for a short time. It will however not be able to resist the attractive pull of a very strong magnetic field resulting from a very high current. This description is greatly simplified but should serve to illustrate how such a safety device operates.

Thermal circuit breakers

Thermal circuit breakers are rarely used in modern X-ray units but may be used in accessory equipment and may still be found on old mobile units where they act as a simple rather unsatisfactory form of overload protection. The unit uses a bi-metal strip. The current drawn by the unit passes through a strip of metal formed from two different metals as shown in Figure 9.3. The two metals are selected because of their marked difference in expansion coefficient. The current passing through the strip causes it to heat and as it heats the two metals expand to a different degree causing the strip to distort. When the degree of distortion reaches a predetermined point it will release a spring-loaded switch which breaks the supply to the unit. It is important to understand the operation of this type of switch as it is not possible to reset the breaker immediately; time must be allowed for the strip to cool and the distortion to be removed.

Interlocks

An interlock is designed to ensure that an action(s) cannot take place until permitted to do so by another quite separate controlling unit. In X-ray equipment their controlling functions are:

1. permitting components to reach optimum performance before they are used. For example, the tube filament must reach its correct temperature before an exposure can commence otherwise the mA value will not be as set.

2. avoiding damage should a component malfunction. For example, an exposure must not be permitted if the anode is not rotating at its correct speed.

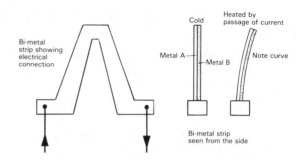

Fig. 9.3 Bi-metal strip thermal cut-out switch.

3. preventing overheating of part or all of the X-ray tube, e.g. overload protection of the tube.

4. controlling of X-radiation, e.g. the screening timer terminating fluoroscopy

5. preventing injury to person or damage to equipment by collision. For example, the tilting table motor drive cuts out when collision with the floor occurs and the movement is allowed to continue.

Interlocks may be mechanical although in X-ray equipment they are now largely electro-mechanical or purely electronic using printed circuit boards or microcomputers.

In their simplest form they may be merely one piece of equipment exerting pressure on a microswitch in the circuit of another piece of equipment. The microswitch is arranged to make or break the continuity of the second circuit. Examples include:

a. the passing of the cassette carrier in an explorator (serial changer) over a microswitch to cause the unit to change from fluoroscopy to radiography not permitting fluoroscopy again until the cassette carriage is returned to its standby position.

b. automatic closing of the undercouch tube collimating diaphragms to match the field size appropriate to a particular focus-to-screen distance. Here the raising or lowering of the explorator operates a microswitch which controls the circuit adjusting the collimator diaphragms.

c. the X-ray tube if sited at the extreme end of the tilting table will operate a microswitch to prevent the table being tilted further in the direction which could damage the tube.

The more complex forms of interlock are found controlling the X-ray circuit itself, for example, where X-rays cannot be generated or continue to be generated safely until other subsidiary circuits are functioning correctly and at their optimum performance. To illustrate the design and function of such a circuit, the exposure interlock circuit will be described and also some of the more important subsidiary circuits. Their purpose is to control the 'make' and 'break' of the exposure contactor so controlling the production of X-rays and the loading of the X-ray tube.

The exposure interlock circuit
Before an exposure can take place, it is necessary to ensure that all components are operating correctly. Therefore before the operator presses the exposure button, the unit enters the 'prepare' period. With the start of the 'prepare' period, the low tension exposure interlock circuit switch is closed. This circuit will not pass current even after it is switched on until an array of switches in its circuit is closed by the operation of a number of relays, each forming part of a subsidiary circuit. Once all the switches are closed the timer circuit which also operates on the exposure interlock circuit takes over and will allow the exposure to commence and continue for the selected time and then terminate the exposure. The timer circuit can be over-ridden and the exposure ended prematurely by the opening of any of the other switches should it be unsafe for the exposure to continue. By this means the patient's safety is assured and the X-ray tube is protected from damage. In fluoroscopy, the screening current will only be present whilst the operator keeps pressure on the screening switch.

The subsidiary circuits are switched at the same time as the exposure interlock circuit and so start to operate at the same time. If there is a fault on any of them, the switch in the interlock circuit will not be closed by the relay in the faulty subsidiary circuit. In other words, each circuit is interlocked with another, each controlling the other's operation.

Subsidiary circuits interlocked with the exposure interlock circuit include:

1. Delay circuits designed to allow time for components to reach peak performance
2. Tube stator circuits
3. Tube overload protection circuits

Figure 9.4 illustrates a simple exposure interlock circuit with its subsidiary circuits. Only three subsidiary circuits are shown but in practice there are many more.

Details of the subsidiary circuits. *A delay circuit (Fig. 9.5).* The purpose of delay circuits is to hold back the operation of another circuit so that the components elsewhere have time to reach their proper operating conditions. For example, it must not be possible to make an exposure immediately after:

a. the unit has been switched on. A delay of about 30 seconds is built in to allow the circuit components to stabilise.

b. the exposure sequence has started. Time is needed for the tube filament to reach its operating temperature and the rotating anode to reach its correct speed of rotation.

A delay circuit has a relay coil which when energised will close a pair of contacts in another circuit, the exposure interlock circuit, and allow this second circuit to start operating. The delay is caused by preventing the immediate operation of the relay. This is brought about by placing a capacitor into the circuit in parallel with the relay coil. Initially the capacitor will draw a large percentage of the current leaving insufficient current to energise the coil to operate the contacts. When the capacitor approaches full charge it draws very little current and the large percentage remaining then passing through the coil will be able to operate the contacts. Control over the time delay is provided by a variable resistance in series with the capacitor, an increase in the amount of the resistance extends the capacitor charging time and hence the delay time. The circuit supply is drawn from the autotransformer rectified to provide the capacitor with a direct current supply.

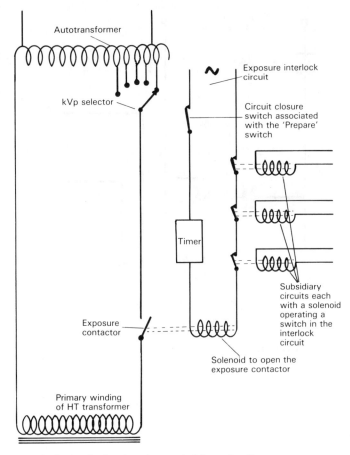

Fig. 9.4 Simple exposure interlock circuit showing three subsidiary circuits.

Tube stator circuits. The X-ray tube overload circuit cannot prevent local overheating of part of the anode target track of a rotating anode X-ray tube since it is designed to respond only to an overload applied to an anode revolving at the correct speed. However, local overheating can occur causing severe damage to a section of the annular track if this receives the full input load delivered by an exposure which was intended to be spread over the full annular track. So protective circuits are necessary to prevent an exposure being made on a stationary or slow running anode. To provide this protection it is essential that an exposure cannot take place unless:

a. Adequate time is given for the anode to reach the required rotation speed, hence the need for a delay circuit described previously.

The delay will need to be longer if a high speed rotation is selected as it will take longer for a speed of 9000 revs per minute to be reached than for 3000.

b. The electrical supply to the stator is present to start the anode rotating and continues to be present for the full exposure time. This requires the inclusion of a stator interlock circuit to operate on the exposure interlock circuit to prevent exposure if rotation is not present. This circuit is described below.

The stator interlock circuit is illustrated in Figure 9.6. To ensure that no load can be applied to a stationary or slow running rotating anode tube two fast operating relays are included in the stator circuit. The relay coils operate contacts in the exposure interlock circuit to prevent initiation of an exposure or termi-

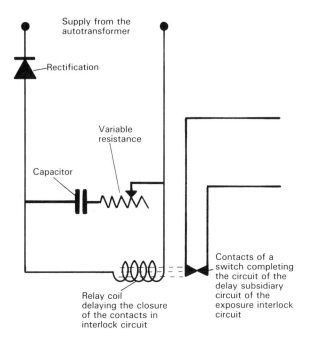

Fig. 9.5 Simple diagram of a delay circuit.

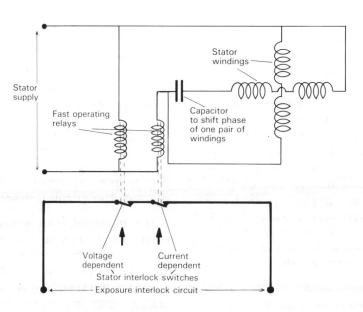

Fig. 9.6 Simple diagram of stator interlock circuit.

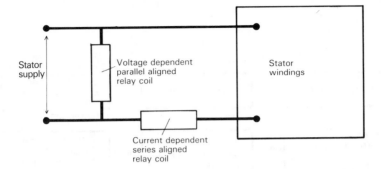

Fig. 9.7 Simple block diagram to show the parallel and series arrangement of the relay coils in a stator interlock circuit.

nation of an already running exposure as quickly as possible in the hope of preventing severe damage to the target surface. The relays are placed in the circuit so that one will be energised as soon as a voltage is applied to the stator winding and the other placed so that it will cease to be energised if there is no current flow through the windings. Relay 1 is placed across the stator supply in parallel with it. Relay 2 is in series with it. Relay 2 will only hold the contacts closed if a current is present and is of sufficient energising value. Figure 9.7 is a simplified block diagram to show the parallel and series position of the two relays.

Tube overload protection circuits

Simple system providing limited protection. In units, such as mobiles or low-powered fixed units, where exposures are not likely to be repeated after a short interval very simple protective systems are adequate. Sometimes there is just a mechanical block to prevent the user selecting a combination of exposure factors which would give an input load in excess of the tube rating for a particular focus. However, these systems do not take into account any heat that may be present in the anode from a previous exposure. The addition of this residual heat to the heat created by the second exposure which was permitted by the mechanical protection may be above the safe level and result in target damage.

The system relies on sufficient cooling tak-

ing place during the time needed for the re-positioning of the patient and film between exposures to avoid overheating. It is important that radiographers know of the importance of the interval between exposures and make sure that they pause between test exposures when undertaking quality assurance tests or on any other occasion when it is necessary to make a series of exposures.

Sophisticated system giving full overload protection. Major units require much more sophisticated systems to provide full overload protection from single or repetitive exposures that are possible on major units.

The easiest system for achieving maximum protection is to arrange for an analogue circuit to be energised concurrently with the X-ray tube and to vary the the value of its components so that it simulates electrically the thermal situation within the X-ray tube and through the exposure interlock circuit terminates the exposure at once should the safe rating be exceeded. The analogue circuit takes into account the single exposure and series of exposures. To simplify the explanation of the circuit it will be considered in two parts. Figure 9.8 indicates the association between the X-ray circuit and the analogue circuit.

Single load protection. This part of the circuit will prevent a single exposure being made if it will overload the target. The circuit may be linked to an indicating system showing the percentage of the maximum permissible load the exposure represents. The display may be

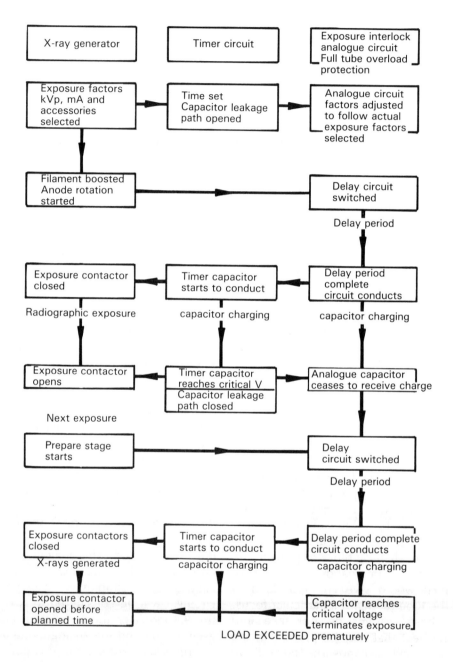

Fig. 9.8 Interaction between circuits ensuring full overload protection for the tube.

by a series of coloured lamps or by a meter with its scale calibrated in percentage of maximum load.

Serial load protection. In this part of the analogue circuit, the thermal condition of the X-ray tube is constantly monitored taking into account the input loading from a series of exposures and the rate at which the heat is dissipated. Should any part of the tube reach its heat capacity, the exposure will be terminated. Indicators are available to allow the current situation at the anode to be known as the sequence of exposures progresses. These monitoring devices will be considered in the section after tube rating.

A simplified analogue circuit. The description and operating principles of this analogue circuit should be read with reference to Figure 9.9. The kVp selected for the exposure is reflected on the isolating transformer primary voltage supply to the analogue circuit. The primary voltage is altered automatically as the exposure kVp is altered. The output supply from the transformer is rectified to provide direct current for the charging of the capacitors in the circuit.

Two variable resistances are placed in series in the circuit to alter the time taken to charge capacitor C_t. One resistance is linked to the mA selector so that as the mA is increased, increasing the rate of heat generation in the tube target, the time taken to charge the capacitor is reduced by cutting the resistance value. The second resistance is linked to the exposure time selector so that as the time is increased the resistance is decreased so again the charging time for the capacitor will decrease.

If the mA or time is decreased the resistance's value will be increased. In this way the analogue circuit follows changes in exposure factors. The current flowing through the circuit gradually builds up the charge on the capacitor C_t. Should the capacitor be charged to the critical value needed to remove the bias on the thyristor, the exposure will be terminated by the opening of the contacts in the exposure interlock circuit by the energising of the relay coil passing current as soon as the thyristor

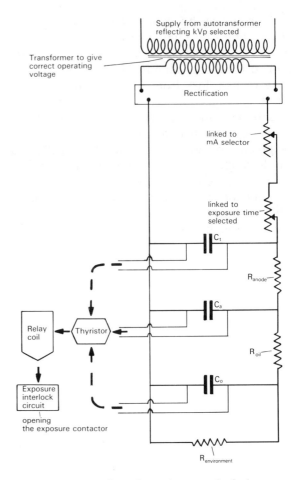

Fig. 9.9 Circuit to show the analogue method of providing full overload protection for the X-ray tube.

conducts. If the exposure factors are within the single load rating, the capacitor will not be charged to the voltage needed to remove the thyristor bias.

The selection of the value of the components has to be carefully made so that exposure termination takes place in accordance with the rating of the particular tube and focus. The charge on the capacitor may be the result of a single exposure or may be built up by several exposures. Therefore protection takes into account the effect of previous exposures, and unless provision is made for the cooling of the tube the system will terminate the exposure unnecessarily early. This difficulty is overcome by adding to the circuit described.

To simulate the cooling taking place in the X-ray tube, the charge on capacitor C_t is allowed to leak away through a resistance labelled R_a whose value is chosen to match the rate of heat loss from the tube anode on to another capacitor C_a.. This capacitor may reach a charge which is great enough to remove the thyristor bias and cause the exposure to end. The capacitor is also allowed to leak charge to yet another capacitor C_o through a resistance R_o whose value is chosen to simulate the rate of cooling of the oil within the tube housing. Again this capacitor leaks away through a resistance R_a which simulates the cooling of the whole tube by the surrounding atmosphere or in some instances by a fan or heat exchanger. The components in the analogue circuit will be particular to a tube and its focus, therefore a unit with three dual focus tubes may require six different circuits to cover the combination of focal spot sizes and different tube characteristics.

In modern units the circuits are formed into printed circuit boards or may have the information handled by a microcomputer. Whatever method is used by the manufacturer the approach to overload protection will be on the lines described above.

10
X-ray tube rating

Tube rating is defined as the maximum input of electrical energy (the load) that may be applied to an X-ray tube by a single exposure, a rapid sequence of exposures or a continuous input of energy, without causing damage by over-heating to any part of the tube assembly.

The rating of a tube is governed entirely by the temperature to which each part of the tube assembly may safely be allowed to rise and by the measures taken in the design and manufacture to minimise and tolerate temperature rise. Each part has its thermal capacity and upper temperature limit which must not be exceeded. Heating of the tube above the maximum safe temperature will cause:

Damage to the tube insert due to:

a. melting of the target — a tungsten focus can tolerate without melting 200 watts per millimetre^2.

b. crazing of the target surface due to differential thermal expansion between the surface and deeper layers of the target.

c. deposition of a tungsten film on the inside of the glass envelope through vaporisation of tungsten.

d. in self-rectified tubes only — damage to the cathode by electron bombardment possible through thermionic emission from a very hot target and available reverse potential across the tube.

e. in rotating anode tubes — failure of the anode rotation through the seizing up of the bearings.

OVERHEATING OF THE OIL WITHIN THE TUBE HOUSING

The factors which influence an X-ray tube loading are:

1. The construction of the tube assembly to enable it to tolerate heat and rapidly remove the heat.

2. Anode characteristics notably:
   a. type of tube — stationary or rotating anode
   b. composition and construction of the anode
   c. focal spot size
   d. angle of the target face
In rotating anode tubes
   e. diameter of the anode target disc
   f. rotation speed of the anode disc.

The magnitude of the electrical energy applied to the X-ray tube controlled by:

a. tube current (mA)
b. potential difference across the tube (kVp)
c. generator type — voltage waveform
d. frequency of the mains supply
e. length of time the target receives the load (exposure time)
f. method of delivering the load — an isolated single delivery or a continuous delivery.

The rate of heat dissipation influenced by:

137

a. design of the tube and the materials used in its construction
b. environment
c. forced cooling by fans or heat exchangers.

RATING OF AN X-RAY TUBE

As the rating of an X-ray tube is dependant upon the method of delivery of the load, each tube has a:

1. *single load rating* where only a single exposure is made with adequate cooling time before the next exposure.

2. *serial load rating* where a rapid sequence of repetitive exposures are made with such short intervals between exposures that the sequence is considered as a continuous exposure.

3. *continuous fluoroscopic rating* where the tube can be energised continuously since the rate of tube cooling is equal to the rate of heat input producing a state of equilibrium.

Single load rating is controlled by the ability of the target face to accept the injection of heat from a single exposure without damage from overheating.

Serial load rating is determined by the ability of each part of the whole tube assembly to tolerate the input of heat and the efficiency with which it is cooled by transfer of the heat from it.

Figure 10.1 shows the heat transfer path of a tube. Heat is lost by radiation, conduction and convection. In the rotating anode tube the principal means of heat removal is by radiation from the target face to the surrounding oil, where the heat is conveyed by conduction and convection to the tube housing, thence passed to the surrounding air. Conduction back from the target is restricted by design to protect the bearings from excessive heat. In the stationary anode tube heat is largely removed from the target by conduction through the copper anode block to the oil. There is some heat loss by radiation but because of the low loading the operating temperature is much lower than the rotating anode tube making heat loss by radiation much less efficient.

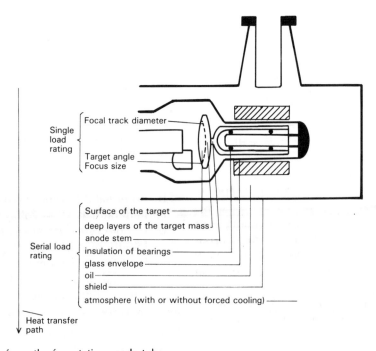

Fig. 10.1   Heat transfer path of a rotating anode tube.

RATING MEASUREMENT

The unit of measurement for rating purposes is the Heat Unit (HU). Anode input is correctly measured in watts but the heat unit being a more convenient unit to measure the heat energy applied to the anode of an X-ray tube is generally used by manufacturers of X-ray equipment.

The heat unit is based on the heat input of a single-phase 2-pulse generator so care must be taken to apply a modifying factor with other types of generator where the heat input is much greater.

Single-phase 2-pulse   Energy in HU
$= kVp \times mAs$

Three-phase 6-pulse   Energy in HU
$= kVp \times mAs \times 1.35$

Three-phase 12-pulse and constant potential   Energy in HU
$= kVp \times mAs \times 1.41$

kVp is used in the formula as the peak kV generates the greatest amount of heat. mA is the tube current average value (the tube current is always quoted in average value).

By using the formulae the input load in HUs can be calculated for a single exposure or a sequence of exposures. If the HUs are calculated for the same exposure for the different types of generator it will be seen that the input load on a tube supplied by a three-phase generator is much greater than from a single-phase. This would at first sight appear to be a disadvantage of three-phase or constant potential units but in practice it does not present a problem because the efficiency of X-ray production is so much greater with three-phase that the required quantity of radiation is produced in a much shorter time. However, it is important to be aware of this when selecting tubes for use with different types of generator.

HU can be converted to watts by applying the following formulae:

Single-phase
2-pulse   Watts = HU/sec $\times$ 0.71
Three-phase
6-pulse   Watts = HU/sec $\times$ 0.96

Three-phase   12-pulse and
Constant potential
    Watts = HU/sec $\times$ 1.00

MANUFACTURERS PROVIDE FOR ALL THEIR TUBES AND THEIR DIFFERENT FOCI THE FOLLOWING INFORMATION:

1. *For the anode*
   a. *Anode thermal (heat) storage capacity* say 300 000 HU
   b. *Maximum cooling rate* say 75 000 HU/minute
2. For the tube housing
   a. *Thermal (heat) storage capacity* say 1 500 000 HU.
   b. *Maximum cooling rate* say 18 000 HU/min without forced cooling, 36 000 HU/min with forced cooling.
3. *Maximum continuous fluoroscopic rating* say 600 HU/sec for 40 minutes.
4. *Radiographic rating* — charts display the maximum load that can be applied by a single exposure using various kVp.
5. *Cineradiographic rating* — charts display the number of frames per second for various lengths of run at different HUs per exposure.
6. *Angiographic rating* — charts display the number of exposures per second, the total number of exposures for different HUs per exposure.
7. *Cooling charts* indicate the cooling process where there is no forced cooling and with forced cooling.

A set of rating charts is shown in Figure 10.2

The information provided by the manufacturers is a guide to the selection of the most suitable tube for use with a particular generator. It allows techniques to be planned within the maximum permissible loading of the anode and the tube housing. Rating charts are used by the engineer to set up the overload protection circuits so that they will permit loading approaching maximum but always terminating the exposure before the rating limit is exceeded.

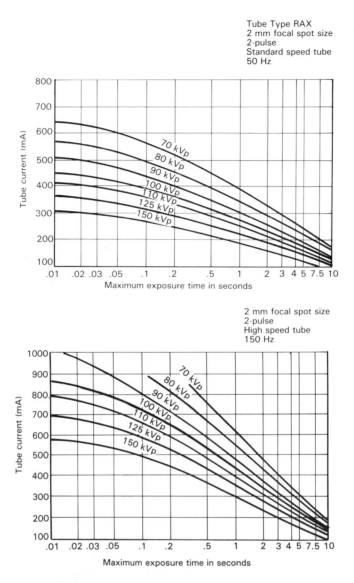

Fig. 10.2a Radiographic rating — 2 mm focus.

EXTRACTING INFORMATION FROM RATING CHARTS

Radiographic rating charts have a series of curves, in which each curve plots the maximum permissible exposure time for different mA and kVp. Provided the exposure factors do not place their intersection point outside the curve the exposure is within the tube loading. The curves are for use with a single exposure made on a cold anode. The maximum rating is determined largely by the temperature of the target track surface. The longer exposure times on the chart are limited by the maximum anode thermal storage capacity.

Since there are many factors affecting the

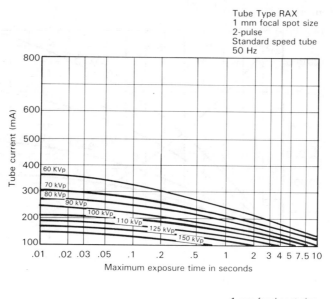

Tube Type RAX
1 mm focal spot size
2-pulse
Standard speed tube
50 Hz

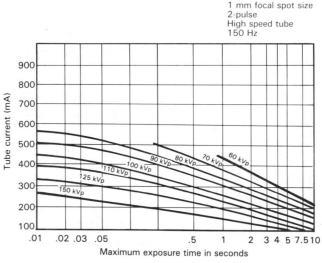

1 mm focal spot size
2-pulse
High speed tube
150 Hz

Fig. 10.2b Radiographic rating — 1 mm focus.

maximum radiographic rating of a tube great care must be taken to select the chart specifying the correct:

Tube type
Focal spot size
Frequency of the mains supply
Rotation speed of the anode
Type of waveform produced by the generator.

Figure 10.3 is a typical radiographic rating chart for a 2-pulse 2 mm focal spot operating at 50 Hz of a particular type (RA 125). To illustrate how such a chart is used, an exposure of 100 mAs at 90 kVp is required. Determine from the chart the highest mA that may be used. First try 500 mA at 0.2 s (Point A) — this is not possible as it is outside the tube loading. Now try 400 mA and 0.25 s (Point B) — this is also outside the loading. Now try 300 mA and 0.4 s (Point C). This is inside the permitted loading and so is safe to use. In practice modern units use microprocessors to indicate

Anode thermal capacity

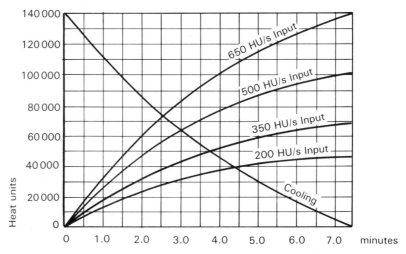

Fig. 10.2c   Anode thermal characteristics chart.

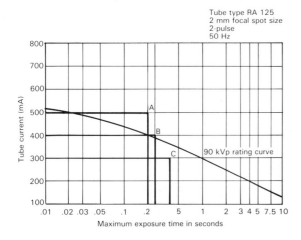

Fig. 10.3   A typical rating chart illustrating how it is used to determine the maximum mA which can be used at a particular kVp.

Anode thermal characteristics charts

Cooling charts have a single curve gradually dropping from the maximum thermal capacity in HU to zero over a period of minutes. From this single curve it is possible to determine how long it is necessary to wait before the anode can accept a further input load without exceeding the maximum thermal storage capacity. Figure 10.4 shows a typical cooling chart. It must be remembered that the chart for the particular tube must be used.

Continuous fluoroscopy input curves are often shown on the same chart as the cooling curve. They are a series of curves for various HU/sec input of continuous fluoroscopy indicating the gradual build up of heat as fluoroscopy continues through a period of time measured in minutes.

Rating for rapid repetitive radiographic exposures can be determined by reference to the

when a combination of exposure factors is outside the limit by displaying a red light and blocking the exposure.

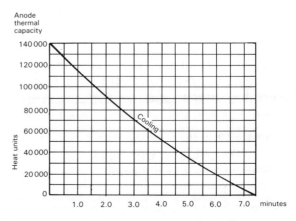

Fig. 10.4   Cooling curve of a typical X-ray tube.

rating charts in Figure 10.2 and described above. Four questions must be asked, these are:

a. Will the individual exposure be within the radiographic rating? Refer to the radiographic rating chart to verify.

b. Will the sequence of exposure and any fluoroscopy be within the thermal storage capacity of anode? Must there be some modification in the technique, perhaps by fewer exposures in the sequence, less fluoroscopy or an interval introduced between the fluoroscopy and the exposure sequence to enable the examination to be performed within the tube rating limit? Calculations using the anode thermal characteristic curves and the cooling curve will provide the information.

c. What length of interval must there be before a repeat sequence can be performed? Reference to the cooling curve will provide the information.

d. Will the total heat units be within the maximum tube housing thermal storage capacity? Reference to the tube data will provide the information.
A worked example is given below:

Technique
10 exposures of 80 kVp, 500 mA, 0.2 s taken in 25 seconds, preceeded by 1.0 minutes of fluoroscopy with an input of 350 HU/sec. The radiographic sequence may have to be repeated.

Process
a. Check that the single exposure of 80 kVp, 500 mA, 0.2 s is within the radiographic rating limit.

b. Trace the fluoroscopy input load by following up the 350 HU/sec anode thermal characteristic curve for 1.0 minutes. This gives an input of 20 000 HU.

c. Calculate the total radiographic input in HU. 80 kVp × 500 mA α 0.2 s × 10 exposures = 80 000 HU

d. Plot the radiographic HU on the cooling chart starting from the point where the fluoroscopy trace ended. The total input HU

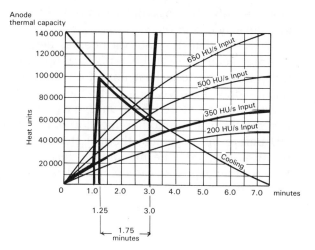

Fig. 10.5 Method of planning a series of exposures within the tube rating.

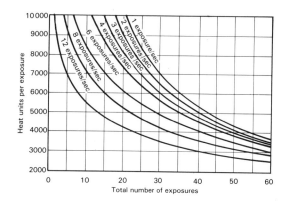

Fig. 10.6 Angiographic rating chart illustrating the layout of a manufacturer's information for planning serial exposure.

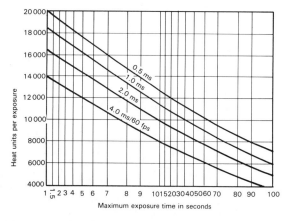

Fig. 10.7 Cineradiographic rating chart to show the manufacturer's method of presenting the information.

must be within the maximum permissible storage capacity of the tube.

   e. To calculate the interval needed before a repeat sequence can be run. Starting from the plot of the total heat units from the exposure draw a curve parallel to the cooling curve until the stored heat units have fallen sufficiently to allow another injection of 80 000 HU before the maximum thermal storage capacity is reached. The minimum interval before another exposure can be made is read off the chart.

3.0 minutes − 1.25 minutes = 1.75 minutes delay.

The chart used for the worked example is shown in Figure 10.5.

   Manufacturers supply angiographic and cineradiographic rating charts to allow technique programmes to be planned without resorting to the tedious method described above. Typical charts are shown in Figures 10.6 and 10.7.

11

Monitoring of X-ray tube loading

When an overload circuit operates, the supply to the X-ray tube is cut off preventing further generation of X-rays. This may occur at a most inconvenient point in the X-ray examination, possibly necessitating a repeat examination adding to the risk, causing additional radiation dose, extra strain on the tube and waste of time and materials. Therefore there is a need for some system of making certain that the operator is aware of the thermal state of the tube so that the examination can be organised when the tube is able to accept the full sequence of exposures without interruption. This system does not replace the need for careful planning of the programme by means of rating charts but serves as another source of information.

To fulfil this need manufacturers have produced monitoring devices which continuously record the level of heat stored in the anode and display the information digitally, by meter or by a series of coloured lights. Audible signals may be incorporated indicating the approach of the rating limit.

EXAMPLES OF CONTINUOUS MONITORING DEVICES

By the use of infra-red heat sensors

The X-ray tube anode gradually builds up heat as the sequence of exposures progresses. This heat is lost by infra-red radiation, the quantity and quality of the radiation increasing as the

temperature of the disc rises. A sample of this infra-red radiation is collected on a photo-electric infra-red sensing device positioned behind the target disc (see Fig. 11.1). The photo-electric device generates a current in proportion to the radiation received. The very

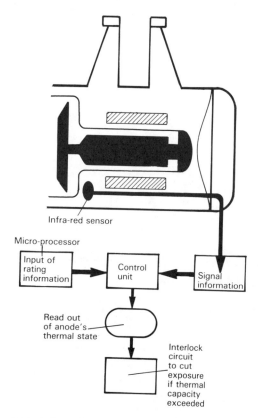

Fig. 11.1 Infra-red monitoring of the thermal state of the anode.

small current is amplified and used to display visually the thermal state of the anode and to terminate the exposure when the heat in the anode reaches the maximum thermal storage capacity. This form of monitoring has the added advantage that it automatically takes into account the cooling taking place.

The display of stored heat may be by a green, yellow and red lamp, lighting up the green light when the anode is cool, the yellow as a warning when the heat is approaching the maximum safe level and red as this point is reached. It is at this point that the exposure is terminated. The actual points at which the lights change are set up by the engineer using the rating charts for the particular tube. As an alternative means of displaying the information the current from the photocell after amplification is connected to a meter, whose scale is calibrated to read the percentage of the maximum thermal capacity.

There is a variation of this system available which uses fibre optic pipes to transfer the light emitted by the disc to a photocell sited outside the tube.

By the use of micro-processors

Micro-processors can be designed to simulate the input of heat to the anode, taking into account the exposure factors, the interval between exposures and the other factors affecting the loading and the cooling of the tube. The processor digitally displays information on the thermal state of the anode. The operator can immediately see when it is necessary to terminate a cine run or when it is safe to repeat a sequence of exposures without reference to rating charts. The micro-processor is linked to the overload protection circuit terminating the exposure if the maximum rating is about to be exceeded.

PART | # TWO

The handling and use of the X-ray beam

12
Introduction

The chapters in this part of the book are concerned with the handling and use of the X-ray beam and with the equipment needed to support the patient and to control the scattered radiation produced by the patient.

The description of the equipment given in this book is limited to its basic features. Students are recommended to examine closely examples of the different types of equipment in their departments. By adding the information gained from their observations of the actual equipment to that given in the text and diagrams, and by studying the manufacturer's data sheets, the student can acquire a depth of knowledge of the equipment they use in their departments and will be able to keep their knowledge updated as new models are introduced.

13

Production and recording of the 'real time' fluorescent image

PRODUCTION OF THE 'REAL TIME' FLUORESCENT IMAGE

In fluoroscopy a dynamic visible image is produced from the beam of X-ray photons. To produce the image the X-ray photons are directed to a layer of material with luminescent properties. The X-ray photons interact with the luminescent material, the phosphor and give up their energy to the outer orbital electrons of the phosphor atoms. This additional energy excites the atom and the atom gives up the surplus energy as visible light. The wavelength of the light is dependent upon the binding energy of the atoms and is specific to the phosphor material. In fluoroscopy the phosphor produces a green light. The luminescent material must have no phosphorescent property as this causes persistence of the image, termed 'after-glow' which will cause loss of image definition in a moving structure by confusing the current image with those preceeding it.

Fluoroscopy may be undertaken by means of a simple fluorescent screen or by the use of an image intensifier and a TV chain. The latter system is almost universally used because of the radiation dose reduction it permits. However, the simple fluorescent screen will be described as it is still in use where the very costly equipment cannot be justified. This simple type of screen may in the future be replaced by a panel-type X-ray image intensifier which has recently been produced. The unit increases the light output from the screen by a factor of about eight over an ordinary fluorescent screen. The degree of image intensification will reduce the dose received by the patient and improve the working conditions of the operator. Details of the unit are not included as they are still being developed.

The image formed on a simple fluorescent sceen can be photographed directly. This is the method used in photo-fluorography of the chest. Details of the unit are given on pages 183–184.

The simple fluorescent screen

Figure 13.1 illustrates the construction of a simple fluorescent screen showing its various layers. The phosphor layer is formed from green emitting zinc cadmium sulphide. An undercoat of magnesium oxide between the phosphor layer and the backing support reflects any backward directed light forward to the front of the screen. The zinc cadmium sulphide layer is covered with a thin cellulose acetate coating to protect its surface before it is mounted behind a sheet of lead glass. The lead glass is necessary to protect the operator from the residual primary beam. The lead equivalent of the glass must conform with the 'Code of Practice' requirements, namely 2 mm l.e. for energies up to 150 kVp. The screen face directed to the X-ray tube is protected by a thin plastic or aluminium sheet. The fluorescent screen with its lead glass front is mounted

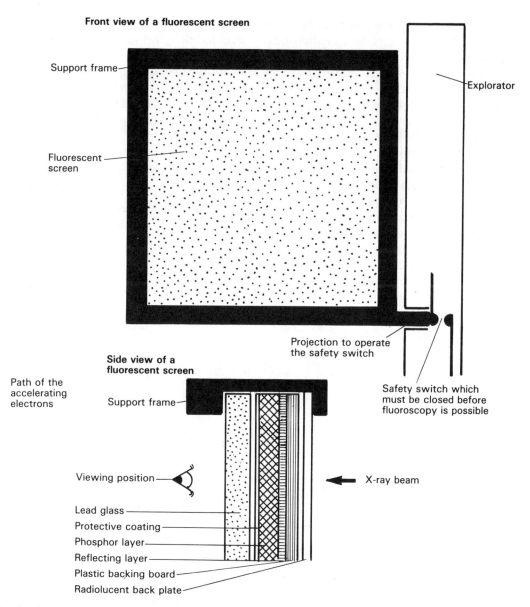

Fig. 13.1 The fluorescent screen.

in a metal frame which forms part of an explorator, which will be described later. An opaque plastic cover is provided so that bright daylight, which would cause deterioration of the phosphor, can be excluded when the screen is not in use.

There is intrinsic unsharpness in the screen due to the phosphor crystal size. The smaller the crystal, the better the resolution, but the greater the quantity of X-radiation needed to provide the required level of image brightness. Therefore a compromise must be drawn between the degree of image unsharpness and the radiation dose delivered to the patient. In most fluoroscopic units the focus-to-film distance is short and the explorator supporting the screen somewhat bulky causing a fairly large object-to-screen distance. These two factors cause increased geometric unsharpness so it is advisable to use a focal spot size which will keep the geometric unsharpness down to the value of the intrinsic screen unsharpness to give the best resolution possible.

Of course the focal spot size must be large enough to permit a tube loading which will allow the examination to be completed.

The level of illumination from a fluorescent screen is very low. The image can only be seen with scotopic (night) vision with its diminished visual acuity, and even when time is allowed for the eyes to become adapted to the dark, the detail perceived by the operator is very limited. This is very inconvenient and time consuming for the operator, and difficult for the patient, so there is obvious advantage in electronically enhancing the fluoroscopic image. Hence the introduction of image intensifier and TV chain which makes it possible to view the fluoroscopic image in normal low-level lighting and to display more image information whilst reducing the radiation dose rate to about 10% of the dose received by fluoroscopy alone. As a result of the improved image quality the examination can be performed more quickly and efficiently.

The image intensifier and TV chain

Figure 13.2 shows the layout and image pathway of an image intensifier and TV chain. Each component shown in the diagram will be considered in detail.

Advantages of an image intensifier and TV chain over a simple fluorescent screen

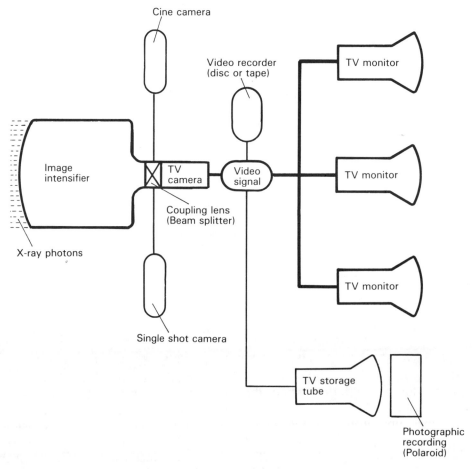

Fig. 13.2 Components and image pathway of an image intensifier and TV chain.

1. Radiation dose reduction.
2. More diagnostic information presented.
3. Less trying for the patient.
4. Quicker examination.
5. Better working environment.
6. Extension of fluoroscopy time permitted because of the reduced power requirement.
7. Electronic manipulation of the image possible, permitting such techniques as image enlargement and enhancement and subtraction.
8. Permits electronic image recording and photofluorography in static or dynamic mode.
9. Allows simultaneous viewing/recording at a number of sites.

Disadvantages

1. Large capital and revenue costs incurred
2. Greatly increased sophistication necessitates regular maintenance and fairly frequent fault correction by specialist engineers.

Image intensification

The purpose of image intensification is to convert an X-ray pattern into a visible image which is several thousand times brighter than the conventional fluoroscopic image produced by a simple fluorescent screen.

Image intensification takes place in an evacuated envelope. A fluorescent screen (the input screen) is placed at the front of the envelope. A photocathode is put in intimate contact with the back of the fluorescent screen. The X-rays falling on the fluorescent screen cause light photons to be produced. The light photons release electrons from the photocathode. The number and distribution of released electrons are proportional to the number of X-rays incident on the screen.

The released electrons are then accelerated and focused by an electric field existing between the photocathode and the electrodes of an electron lens system to form an image on an output phosphor at the opposite end, the back, of the image intensifier tube. The acceleration of the electrons is caused by a potential difference of about 25 kVp between the input and output screen. This gives the electrons greatly increased energy which causes the output screen to fluoresce brightly under their impact. Figure 13.3 outlines the system.

Details of the design and function of an image intensifier

The housing (shield) and support plate. The shield is a strong metal cover which protects

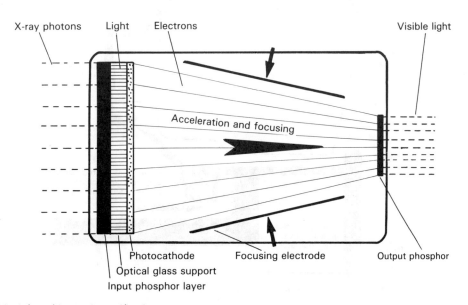

Fig. 13.3 Principles of image intensification.

the insert from damage and it protects the operator and patient from injury should the insert envelope implode. The housing is lined with lead to ensure that the primary radiation is reduced to a level which provides adequate protection as required by the 'Code of Practice' for the operator. The output phosphor is covered with lead glass for the same reason.

The intensifier housing is fitted to the X-ray table by a strong base plate. The plate is made of metal, usually steel to give it strength and to provide a primary radiation barrier. It has a central circular opening to allow the X-radiation to reach the input screen of the image intensifier. Care is taken to ensure that there is an overlap between the radiation barrier provided by the intensifier housing and the base plate. The opening in the base plate is covered with a radiolucent sheet of plastic or aluminium to protect the input face of the intensifier.

The shield and its contents with its base plate are very heavy and must be mounted on a sturdy support suspended from an overhead mounting or attached to the X-ray table to allow either an over or under table position. Whichever way the unit is supported it must be adequately counterweighted to facilitate movement. As the support plate and the intensifier housing provide essential radiation protection it is important to provide an interlock circuit which makes it impossible to generate radiation from the X-ray tube directed towards the intensifier without the intensifier and its support plate correctly positioned in front of the X-ray beam. Figure 13.4 shows a section through the housing and its support plate, and indicates a form of interlock switch associated with the control of X-ray generation.

The intensifier insert. *The envelope.* The intensifier tube insert envelope is made of metal or glass. The input face must offer little attenuation to the X-ray beam and so is formed from thin glass or in some modern units from

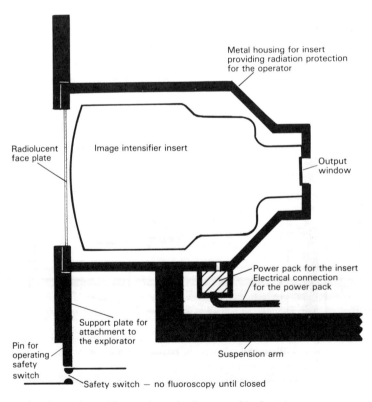

Fig. 13.4 Cross-section of an image intensifier to show the insert and its housing.

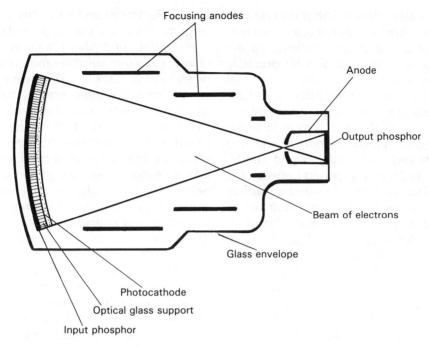

Fig. 13.5 Section of an image intensifier.

titanium. It is cylindrical in shape with a domed input face and a narrowed output end with a small diameter output. Figure 13.5 shows the shape of the insert and the location of its contents.

The input phosphor. This is a dome-shaped fluorescent screen, the actual shape being important as it affects the quality of the image. It is sometimes formed on a titanium base which is made to precise dimensions calculated by a computer to give exact focusing across the whole of the output fluorescent screen. The phosphor coating used is caesium iodide whose rod-like crystals are deposited vertically on the backing support. This alignment of crystals increases the absorption of X-radiation by the increased thickness of the layer; the small cross-section of the crystals provides a resolution of about 5 line pairs/mm (Fig. 13.6).

The photocathode is a coating of caesium or antimony or other material which will release electrons when struck by light. For efficiency the input phosphor and the photocathode must be placed very close together. This is

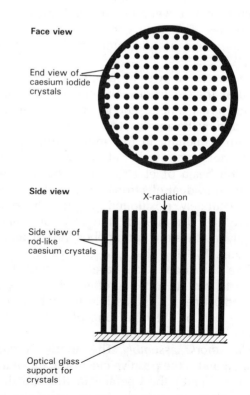

Fig. 13.6 End-on position of the caesium iodide crystals on their optical glass support (greatly enlarged).

achieved by coating the phosphor on one side of a very thin sheet of optical glass, 0.2 mm thick, and the photocathode material on the other. The glass plate must also be precisely shaped. There is a reflecting layer in front of the phosphor to increase the number of light photons interacting with the photocathode.

The electron-optical system is formed by the input fluorescent screen, cylindrical and ring shaped electrodes and a cup-shaped anode. The potential of 25 kVp is applied between the input phosphor and the cup-shaped anode and this accelerates the electrons produced by the photocathode to the output phosphor. The electrons leave the dome-shaped photocathode at right angles to its surface and during their passage to the output phosphor, they are focused electrostatically by a series of electrodes. The dome shape causes the electron stream to reduce in diameter and the electrostatic field at the first anode reinforces this effect. Drawn by the anode potential, the electrons continue to move back influenced by the electric field between the first and the second electrodes. This field continues to reinforce the reduction in diameter of the electron image.

Figure 13.7 shows the electric fields developed by the electrodes. The electrons, having gained great kinetic energy, continue to be attracted by the anode and finally pass through a central opening in the anode cup. At this point there is no further electrostatic focusing and the beam of electrons by repulsion between individual electrons diverges to fall on the accurately positioned output phosphor where the diameter of the electron image exactly matches the output phosphor diameter (25 mm). The ring electrode, the last electrode before the anode, can have its potential altered to vary its focusing effect. By means of this adjustment it is possible to magnify the centre part of the input phosphor to fill the whole output phosphor.

The anode assembly. The anode is cup-shaped and is the positive electrode. Once the electrons enter the opening in the cup they are no longer under the influence of the fo-

cusing electrodes and so at this point they diverge to cover the output phosphor.

The output phosphor is a fluorescent screen of zinc cadmium sulphide mounted on a glass or glass fibre backing. The diameter is much smaller than the input screen, about 25 mm, which matches the size of the input face of the TV camera. The reduction in size gives a much brighter image because the same number of electrons that were generated by the much larger photocathode fall on the output phosphor. This minification of the image is one of the ways of producing the intensified image; the other is of course the result of the kinetic energy acquired by the electrons as they are accelerated across the intensifier tube by the potential difference. The output phosphor is backed on the vacuum side by a very thin sheet of aluminium to prevent the light from the output phosphor falling back on to the photocathode to produce spurious electrons which will degrade the image. The sheet is so thin that it does not obstruct the passage of the electrons to the fluorescent screen

The power supply. The intensifier insert requires a high voltage supply (25 kV) to accelerate the electrons and a supply for the electrostatic focusing of the electrons. This is provided by a power-pack which may be placed within the housing or mounted on it. The supply cable for this unit is brought from a control unit at low voltage, the power pack generating the stable, rectified, output required.

Operator controls. The housing is used to support a control box which allows the operator to select the factors and accessories required during the fluoroscopic investigation and allows the intensifier field size to be altered if the unit provides this facility. The connections from this unit travel back to the control unit beside the power pack supply.

Intensifier input sizes. Image intensifiers are available in three sizes: 5 in (17 cm), 9 in (25 cm) and 14 in (35 cm) input phosphor diameter. The 9 in (25 cm) is the most commonly used size for general fluoroscopic purposes

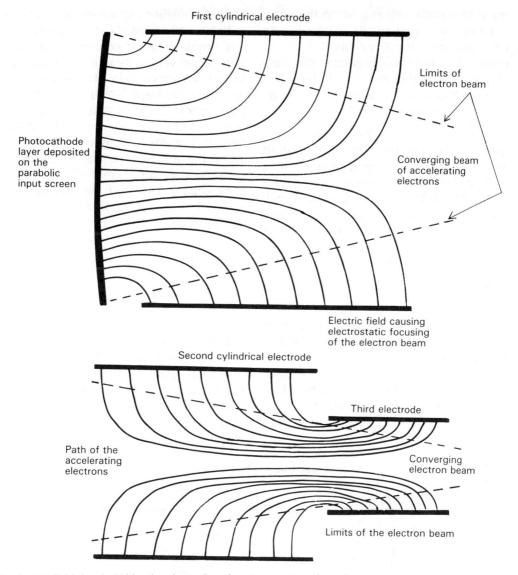

First cylindrical electrode

Limits of
electron beam

Photocathode
layer deposited
on the
parabolic
input screen

Converging beam
of accelerating
electrons

Electric field causing
electrostatic focusing
of the electron beam

Second cylindrical electrode

Third electrode

Path of the
accelerating
electrons

Converging
electron beam

Limits of the electron beam

Fig. 13.7 Electric field developed by the electrodes of an image intensifier tube.

although the larger 14 in (35 cm) field size is obviously more convenient for abdominal and thoracic cavity coverage, but these units are much more expensive and hard to justify for general work. As the 5 in (17 cm) unit is very compact, it is ideal for mobile units.

The output image. Some characteristics of the image can be assessed visually by the operator either on the TV monitor or from a photofluorographic film. These include:

1. The area of the object displayed by the intensifier. This is governed by three factors:
a. input phosphor size
b. geometric enlargement of the object due to the ratio of the object-input phosphor distance to the focus-input phosphor distance. The ratio should be as large as possible but will depend upon the proximity of the entry plate of the intensifier to the patient's skin, the location of the

input phosphor with respect to the entry plate of the mounting and, of course, to the position of the X-ray tube.

c. potential difference between the ring electrode and the anode cylinder. Variation in this value will alter the focussing effect on the beam.

Figure 13.8 shows how the centre of the input phosphor can be made to fill the output phosphor giving an enlarged image of a smaller field. The exposure must be increased when a smaller field is selected as there will be fewer photons reaching the output phosphor since they are only derived from a reduced area of photocathode and will be insufficient in number to generate an acceptable level of light output. Units are available which provide two or three field sizes. For example a 9 in (25 cm) intensifier tube may allow a 5 in (12.5 cm) field, or if it is a three field type, a 4, 6 and 9 in (10, 15 and 25 cm) field.

2. Brightness gain

The output phosphor is much brighter than the input phosphor and the amount by which it is brighter is the brightness gain. Therefore the term gain was used to describe efficiency of the intensifier and values of $\times$ 6000 or even $\times$ 10 000 were quoted for new units. However, this simple method of measuring the output gain is not very satisfactory because so many factors influence gain. Therefore, recently a new term has been introduced — the 'conversion factor' — it is the ratio of the light output of the intensifier to the input exposure rate. It is measured in candelas per square metre per mR per second (cdm^{-2}/mRs^{-1}). The conversion factor numerically is about 1% of the old gain. That is if the unit had a gain of $\times$ 6000 the conversion factor is about 60 cdm^{-2}/mRs^{-1}. The conversion factor is affected by:

a. the quantity and quality of the input exposure
b. the photocathode emission level
c. the ratio of the input screen area to the output screen area
d. the accelerating potential between the input and output phosphor.

3. Resolution

Resolution is the fineness of a line pattern that can be visually observed. It is measured in line pairs per millimetre (l p/mm). A modern

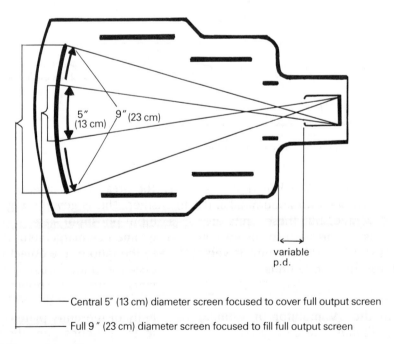

5″ (13 cm)   9″ (23 cm)

variable p.d.

Central 5″ (13 cm) diameter screen focused to cover full output screen

Full 9″ (23 cm) diameter screen focused to fill full output screen

Fig. 13.8 Dual field image intensifier.

image intensifier will allow resolution of 4–5 l p/mm. This value when measured in the most ideal conditions is described as the limiting resolution of the intensifier. However many factors influence the resolution, including:

a. the phosphor
b. the quality of the radiation
c. the input exposure rate
d. focal spot size
e. focus-input phosphor distance
f. object-input phosphor distance
g. subject contrast
h. scatter.

Therefore, resolution measured by line pairs is perhaps not the ideal method of comparing the maximum resolution of one unit with another under normal working conditions. Modulation transfer function (MTF) is much better since it is a measure of the percentage of input information delivered at the output and is determined at different values of contrast. Figure 13.9 is a graph to show the MTF of the three fields of a triple-field image intensifier unit. It can be seen from the graph that the l p/mm vary with the different field sizes and with relative contrast.

Quantum noise, both spatial and temporal arising from the random fluctuation in the emission and absorption of X-ray photons due to variations in voltage and luminance, will affect the quality of the image, as will contrast

loss resulting from the lateral spread of X-rays, light and electrons.

4. Vignetting

Vignetting is the progressive decrease in luminance of the image from the centre to the periphery of the image. It results from the energy distribution across the input screen through variation in focus to screen distance at the centre and at the periphery of the screen and the optical system. The best units will show an evenness of luminance across the field.

5. Lag

Lag is defined as the persistance of luminance after the exciting radiation has ended. This persisting image becomes confused with the new image being formed. Any phosphor takes time to produce the luminance and time for it to decay, the modern phosphors have a lag of less than 1 ms where the older types could be up to 30 ms or even more. Lag becomes most important in the fluoroscopy of rapidly moving structures since their images are changing at very high speed.

Assessment of the intensifier. The operator can make a subjective assessment of the output image from the image intensifier, but regular objective tests must be undertaken to monitor performance since patient dose increases and image quality deteriorates with age or malfunction. The operator may not be aware of the gradual fall off in efficiency if relying on subjective assessment alone. The fall off results from deterioration of the phosphor and reduction in the potential difference across the tube. Any gas produced within the insert will be held in the centre of the field and will increase the brilliance of the image in the centre of the field. In time it will burn out this part of the phosphor and leave the centre of the field with no image or a very poor quality image.

The operator must take note of the tube current required to produce a good image, for if the conversion factor reduces, the input exposure must be increased to offset the loss. This will increase the radiation dose to the patient. With automatic exposure control this

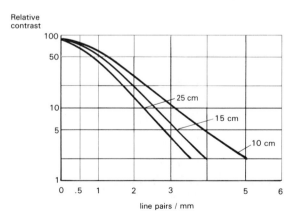

Fig. 13.9 Different degrees of resolution at different contrast values for three images intensifier fields (MTF).

can pass unnoticed if the operator is not alert to the possibility.

The effect of varying the input exposure factors. An increase in tube current (mA) will enhance the image by providing extra X-ray photons to be intensified but will increase the patient dose. The output phosphor will be more brilliant.

Automatic brightness control. In order to maintain maximum image quality on the TV monitor and/or video recording and to provide constant exposure factors for the photographic recording of the image intensifier image, it is necessary to ensure that the level of illumination of the intensifier output phosphor remains constant. Therefore a system of automatic brightness control is provided as an alternative to manual control (Fig. 13.28).

Automatic brightness control operates by comparing the level of illumination from the output phosphor with a standard. If the monitored value differs from the standard, the fluorsocopy factors controlling the X-ray output of the tube are automatically adjusted until the output phosphor illumination level is restored to the normal standard value. Since it is important that the radiation dose delivered to the patient is kept as low as possible, the modern automatic control will adjust the kV and the mA to correct the output phosphor illumination.

An increase in kV will not increase the radiation dose as much as a comparable mA increase, but it must be remembered that an increase in kV will reduce contrast, so it is best to compromise by adjusting both. Generally the fluoroscopy mA is increased to provide additional photons until a top value is reached, say 1 mA, and then, if sufficient photons are still not available, the kV is automatically increased by 10, the mA being cut back to a lower value. Automatic brightness control operates throughout the fluoroscopic examination changing the factors as the patient turns or the area under examination is changed.

It is most important when using automatic control that the operator keeps a close watch on the mA values demanded by the control by watching the mA meter. If the mA values are consistently higher than the normal values required when the image intensifier and TV system was installed, checks must be made on the conversion factor. If this factor has fallen off, the unit will automatically increase the input exposure rate to compensate, and the patient dose may reach unacceptable levels. Proof of this will justify replacement of the image intensifier and/or the TV tube.

There are occasions when automatic brightness control may need to be switched off and manual control substituted, for instance when opaque contrast agents are being used but recording of the non-opacified structures are to be optimally exposed.

Coupling of the image intensifier to the TV camera. The light image formed on the output phosphor of the image intensifier must be conveyed to the input face of the TV camera without distortion and with minimal loss of light intensity. There are two methods of coupling: by simple direct fibre-optic coupling or by an optical system.

The fibre-optic coupling. The fibre-optic system is simple, comparatively cheap and

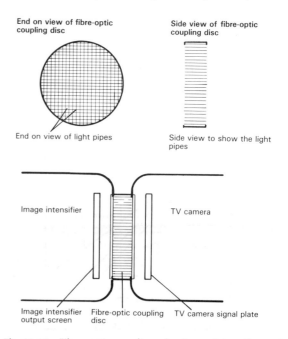

Fig. 13.10 Fibre-optic coupling of an image intensifier and a TV camera.

very compact. It is a coin-shaped disc formed of very fine light pipes tightly packed into a circular frame of about 25 mm diameter and 5 mm thick. Each pipe conveys the light incident from one end to the other end where it interfaces with the TV camera input. Figure 13.10 illustrates the construction of the disc and its location. The walls of the pipe prevent any lateral spread of the light and the loss of intensity between the ends is minimal. The fineness of detail conveyed in this way depends upon the diameter of the pipes. It is a very efficient form of coupling but can only be used in systems where photofluorography is not required since the image pathway from the image intensifier output phosphor to the TV camera cannot be interrupted.

The optical system of coupling. The optical coupling of the image intensifier and the TV camera is provided by a lens system. This is a very expensive system and much more bulky than the fibre-optic coupling but it does provide a more versatile system of coupling. The optical system must transmit the maximum amount of light possible from the image intensifier output to the input of the TV camera. Therefore two very high quality fast lenses are used in a tandem arrangement (see Fig. 13.11). The input image and the output image receptor must be accurately positioned so that they are located on the focal planes of the lenses. The focal length of the lens is usually 50 mm. The size of the output image transmitted by the lens system is the same as the input.

Coupling of two lenses allows transmission of four times as much light as a single lens. In addition the use of two lenses provides a parallel (telecentric) beam between the two, permitting the introduction of a beam-splitting mirror (see Fig. 13.11).

In assessing an optical system the following factors must be considered:

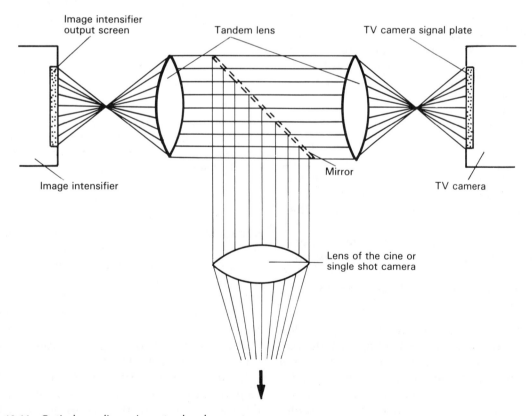

Fig. 13.11 Optical coupling using a tandem lens system.

a. Percentage transmission

Percentage transmission is an indication of the efficiency of the system in transmitting light. It is dependent upon the quality of the lens system

b. Relative aperture (speed)

The aperture size controls the amount of light entering the system. In optical coupling of the TV camera to the image intensifier an aperture of f.0.75 is most commonly used. The very large aperture gives a very narrow depth of field but does allow a great deal of light to enter the system. The narrow depth of field does not present focusing problems since the input and output images are produced on flat plates, and providing the components of the system are very accurately positioned and secured in place, there will be no difficulty. If malalignment of any part of the system should occur, the output image will become unsharp.

c. Resolution

The resolution of the system must be equal or better than the image it is to transmit. The optical system described resolves at 8–9 l p/mm and this is very adequate as the modern image intensifier has a resolution of about 5 lp/mm. It is important that this level of resolution is maintained across the whole field and not just in the centre, a common failing of poor quality lens systems.

d. Vignetting

Vignetting, the loss in brightness towards the periphery of the lens, is evident in most optical coupling systems. It is more obvious when a large aperture and a tandem lens with a wide gap between the lenses is used. These features are necessary in the coupling of an image intensifier and a TV camera, so vignetting could be a problem. However, with a high quality TV system compensation can be made for any loss of peripheral light from the lens.

The beam-splitting mirror. This is a mirror which reflects a percentage of the light falling on it and allows the remaining light to pass through it. This feature permits the recording on photographic film of an image whilst it is still in the operator's view, so the image intensifier image can be simultaneously presented to two recording systems. A cine or single-shot camera records the reflected image. The transmitted image is picked up by the TV camera for immediate display on the TV monitors. The percentage of reflected light ranges between 75 and 90%, leaving 10 to 25% to form the TV image. This amount of light is inadequate for the display of a satisfactory image, therefore the input X-ray exposure rate must be increased to make up for the loss due to reflection. The increased exposure will increase the patient's radiation dose so it is most important that the mirror is removed from the telecentric beam when photofluorography is not required. In practice the mirror must be deliberately introduced by the operator either manually or automatically on selection of photofluorography.

Some installations allow the recording of the image by a single-shot camera or by a cine camera. This necessitates the introduction of a rotating mirror support to allow the mirror to be rotated through 180° to direct the reflected light towards either the single-shot or the cine-camera.

The television camera

The optical image formed on the image intensifier output screen is conveyed through the coupling system to the input face of the TV camera where the image is transformed into an electrical charge pattern which is periodically scanned and neutralised by an electron beam. The scanning operation takes place from top to bottom along a number of parallel horizontal lines, and once the scanning beam reaches the bottom of the charge pattern it starts scanning from the top again. One scanning of all the lines, generally 625 lines or sometimes 1249, is described as a frame. There are 25 frames per second in systems operating on a 50 Hz supply.

The components of a typical TV camera tube are shown in Figure 13.12.

During its scan, a beam of electrons in the camera tube continuously falls on a plate of electrical charges whose values are modified

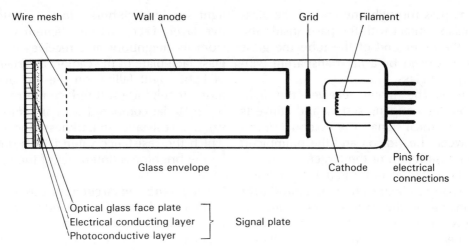

Fig. 13.12 Vidicon TV camera tube.

by the optical image falling upon them. The electrical charge therefore models the light image by being in proportion to the amount of light incident upon the corresponding point in the image receiving layer. The beam neutralises these charges, and the discharge current forms an electrical signal which is proportional to the brightness of the optical image at the point corresponding to the momentary position of the scanning beam.

Types of camera tubes used in X-ray TV chains
There are two types of TV camera tubes in general use today: the vidicon and the plumbicon. In design they are very similar, as both convert the light image falling on their face to an electrical signal which can be transmitted immediately to the TV monitor.

The vidicon tube. The main drawback of the vidicon tube is its image persistance, lag, which is particularly noticeable at low lighting levels. This is a definite disadvantage when displaying rapidly moving objects, but is an advantage when slow moving objects are to be examined for it helps to suppress some of the random fluctuations in the X-ray pattern which create irritating noise in the image especially at low dose rates.

The plumbicon tube. This tube, on the other hand, has no perceptible persistance which makes it ideal for recording rapidly moving structures, but it does have a higher noise level at low light levels. Additionally it has the advantage of a proportional response to all values of light input.

Desirable features in a TV camera tube
Whichever type of tube selected it must be:

small in size, low in weight
simple in design
robust in construction
easy to operate
reasonably long lived
not too expensive
having:

high sensitivity
low dark current
low noise level
high response speed
large dynamic range
good resolution.

The components of the TV tube (see Fig. 13.12)
The glass envelope. The contents of the camera tube are housed within an evacuated cylindrical glass envelope which is about 25 mm in diameter and 160–200 mm in length.

Metal pins pass through one end of the glass wall to make contact with the parts inside the tube. At the other end of the tube the glass envelope is closed by a flat transparent window of optical glass.

The target. The target receives the light image from the coupling system and converts it into an electrical signal. The essential difference between the vidicon and the plumbicon is in the construction of the target.

The *vidicon target* is formed by coating a semi-transparent electrically conducting layer on the inside of the optical glass window. Graphite is often used for this layer. An electrical connection is made with this layer which is known as the signal plate (Fig. 13.13).

On top of the conducting surface is a layer of photoconductive material, made of antimony trisulphide. This layer forms the light sensitive or photoconductive layer, for it is here that the light image is converted into an image formed of electric charge. The layer is a mosaic built up of millions of light sensitive globules, each insulated from its neighbour.

The layer of antimony trisulphide has the property of varying in resistivity according to the light level incident upon it. The image is built up from millions of picture elements, the light sensitive globules, in the photoconductive layer. Each picture element is insulated from its neighbour and receives through the glass face-plate of the camera a certain amount of light. Light falling on the globule of antimony trisulphide will reduce the resistance of the material compared with an almost infinite value of resistance in darkness. The amount by which the resistance value falls is determined by the brightness (intensity) of the light falling on it.

The *plumbicon target* has a semi-transparent conducting layer of zinc oxide coated on the glass face. The photoconductive layer is lead monoxide, as its structure allows the formation of a semi-conductor p-i-n junction. By doping the lead monoxide an n-type material is formed in the outer surface layer of the target and a p-type in the inner surface layer. Figure 13.14 is a section through a lead monoxide target showing the layers. The presence of the p-type material distinguishes lead monoxide from other target materials.

When there is no light incident on the target there can be no current through the target because the p-i-n junction is reverse biased, hence the absence of any dark current. When illuminated electron/hole pairs are created in

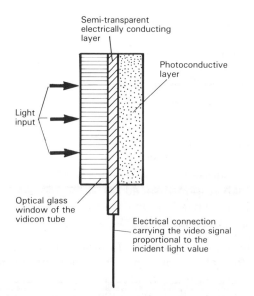

Fig. 13.13 Schematic diagram of the vidicon signal plate of a vidicon camera tube.

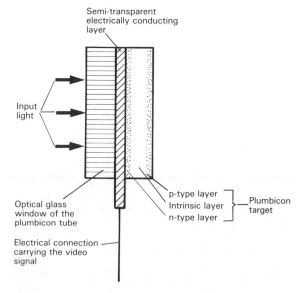

Fig. 13.14 Schematic diagram of a plumbicon tube target plat (signal plate).

the centre of the photoconductive layer (the intrinsic layer) they are quickly transported to the surfaces of the layer giving rise to the electrical signal. The electron/hole pairs are produced in linear proportion to the incident light, which, with the absence of a dark-current, are the main advantages of the plumbicon over the vidicon camera tube.

The electron gun. The electron gun provides a very fine stream of electrons needed to scan the target to convert the optical image falling on the camera face into an electrical signal suitable for transmission. The resolution of the system is partly dependent upon the cross-sectional area of the electron stream and the precision of the scanning.

The electrons are released by thermionic emission at the cathode filament and the stream of electrons is drawn away from the cathode by the anode voltage, the anode being about 200 V positive to the cathode. The electron stream is focused as it passes through a central aperture of a negatively charged grid placed just in front of the cathode.

A cylindrically-shaped wall anode extends the full length of the tube forming the final electrode of the gun. It gives a uniform accelerating field. A wire mesh covers the far end of the wall anode to trap any slow moving negative ions which may be present but it

does not obstruct the passage of the fast moving electron stream

The TV camera assembly
Outside the evacuated glass camera tube are two sets of coils (Fig. 13.15). These are concerned with the alignment of the electron stream and with its scanning.

Alignment coils. The alignment of the electron stream is maintained by two coils:

a. A coil surrounding the outside of the camera tube at the point where the electron stream passes through the grid aperture. The magnetic field produced by the coil exerts a compressing effect on the stream reducing its cross-sectional diameter.
b. A long focusing coil forms a sleeve-like structure over the whole length of the tube. This ensures that the electron stream remains extremely fine.

Scanning coils. Two pairs of scanning coils are provided to bring about horizontal and vertical deflection of the electron stream. They are positioned about half way along the tube. Once the stream is deflected towards its correct position on the target's photoconductive layer, the long focusing coil ensures that the electrons pass perpendicular to the grid to strike the target at right-angles.

The two pairs of scanning coils are set at

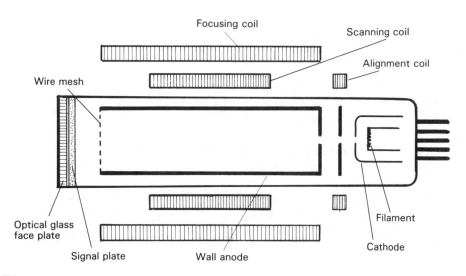

Fig. 13.15 TV camera.

right-angles to each other. The horizontally positioned pair cause the electron stream to move across the target and the other pair vertically positioned move the transversely positioned electron stream to a different vertical level.

The principle of scanning. If the magnetic field produced by two coils forming a pair is equal, the force on an electron stream moving between them will cause the stream to take up the central position between the two coils. If the current flowing through the coils is different, the strength of the magnetic field developed by each coil will be different causing the electron stream to move until it reaches a position where the forces on it are equal. Thus by delivering a changing supply to the coils it is possible to cause the electron stream to scan the target, in an action rather like reading a book, i.e. by starting to read at the left-hand end of the top line, reading across the line from left to right, and then returning almost instantly to the second line, and so on until the last line is read. The eye then returns to start the process again on the next page. The left to right movement is the scan, the rapid return from right to left the flyback and the page the frame. The horizontally placed coils cause each line to be scanned followed by another line below it. The vertically placed coils cause this line of scanning to be positioned immediately below the previous line, so eventually the whole target is scanned.

In the majority of television systems there are 625 lines of horizontal scanning in each frame. There are 25 frames per second. It takes 60×10^{-6} s to scan one line from left to right and 5×10^{-6} s to flyback. Some very expensive systems scan 1249 lines in a frame. The increased number of lines providing an image with better resolution and this is essential if all the fine detail displayed by the image intensifier is to be recorded by the TV system. This is the reason why a 1249 line system is specified for the image intensifier/TV chain of a unit for digital vascular imaging where it is the TV image which must be electronically manipulated.

25 frames per second may display some degree of flickering on the TV monitor so it is usual for alternate (odd) lines to be scanned in one frame and then to scan the others (even) lines. This is termed interlaced scanning. It offers a greatly improved image, the result of halving the time between scanning one part of the frame and scanning again almost the same part.

It is important to remember that the brain builds up the image by recording the many hundreds of positions of a single spot (pixel) of light produced by each target globule as the electron stream scans the target. As all the 625 lines are scanned in 1/25 s, the nerve endings in the eye gather information from each spot and the visual centre of the brain holds the information by persistance of vision so that a complete frame is 'seen'. Figure 13.16 shows the raster pattern of simple and interlaced

Simple scanning

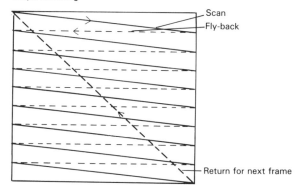

Interlaced scanning

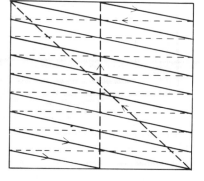

Fig. 13.16 Raster patterns.

scanning. Interlaced scanning reinforces the image by covering the area twice in the same time as a simple scan.

Synchronising signals. For accurate reproduction of the image on the TV monitor, it is essential that the signal produced by the electron stream as it scans the camera target is correctly located on the screen of the TV monitor (Fig. 13.17). To achieve this a synchronising signal is added at the end of each line of picture information. The combined signal containing the picture information signal and the synchronising signal is transmitted to the monitor where the two signals are separated so that the synchronising signal can ensure that the picture line is correctly orientated.

Picture formation. The image is built up from millions of picture elements (pixels) on the target photocathode. The light from the intensifier output phosphor passes through the glass face-plate of the camera on to the target. The vidicon or plumbicon camera tubes produce an electrical signal because the action of the light on the photocathode causes the charge on the pixel of the target to leak away in proportion to the quantity of the light falling upon it. The first coating on the back of the glass face-plate is an electrical conducting layer which has a positive potential of 30 V when measured in darkness. The stream of electrons from the electron gun scans each line of picture elements. Where light has fallen on a picture element, the resistance across the target is low allowing the electrons to traverse the layer more freely. As the level of light illumination across the line varies so does the resistance offered by the target. Thus the current flowing across the target will vary providing a variable current which is an electrical record of the light levels forming the picture.

The 30 V on the target provides the potential difference needed to cause the current to flow. This current is known as the video signal which, after it has been suitably amplified, is carried by conductors to the control box and on to the TV monitor. The video signal may be reproduced at once on the monitor or it may be diverted to a video recording unit for storage before being transmitted at another time to the TV monitor. The signal may be divided to allow immediate display and storage to take place simultaneously. Recently equipment has been developed to digitise the video signal to allow it to be put into a computer where the image can be manipulated to provide an enhanced image.

The television monitor

The television monitor converts the signal produced by the television camera back into a visible image. It consists of a cathode ray tube and its associated circuits. The whole is enclosed in a housing to prevent injury from an imploding glass envelope or from the electrical hazard from the high voltage circuits and to absorb any low energy X-radiation produced by the high energy electrons produced by the tube.

The cathode ray tube
The tube is funnel-shaped with a convex front. The expanded front provides a good sized image for easy viewing. It consists of an evacuated glass envelope containing a cathode with an electron gun and an associated controlling grid, an anode and a fluorescent screen. Figure 13.18 illustrates the layout of the cathode ray tube components.

The cathode is formed from a nickel cup supporting a filament helix in a precise position.

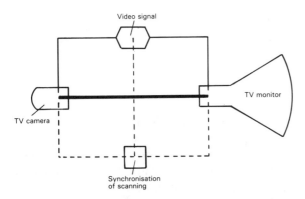

Fig. 13.17 Linking of the TV camera to the monitor showing the relationship of the raster scanning with the video signal.

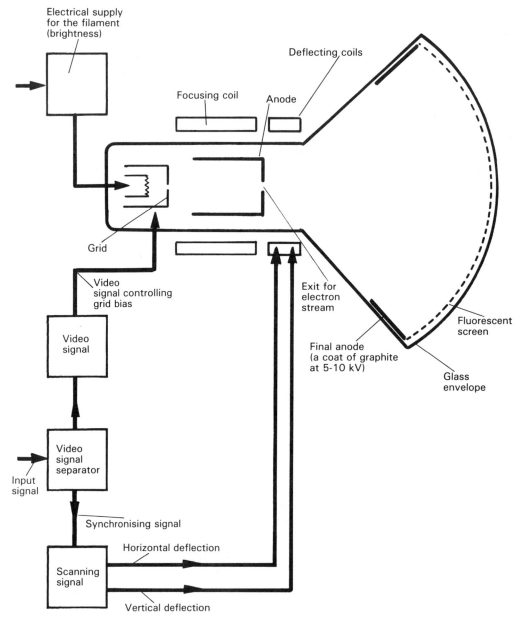

Fig. 13.18 TV monitor.

This filament when heated produces electrons which are focused electrostatically into a very fine stream. The number of electrons leaving the cathode is modulated by the grid placed in front of the cathode. The bias on the grid is varied by the strength of the picture information part of the video signal. When the video signal is high, because the light falling on the particular picture element of the camera target is bright, the bias on the grid of the monitor is low, so more electrons are permitted to leave the cathode to produce a brighter spot on the monitor screen.

The anode. The first anode is set in front of the cathode gun. It has a central aperture through which the electrons accelerated by the anode can pass to reach the fluorescent screen. The inside of the funnel walls are coated with graphite acting as a second anode.

The fluorescent screen. This is formed by coating the inside of the convex front of the glass envelope with a fluorescent material. The intensity of the fluorescence produced depends upon the intensity of the electron stream falling upon it. The glass front of the tube is thick enough to attenuate the low energy X-rays produced by the deceleration of the high speed electrons.

The cathode ray assembly. Surrounding the glass envelope are two sets of coils: the focusing and deflecting coils. The magnetic fields produced by these coils apply forces on the electron stream as it leaves the cathode to emerge through the anode aperture.

The focusing coil is mounted round the glass envelope in its narrow part as shown in Figure 13.18. This coil keeps the electron stream compressed to a small cross-sectional area and correctly centred before it comes under the influence of the deflecting coils.

The deflecting coils are mounted around the glass envelope's narrow part just before it expands to form the funnel-shape. Two pairs of coils are arranged around the camera tube. They receive the synchronising signal from the TV camera which modifies their current so that the magnetic field produced deflects the centrally placed electron stream to the exact position on the fluorescent screen to match the position on the camera target where the picture information was collected.

The controls provided for the operator's use. On the housing of the TV monitor is a set of controls which allows the operator to vary the brightness and contrast of the image. Manual operation of these controls should not normally be necessary if the unit is correctly set up to give an optimum image and regular servicing is carried out. The operation of these controls does become necessary when the monitor has deteriorated and needs adjustment to return to optimum performance. The operator cannot improve the quality of the image by changing these controls if the video signal is poor.

When the brightness control is adjusted it increases or decreases the current through the filament, altering its temperature and causing the release of more or less electrons.

The image contrast control alters the amplification on the grid bias, so exaggerating the difference between the bright areas and the dark areas.

Vertical and horizontal controls are provided on the back of the unit. These are only used to adjust the supply to the deflecting coils. Should the picture roll, this is corrected by adjustment to the vertical hold, and if the picture is displaced sideways this requires an adjustment of the horizontal hold.

The mounting of a TV monitor
The TV monitor must be mounted on an overhead support or on a trolley so that the image can be viewed at eye level and in a convenient position some 3 or 4 feet from the viewer. It is important not to view the image from too short a distance as the lines which form the image become more obvious and distracting to the viewer. Whichever method of mounting is selected, the cables connecting the monitor to the rest of the system must be long enough to allow unrestricted movement, supported throughout their length and protected from mechanical damage.

Care and maintenance of the image intensifier and TV chain

Care in the handling, in the use and in the regular servicing of the image intensifier and TV chain will extend the useful life of the system and ensure that maximum information is transmitted.

The following procedures will prolong the useful life of the image intensifier, TV camera and TV monitor:

1. Switch the system off when it is not in use, remembering to switch off units which are directly connected to the mains supply and not through the X-ray unit. The reduction in running hours will extend the life of the filaments, reduce the wear on the fluorescent

screen and reduce the amount of heat generated.

2. Run the image intensifier occasionally, if it is not used frequently as this will eliminate any gas molecule that may be present in the glass envelope — a gettering mechanism to burn up the gas is provided by the manufacturers to operate when the system is energised. Should gas molecules be present in the glass envelope, the electron control in the image intensifier is less efficient. Image resolution is impaired and the gas ions are focused giving a very high intensity central spot which will damage the central part of the screen just where the maximum information is to be found.

3. Avoid the projection of any intense light on the TV camera target — radiographic exposures should not be made directly on the intensifier without an attenuating medium interposed between the X-ray source and the intensifier input phosphor. If high tube currents are required for radiographic exposures, it is common to find an iris diaphragm placed in front of the TV camera face which closes down when radiography is selected. A biasing current to cut off excessively high video currents may be supplied which automatically operates when radiographic exposures are selected. The metal back of the cassette adequately protects the system and when photofluorography is selected the beam splitting mirror prevents excessive light reaching the TV camera face.

4. Position the TV monitor when it is not in use in a position where it is not in direct sunlight. Bright sunlight causes even the less sensitive modern phosphors to deteriorate.

Mechanical damage must be avoided and the following will reduce the likelihood of damage:

1. Ensure that the image intensifier and TV camera are securely attached to their support by checking frequently for evidence of worn parts.

2. Store the image intensifier and TV camera and the monitor in the sites designed for them and secure them in position.

3. Keep the TV monitor correctly positioned on its trolley or well secured to the overhead support, ensuring that it cannot collide with any other equipment. If a trolley is used the wheels must be checked regularly and kept free moving for a seized wheel can cause the trolley to be pushed over.

4. Never leave trailing or twisted cables.

5. See that the air circulates freely around the units to avoid a build up of heat. Pillows and blankets should never be put on top of the monitor.

It is important to keep the equipment clean. By its electrostatic charge the TV monitor screen will attract dust. A layer of dust will absorb quite a lot of generated light and may, if not removed, cause the exposure factors to be increased to overcome the light loss by absorption in the dust layer. This is to be deplored as it will give the patient an unjustifiable increase in radiation dose.

The appearance of deterioration in an image intensifier and TV chain
Deterioration will be apparent to the operator by:

1. A need to increase the exposure factors to provide a satisfactory image on the TV monitor. This is the result of loss of amplification somewhere in the system.

2. A loss of resolution in the TV image.

3. A loss of image contrast.

4. The presence of a black central spot on the screen due to phosphor damage.

These changes can be insidious, making it very important to undertake regular routine checks on the performance of the unit. When automatic brightness control is installed, exposures are increased automatically to overcome a loss in amplification — a real radiation hazard.

Evaluation of a TV chain and the location of malfunctioning parts
Evaluation of the whole TV chain and its component parts must be approached methodically. It can be undertaken by the operator without engineering knowledge.

A phantom is used which allows objective assessments to be made. The design of the phantom must ensure that its characteristics are always the same so that the image taken on one occasion can be compared with one taken on a previous occasion. It must contain structures which will allow the density, contrast, resolution, magnification, distortion and the uniformity of screen luminance of the system to be assessed.

It is important that the phantom is used to produce a base-line record of the TV chain's performance as soon as the system is installed and after any resetting of the system. Then the performance of the system can be matched against this base-line for any evidence of deterioration. The test procedure must be very fully recorded, giving details of the exposure factors and other relevant information necessary to allow a repeat examination to performed under exactly similar circumstances. If possible, the incident radiation dose should be measured and recorded. In addition an image of the phantom should be taken and retained for comparative purposes.

By utilising all the image outlets provided by the system it is possible to determine which part of the system is responsible for the loss or deterioration in output.

The network diagram shown in Figure 13.28 (p. 184) outlines one method of assessing performance. It must be remembered that all TV chains fall off in performance from the day they are installed. Some of these changes are reversible but some are not. The unacceptable increase in radiation dose to the patient is one

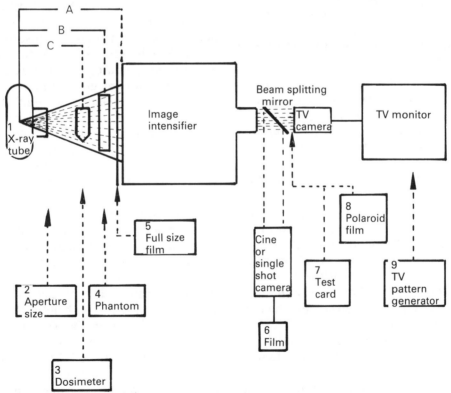

Fig. 13.19 Layout of system for checking the performance of an image intensifier and TV chain.

Key
1 Exposure factors
2 Aperture size (degree of collimation)
3 Dosimeter
4 Phantom
5 Full size film in cassette
6 Film taken of image intensifier output
7 Test card
8 Polaroid film taken of monitor image
9 TV pattern generator
A Focus-to-image intensifier input face distance
B Focus-to-phantom distance
C Focus-to-dosimeter distance

of the criteria on which replacement of a component must be made. and another is poor image quality which lowers the diagnostic value of the examination. The value of a regular assessment of image quality and the availability of unequivocal evidence of deterioration will facilitate the acceptance of the need for replacement of components which are operating at an unacceptable standard.

The method of checking the performance of the image intensifier and TV chain

Preparation. Set up the equipment as shown in Figure 13.19 making sure that:

a. the distance between the focus and the intensifier face and the distance between the focus and the phantom are exact and reproducible on other occasions.
b. films, cassette and intensifying screens are of the type and speed specified.
c. TV, cine, single shot or polaroid camera apertures are correctly set.

The exposure factors for the phantom are initially selected empirically to provide an optimum image of the phantom. Similarly the exposure factors for the full size film, exposed in the serial changer of the explorator, are adjusted to give optimum image quality. The shutter times for the cameras must also be set to give good results. These factors should match as closely as possible the exposure factors used on patients. The details are recorded and used for all subsequent assessments.

The incident radiation dose received at the input face of the image intensifier should be measured for the base-line exposure. Care must be taken to place the dosimeter chamber in a repeatable position.

The X-ray beam should be collimated to a particular size so that the scattering volume is always the same.

Procedure. With the base-line exposure factors and all other factors set up to the test requirement, a polaroid film is taken of the TV monitor image of the phantom. If this facility is not available a visual assessment of the image on the monitor is made, and although this introduces some subjective assessment

,objective measurements can be made if the phantom contains components which permit measurements to be taken from the image. The image contrast, density, resolution, distortion, magnification and the uniformity of the image brightness across the field are compared with the base-line image taken at the time of installation or after optimisation. If the result does not compare with the base-line standard, the cause of the change is sought by a process of elimination.

The components of the system are checked individually:

1. by exposing a full size film in the serial changer using the base-line exposure. If this film does not compare with the base-line standard film, the X-ray output from the tube has changed and is responsible at least in part for the fall-off in performance. The dose measurement will confirm. If the exposure delivered to the film is adjusted to restore the input dose to the standard, a further assessment of the TV monitor image is made to see if the base-line image quality is restored. If this is so, the problem does not in any way involve the TV system and any automatic increase of exposure factors will not increase the patient's dose but merely restore the normal dose. However, the tube will be subjected to an increased loading.

2. If the full size film shows no change from the standard, a photofluorographic film is taken with the cine or single shot camera, and this is compared with the standard. If there is a change, the fault must lie with the intensifier. If no beam splitting facility is available, it is difficult to separate a fault in the image intensifier from one in the TV camera without the help of an engineer. However, if the TV camera can be removed from the intensifier the image of a test card with standard illumination can be assessed. The test card used by X-ray engineers is similar to the card displayed on domestic television monitors. If the monitor displays a good image the fault cannot be in the TV system and therefore must be in the intensifier.

3. Alternative monitors are generally avail-

able and the use of another monitor will settle whether the fault is in the camera or the monitor.

TV cameras and monitors are set up to optimum performance and tested by means of a TV pattern generator which is brought by the engineer. It is important that the radiographer is in a position to indicate to the engineer the location of a fault so that he can bring the special test equipment with him on his first visit.

Testing as described here will ensure that the maximum performance of the system is achieved and maintained and that the system is repaired or replaced as soon as the patient dose rises to an unacceptable level or the information loss makes diagnosis insecure. The test results must be carefully recorded and the films retained so that changes can be demonstrated and the case for replacement based on secure documented evidence.

RECORDING OF THE INTENSIFIED FLUOROSCOPIC IMAGE

Intensified fluoroscopic images can be recorded from:

a. the video signal generated by the TV camera on to video tape or video disc. The signal may be reproduced as it was recorded or it may be enhanced digitally by a computer.
b. the output phosphor of the image intensifier by a cine or single-shot camera on to photographic film.

The recording of an intensified image has many advantages over the simple full size film exposed in the serial changer of the explorator. This image is merely a static record of a single image displaying the features observed by the operator which are required to support the diagnosis.

The advantages are:

1. The record can be made at the same time as the fluoroscopic image is viewed by the operator.

2. Radiation dose is much less for an individual image because of the intensification which has taken place.
3. Cost of recording is less.
4. System permits greater versatility in the recording of the image, allowing dynamic as well as static images to be recorded.
5. The recording equipment is less bulky than that required for full size film recording.

The disadvantages are:

1. Much higher capital and revenue costs.
2. More operating time lost through maintenance or failure of sophisticated electronic components.
3. Image quality is not as good as that produced on a full size film, although new technology has brought about such great improvement in image quality that there is now little perceivable difference between the two systems.

Recording of the video image

The closed circuit TV system between the TV camera and the TV monitor can be interrupted so that the video signal may be recorded on magnetic tape or disc for future display on the monitor whilst the image continues to be displayed on the monitor. The video recording may be reproduced as a dynamic (moving) or static image on the TV monitor.

The dynamic image
The dynamic image is collected from the video signal by magnetising a track on a tape or disc to varying levels of intensity in accord with the amplitude of the video signal. The magnetic record is retained on the tape or disc and can be recalled by passing the magnetised track in front of a play-back head which recreates the electrical signal. This is then applied to the TV monitor cathode grid to modulate the cathode stream to reproduce a fluorescent image exactly as the original TV image.

The video tape is a reasonably cheap method of recording images collected over a long period, up to 3 hours, but the system

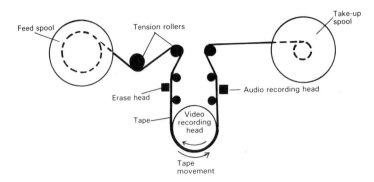

Fig. 13.20a Video tape recorder.

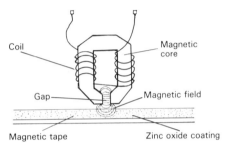

Fig. 13.20b Enlarged view of the video head of a video recorder.

does not permit easy recall of a particular section of the tape nor does it allow rapid review of a preceeding image.

The video disc on the other hand does provide easy recall and allows for slow motion projection or static display of a frame. It also permits the coupling to other electronic devices, such as digital image enhancement and subtraction units. The disc has some disadvantages when compared with tape and these include a shorter maximum recording time and greater cost of the equipment.

The video recorder

For simplicity the video tape recorder will be described and its operation explained. The disc unit is in principle the same but has a spiral track formed as the disc rotates below the recording/play-back head instead of a the linear track of the tape. The essential components are shown in Figure 13.20a.

The video head is a closed core of magnetic material such as ferrite with a very narrow gap across which a magnetic field develops. A coil is wound around the core as shown in Figure 13.20b. The coil receives the video signal which varies in amplitude, the different levels of intensity in the current causing the magnetic field across the core gap to vary in strength. This changing magnetic field is retained on the magnetic tape as varying levels of magnetism. To recall the signal from the tape, the magnetic signal induces magnetism within the core and the lines of force developed cut the turns of the coil around it to produce a current which being an exact copy of the original video signal is used to produce the image on the monitor. Therefore the video head provides the recording and playback facility. To reconstruct accurately the image one border of the tape carries the synchronising signal to indicate the location of the particular part of the video signal within the raster pattern.

The audio head is an additional head aligned to the other border of the tape. This is used to record the sound from a microphone which is synchronised with the video tape so that sound can be reproduced alongside the image. This is useful for identifying the particular part of the record of a series of examinations that belongs to a particular patient. It is also useful when teaching tapes are being produced.

The magnetic tape is made of thin plastic material coated on one side with a layer of magnetisable material such as chrome oxide.

The tape is carried on a feed spool and drawn between tension rollers which prevent the tape pulling too tight as it passes around the recording head to be wound on to the take-up spool. The tape runs obliquely in front of the recording head so that a very long track can be formed on a fairly short tape, of 1 in width (Fig. 13.21).

As the tape passes in front of the video head, the magnetic domains in the tape coating which are normally randomly positioned are aligned by the magnetic field; the number aligned depends upon the strength of the magnitising field which is dependent upon the amplitude of the electric current creating the field. By moving the tape the pattern of aligned domains carrying the detailed picture information is spread along the tape as the video signal proceeds. The rapid movement of the tape in front of the head is increased by rotating the head in the opposite direction to the tape movement as illustrated in Figure 13.21. Air is passed between the tape and the head to produce an air cushion between them to prevent friction.

The erase head is sited between the feed spool and the video head. The tape is cleared of any residual picture information by a current generated in the erase head which causes all the magnetic domains in the tape remaining to lose any alignment with each other. The alignment then is totally randomised ready to collect fresh picture information.

The housing of the video recording unit is plastic. It serves two purposes: to prevent the operator touching live electrical components and to shield the equipment from dust or damage. Any dust collecting around the heads will reduce the coupling of the magnetic field with the magnetic domains in the tape. If the outflow of the anti-friction air cushion is restricted by dust, the separation of the tape and head will be in excess of normal also reducing the coupling.

The operator controls are mounted on the outside of the housing and are similar to any video tape recorder. These include:

Mains On/Off switch

Record — this control must have some additional interlock to ensure that it cannot be operated accidently and perhaps erase a previously recorded signal

Play-back

Rapid rewind

Fast forward drive

Freeze — holds a frame for inspection of a static image

Slow motion — allows the detail of a fast moving object to be examined more closely

Erase

Index counter to allow easy location of a part of the tape

Brilliance and contrast control.

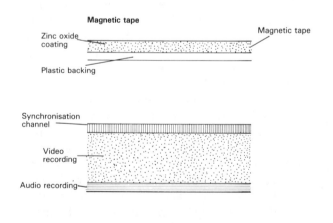

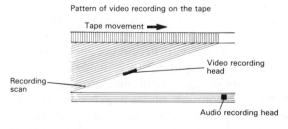

Fig. 13.21 Video tape.

Advantages of video recording compared with cine radiography

1. No special accessory equipment required to project the image.

2. No delay between recording and viewing (no processing).

3. Radiation dose not increased as the video signal is used to provide the normal image on

the monitor and without any additional signal, the image can be stored by the video recorder.

4. The magnetic tape can be re-used time and time again or stored as a permanent record.

5. Contrast and brightness of the image can be adjusted on the recorded image.

Disadvantages

1. The resolution is not as good although the modern units with 1249 lines to the frame closely match the cine film after it has been magnified by the optical projector to a conveniently viewable size.

2. Continuous tape makes the location of particular parts of its length difficult to find. The video disc does not present this problem to the same extent as the recorded track is shorter.

The storing of a static image formed from the fluoroscopic image displayed by the TV chain

Most commonly today a static image from a TV signal is obtained from the image stored on a magnetic disc.

The unit is designed to store the information from a few frames and then by repeatedly playing back these frames on the monitor produce an apparently static image which remains on the TV monitor until it is returned to store or erased by the recommencement of fluoroscopy.

This image will not have the resolution normally produced by the video system for it is formed from the raster of a few frames whose images may be slightly out of register with each other; the ordinary video image is continuously updated by the scanning of the camera target.

There are many uses for this equipment:

1. In theatre work where the TV image is used to align immobilising pins, to locate stones or verify the patency of ducts. These procedures can be satisfactorily undertaken with the use of a series of static images giving

great reduction in radiation dose since the image is formed by a few frames and there is no further screening current until a change of image is required.

2. In departmental radiography it is possible to check the position and projection of the part before the actual radiographic exposure is made. This will reduce the number of reject films reducing the patient dose and the cost of the examination.

The electronic manipulation of the video image

The video image can be manipulated to reduce the radiation dose or enhance the image:

1. Radiation dose reduction. The radiation dose received during a fluoroscopic examination can be reduced by providing very rapid switching of the tube current. The rapid switching permits the pulsing of the fluoroscopy. The fluoroscopy pulse continues for the time taken to scan one frame, then it is switched off for the time taken for a further three frames and then switched on again for one frame and so on throughout the screening period. In this way the radiation dose is reduced to a quarter. The image displayed on the monitor does not show the gaps between the pulses of fluoroscopy as they are filled by repetition of the exposed frames.

2. Image enhancement. The image can be enhanced by digitising the the video signal by passing it through a computer. Once the signal is digitised it can be amplified and if required further manipulated before it is applied to the monitor for visual display. The great advantage of this technique is the speed with which it can take place, its versatility and the fact that the image improvement is obtained without additional radiation dose.

Electronic enhancement is most valuable in vascular imaging. A display rate of 25 images per second avoids irritating image flicker and is sufficiently rapid to prevent obvious blurring of the images of pulsating structures. The level of resolution of such a system should allow the visualisation of blood vessels of 1 mm in diameter which contain 1% of added

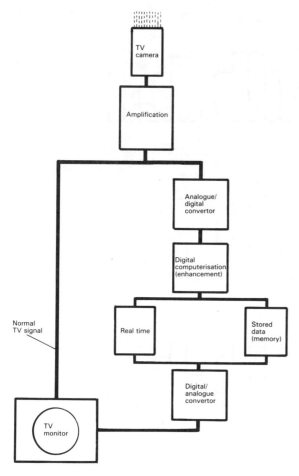

Fig. 13. 22 Principles of digital imaging.

radiographic contrast agent. The additional facility for image subtraction further increases the value of the system. Details of the systems are not considered in this text as further information is readily available in specialist literature provided by equipment manufacturers.

However, Figure 13.22 indicates in simple form the layout of the system's components and Figure 13.23 attempts to show how a signal is modified by digitisation and amplification — in this example the amplification doubles the signal. The final curve shows how the contrast of the final image is greater than the original curve. Subtraction is also undertaken by the system's computer. Figure 13.24 also attempts to indicate the effect of subtracting one image from another and how by elimination of part of the image the remainder containing the useful information is much more clearly displayed.

The images produced by this technique can be displayed in real time, stored on video disc for later display or recorded photographically.

Recording of the image intensifier image

Photofluorography is photography of the fluoroscopic image to produce either a cine or static image. The image formed on the output screen of the image intensifier is recorded on photographic film by a camera focused on the image formed on the beam-splitting mirror

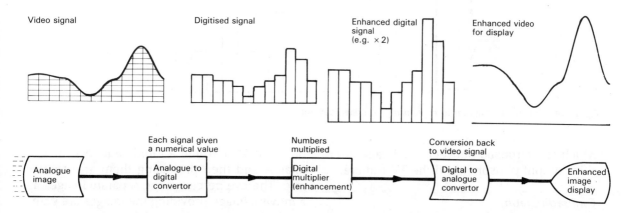

Fig. 13.23 A layout diagram to show how a video signal from a TV camera can be digitised to produce an enhanced image on a TV monitor.

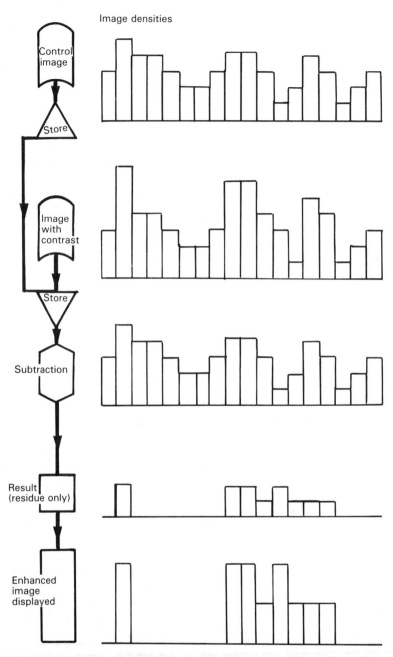

Fig. 13.24 Schematic diagram to explain digital image subtraction.

which is interposed between the image intensifier output phosphor and the TV camera.

Cineradiography

The display of a dynamic image by photography is obtained by photographically recording on 35 or 16 mm film a rapid sequence of still images and then projecting them at a similar rate. The eye perceives the separate images as a moving image providing the images are gathered at a rate in excess of 16 frames per second. This speed of repetition is too great for the eye to register as separate images. The eye will begin to perceive separate images as a flickering image if the repetition rate falls below the 16 frames a second. Higher repetition rate will be required for rapidly moving structures to prevent blurring of the image.

The spectral sensitivity of the photographic emulsion of the film must record the green colour of the output phosphor. Therefore for cine radiography an ortho or panchromatic film is used.

The advantages of cineradiography compared with video recording

The resolution of the film can easily record the detail of the image produced by the image intensifier whereas the TV camera may not be able to record the detail because of the coarseness of the raster pattern. However with high resolution TV systems the disparity between the film and the video record will become less apparent.

Disadvantages

The radiation dose to the patient is greater in cineradiography than in video recording. The video recorder shares the same video signal as the real time display on the monitor, whereas the high resolution film requires a much higher input dose to expose the film adequately. In addition, the camera receives only some 75–90% of the light emitted by the phosphor, the remaining 10–25% is directed on to the TV camera by the beam-splitting mirror necessitating still more input dose to offset this loss.

Cineradiography requires a projector to display the image. The projector enlarges the image which may then display graininess and without a very expensive unit it is difficult to freeze a frame for closer inspection. It is not practical to manipulate the photographic image to give an enhanced image or allow for subtraction.

Basic design of a cine camera

Figure 13.25 shows the layout of basic cine camera. The film is 16 or 35 mm in width and 66 m in length. On some cameras it is possible to add accessory spools to allow a longer film to be fitted. The film runs off a feed spool to pass behind the lens and the shutter where it is held in the correct focal plane by a pressure plate. This region is called the 'gate'. The film on leaving the gate is wound on to the take-up spool.

The film has a series of regularly spaced perforations along one or both edges. These perforations provide the means of moving the film through the gate and around the drive sprocket. The drive sprocket and take-up spool are rotated by a small motor, which moves the film on at a preselected speed. The notches on the drive sprocket lock on to the perforations on the film and ensure a positive drive through the gate.

The speed of the motor drive controls the number of frames that may be exposed in one second. A frame is the image exposed by the opening of the shutter. Frame speeds of up to 120 per second are possible although in cineradiography speeds in excess of 60 frames are rarely used. The duration of the exposure of a frame is governed by the time that the shutter remains open. The number of frames per second and the shutter times are interrelated, for if the shutter is open for a long time there cannot be as many frames exposed in one second. A chart supplied by the camera manufacturer indicates the number of exposed frames per second obtainable at a particular shutter speed.

The shutter is often just a circular plate with a 180° cut out from its border. The plate rotates between the lens and the camera opening called the aperture. As the shutter rotates, it alternately covers and uncovers the aperture letting the image fall upon the film. When the aperture is open, the film is held very firmly by the pressure plate. In this position it cannot move; once the pressure is released, the film is moved on by a pull-down mechanism which engages the perforations on the film edge. Because of this mechanism, the movement of the film in front of the aperture is intermittent even though the film drive sprocket and the take-up spool move continuously. The differences in movement in the camera necessitate

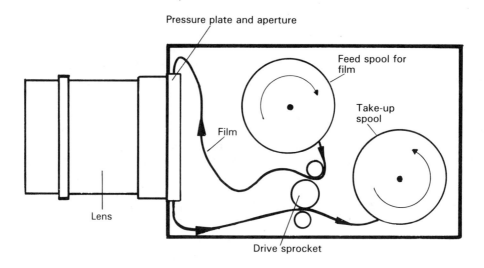

Pressure plate and aperture

Feed spool for film

Take-up spool

Film

Lens

Drive sprocket

Enlarged view of camera shutter

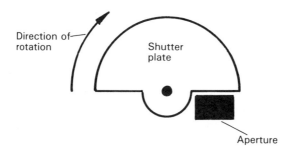

Direction of rotation

Shutter plate

Aperture

Fig. 13.25 Basic design of a cine camera.

a slack loop of film on either side of the aperture in which the change of movement from continuous to intermittent may take place without damage to the film. In many cameras there is a safety contact which operates if this slackness is lost. The contact cuts off the motor drive to the camera.

The camera receives the reflected image from the beam-splitting mirror.

The selection of a suitable lens for the cine camera is governed by its position in relation to the mirror and by the degree of image size reduction or enlargement required to fill the film frame.

The camera aperture should be as large as compatible with the system to enable as much light as possible to reach the film; any reduction in aperture size will require a brighter

image to expose the film to the same level of illumination. To obtain the brighter image, the exposure factors must be increased with a resultant increase in radiation dose to the patient. The maximum aperture size is controlled by the depth of field to be recorded. In cineradiography there is little or no depth of field to be accommodated as it is recording the image reflected by the mirror surface; even if the camera is directed at 45° to the mirror or perpendicular to it, the aperture can be as large as f2.

Accessories. A number of accessories are available, including:

1. automatic exposure control operating on the camera aperture or shutter
2. exposure pulsing controlled by the cam-

era to synchronise with the opening of the shutter

3. chronological marking to aid identification of the film.

Factors controlling the exposure reaching the film. The exposure reaching the film is controlled by the following:

1. brightness of the intensified image
2. percentage of the total light reflected by the mirror.
3. radiographic exposure arrangements, pulsed or continuous
4. aperture size of the camera
5. length of time the shutter is open and the speed of the camera motor (frames per second).

Exposure rating. Cineradiography applies a very high load to the tube, and every frame exposed is a radiographic exposure delivering an increment of heat to the tube. Because of the rapid repetition rate, a cine run is classed as a continuous exposure and is governed by the continuous rating value for the tube. The factors which govern the exposure are:

1. mAs for each exposure and the kVp (heat units per exposure)

2. rate of cooling of the tube
3. generator waveforom
4. focal spot size
5. whether exposure pulsed or continuous
6. length of cine run
7. number of frames per second
8. form of cooling forced or natural
9. tube loading characteristics.

Pulsed cine. Before pulsed cine was introduced, X-rays were generated continuously throughout the whole of the cine run, whether the camera shutter was open or closed. Therefore the patient received radiation during the time when no record could be made of the fluoroscopic image as the shutter was closed. With pulsed cine, X-rays are only generated when the shutter is open. Once the shutter is closed, no further X-rays are generated until the shutter opens again (see Fig. 13.26).

In one system the X-ray switching is controlled by a contact in the cine camera, which is operated by the shutter. When the shutter plate has rotated to the position which will expose the camera opening, the contact is closed and the radiographic exposure commences. Once the plate has rotated on further to close the opening, the contact opens

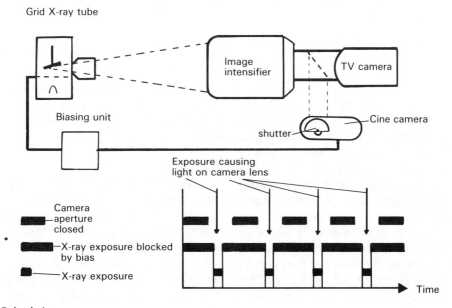

Fig. 13.26 Pulsed cine.

and the radiographic exposure ceases. Therefore the exposure time is controlled by the shutter, but for safety a millisecond timer set with an exposure in excess of the shutter time is provided to operate should there be a failure in the automatic system.

In normal circumstances the shutter contact will override the millisecond timer. The cine camera shutter contact may be linked to the X-ray unit exposure contactor, or ideally operating on the secondary circuit of the HT transformer. The secondary switching is by a grid controlled tube or in highly rated units, allowing the use of very high tube currents, by triode or pentode valves which provide more effective switching of very high mA values.

Advantages of pulsed cine over non-pulsed cine are:

1. Lower dose to the patient.
2. Reduced load on the X-ray tube. This will allow the cine run to be extended in length and still remain within the rating of the tube or may allow the use of a smaller focal spot to improve image quality.
3. The film density of individual frames will be more consistent. The cut-off of the light in response to the shutter contact will be more positive than relying on the gradual obstruction to the light by the shutter as it moves across the camera opening.

Spot-film photofluorography. In cineradiography it is necessary to move the film very rapidly to allow the structures to be recorded without jerky movements. The production of this movement has restricted the width of the film to a maximum of 35 mm. An image of this size requires enlargement before viewing is possible. The small frame size and its subsequent enlargement does not allow the high definition of the image intensifier output phosphor to be adequately recorded. Therefore spot-film cameras have been developed which record on 100 or 105 mm wide film with a repetition rate restricted to a maximum of 6 frames per second on 100 mm cut film and 12 frames per second on 105 mm roll film. This repetition rate is adequate for most techniques although they are only a series of static images. The film is stored in a magazine in a pack of cut film or on a roll. Once exposed the film is collected in another magazine. Both magazines can be removed from the camera and taken to the darkroom for processing and reloading.

The camera operates without a conventional shutter; the film exposure is controlled by the time during which X-rays are emitted by the X-ray tube. Additional limited control can be obtained by varying the lens aperture. However, any change in aperture size will vary the depth of field recorded and the amount of light reaching the film. As the aperture is enlarged, the depth of field will decrease and parts of the image will pass out of focus. The depth of field will not be affected by a decrease in aperture size but the dose to the patient will increase to provide the additional light intensity needed to give the same film density.

The programming of the number of exposures, the interval between exposures and the moving on of the film between exposures is through a camera control unit which is linked to the X-ray generator timing circuit ideally incorporating a photo-timer.

In order that the film does not receive light during fluoroscopy, the beam-splitting mirror reflecting the light into the camera is automatically turned away when fluoroscopy is selected.

The advantages of spot-film photofluography compared with full-size film radiography:
1. Reduced patient dose. The spot-film requires only 25% of the radiation dose. This reduces the tube loading, permitting the use of a smaller focal spot and shorter exposure times
2. Reduced staff dose, less exposure means less scatter.
3. Time is saved between exposures as there are no cassettes to change.
4. The camera operates more quietly than a serial changer and so is less alarming to patients.
5. Exposure repetition rate is much greater than can be achieved manually using cassettes.
6. Allows for the efficient production of stereo pairs.

7. Reduced film costs.
8. Uses less silver.
9. Reduced storage space required.
10. Small format gives apparently sharper image contours because the small size excludes the area of reduced lateral visual acuity.

Disadvantages:

1. Lower image contrast, the single coated film has reduced gamma.
2. May show evidence of vignetting.
3. Possible geometric distortion across the field.
4. Resolution less than the full-size film.
5. Film identification is less clear. Patient's name and other details are reduced before being recorded on the film.

PHOTOFLUOROGRAPHY OF THE CHEST

There is another method of producing a minified image on 100 mm film. The method involves photography of a fluorescent screen image. As the system does not include an image intensifier, the radiation dose received by the patient is more than that received

for a full-size film, and a great deal more than that for a film taken with an amplified image from an image intensifier output screen by a single shot camera. Because of the high radiation dose only chest radiography is undertaken with this equipment and even here the technique must not be used to examine children or patients who may be pregnant.

Figure 13.27 shows the main features of the equipment. The radiographic image transmitted by the patient is converted to a light image by a fluorescent screen having a blue or a green emitting phosphor. This image is reduced in size and focused on to a 100 × 100 mm film by a mirror lens system. The films are automatically fed from a feeder cassette into the gate where they are held for exposure. The light from one part of the fluorescent screen can take many paths to one point on the film so the film transport mechanism can be placed in the beam of light without producing problems. Once the exposure is complete the film automatically feeds into a reception cassette. This cassette can be removed periodically for processing of the films. Alternatively, the films may be fed directly into an automatic processor.

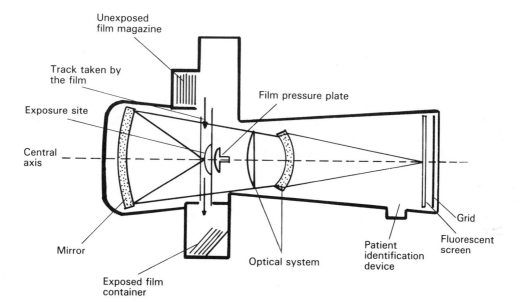

Fig. 13.27 Diagram of 100 mm film camera unit for chest radiography showing the position of the mirror optics and film pathway.

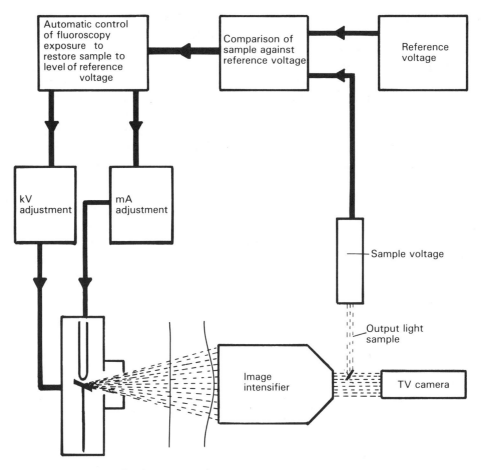

Fig. 13.28 Layout of the automatic brightness control.

The films of patients are identified by means of a card giving patient details which is introduced into the unit where it is reflected by a mirror on to a small part of the film.

The exposure is normally controlled automatically by a photo-electric timer linked to the X-ray unit. The kV and the mA are selected by the operator, and the photographic density is controlled to a pre-fixed level by the auto-timer. The timer operates by monitoring the number of light photons produced from a rectangular part of the fluorescent screen across the lung apices.

14

Interaction of X-rays with the body

The beam of X-radiation leaving the tube port interacts with any material in its path causing the beam to be attenuated.

Attenuation is defined as the removal of energy from an X-ray beam by the process of absorption and/or scatter. The amount of attenuation depends on the thickness and composition of the material in the pathway of the beam and the quality of the radiation.

The thicker the tissue traversed, the greater will be the attenuation. Hence the need to increase exposure factors to maintain the same quantity of transmitted radiation necessary for image production of a thicker patient.

Different tissue composition gives rise to variation in the amount of attenuation taking place. The main constituents of the human body can be grouped for radiographic purposes as:

a. muscle or muscle-like tissue with an effective atomic number of 7.4

b. bone, dependent largely on its calcium content with an effective atomic number of 13.8

c. air-filled cavities with an effective atomic number of 7.6.

These three groups differ in density and atomic number, and it is these differences which give rise to variation in attenuation for every centimetre of tissue traversed.

The quality of radiation, controlled by the kVp, influences tissue attenuation. A change in kVp will cause a change in absorbed dose and image contrast. A higher kV will reduce the proportion of attenuation occurring and alter the distribution of absorbed dose through the thickness of tissue traversed. For the same effect on the recorded image and the same transmitted dose, the higher kV will give a smaller percentage skin dose than will arise with a lower kVp and a lowered absorbed dose.

In attenuation some of the energy is absorbed giving rise to the absorbed dose and some of the X-ray photons change their direction through interaction with the tissue and are described as scatter.

Absorption is the complete removal of the X-ray photon with deposition of its energy into the tissue, or in the case of Compton scatter, absorption of a portion of the energy of the incident photon.

Scatter is radiation which is changed in direction as a result of interaction with some medium. Some of the photon's energy is absorbed in the interaction so leaving the resultant photon not only changed in its direction but with less energy than it had initially. Scatter not only degrades the photographic image but increases the dose to the patient and any other person standing nearby as well as impairing the function of automatic exposure timers.

The effect of scattered radiation on the contrast of the radiograph

Scatter must be kept to a minimum since it increases dose and degrades the X-ray image by

185

adding an overall unwanted density, which contains no useful image information and serves only to reduce subjective contrast of the image. Subjective contrast is difference in density, and density is an expression of the light transmitting ability of areas of film. Therefore it can be seen that an overall density which decreases light transmission over the whole radiograph is bound to affect contrast.

The control of scatter

Scatter is controlled by careful attention to all the factors which help in the reduction of:

1. amount of scatter produced
2. amount of scatter reaching the film and intensifying screen
3. amount of scattered radiation affecting the film

1. Reduction in the amount of scattered radiation produced is obtained by:
A. close control of extra-focal radiation
B. restriction in the volume of tissue irradiated by:
 (i) reducing the surface area of tissue covered by the X-ray beam by closely collimating the beam;
 (ii) reducing where possible the thickness of tissue irradiated.
C. careful selection of exposure factors.

A. Close collimation to reduce extra-focal radiation. The effect of extra-focal radiation can be minimised by using a diaphragm with the smallest aperture to cover the largest field size required and by positioning the diaphragm as close as possible to the focal spot. This is most easily achieved by a 'top-hat' type of lead diaphragm fitted up into the X-ray tube port. Fig-

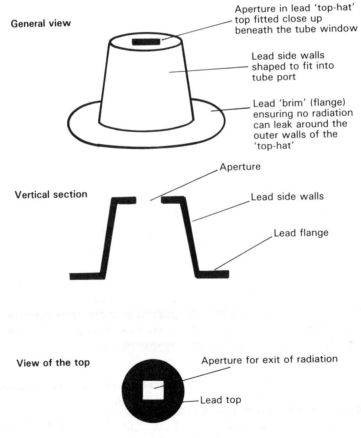

General view

Aperture in lead 'top-hat' top fitted close up beneath the tube window

Lead side walls shaped to fit into tube port

Lead 'brim' (flange) ensuring no radiation can leak around the outer walls of the 'top-hat'

Vertical section

Aperture

Lead side walls

Lead flange

View of the top

Aperture for exit of radiation

Lead top

Fig. 14.1 Detail of the lead 'top-hat' which is inserted into the tube port.

ure 14.1 shows the detail of a 'top-hat' diaphragm. More information on the production and reduction of extra-focal radiation is given in the section on the X-ray tube housing.

The influence of extra-focal radiation on image quality is insignificant when the X-ray beam is collimated closely, and what little remains having lower mean energy than the useful beam will be absorbed by the patient and will not reach the film. It will of course add to the patient dose, especially the skin dose.

B. Restriction in the area of tissue irradiated. It is essential to restrict the size of the primary beam to cover the smallest area possible consistent with the requirements of the X-ray examination and to ensure that the beam limiting equipment removes extra-focal radiation effectively and provides a clean cut-off of the radiation at the borders of the field.

The size of the primary beam can be controlled by a simple metal diaphragm with a central aperture, a movable diaphragm, beam limiting cones or a combination of all three. The majority of X-ray units use a tandem arrangement of all three but there are some specialised units, such as dental units, where a cone and fixed diaphragm is the most practical method of limiting the beam.

(i) Effect on exposure of close collimation — since much scatter is eliminated from the film by close collimation, it is necessary to replace this removed radiation by additional primary radiation by increasing the exposure factors to maintain adequate density of the radiograph. This will of course increase the radiation dose but this radiation will be useful to the image production and a certain amount of additional radiation can be justified. This dose increase can be reduced by increasing the kV rather than the mA. An increase of 5–10 kV may be necessary if the field is much restricted from what was a reasonable large field area.

The geometry of beam collimation. The X-ray photons produced at the tube focus radiate in all directions but because of the barrier provided by the lead lined shield of the tube housing only a useful cone of radiation leaves the tube through the port. The dimen-

sions of the cone of radiation increase as the distance from the source increases, therefore if collimation is to be effective all apertures must be made to limit the beam's dimensions correctly at the distance they are from the source of radiation. Before fixed apertures can be cut, moving diaphragm scales calibrated or cone factors determined, it is necessary to know the maximum field size to be covered by the beam at the normal focus-to-film distance so that the outer limits of the collimating diaphragm can be determined. The diverging beam of radiation forms a series of similar triangles. The length of the base of each triangle is proportional to its height. The formula for calculating the dimensions is given below and Figure 14.3 shows the location of the points on the triangles. It should be remembered that provision has to be made for the axis of the cassette to be turned through 90°, hence the square rather than rectangular diaphragm aperture seen in the tube port.

$$\frac{CD \text{ (diaphragm aperture)}}{AB \text{ (max. field/film size)}} = \frac{FX \text{ (focus-to-diaphragm distance)}}{FY \text{(focus-to-film distance)}}$$

In Figure 14.2, the maximum field size and the focus-to-film distance control the dimensions of the apertures of a series of diaphragms A, B, C and D. The length of the base of each triangle is the aperture size. To calculate the size of each aperture the formula is applied, giving, as an example:

$$\text{Aperture A (CD)} = \frac{43 \times 4.5 \text{ cm}}{100 \text{ cm}}$$

Where the maximum film (field) size is given as 43 cm, Focus-to-diaphragm A distance is given as 4.5 cm, Focus-to-film distance is given as 100 cm.

(i) The fixed diameter diaphragm is a simple steel or brass plate with an aperture which will limit the area covered by the X-ray beam to a specific size at a particular distance.

These devices are used to limit the beam in sites where there is insufficient space to fit any other form of collimator, or where the irradi-

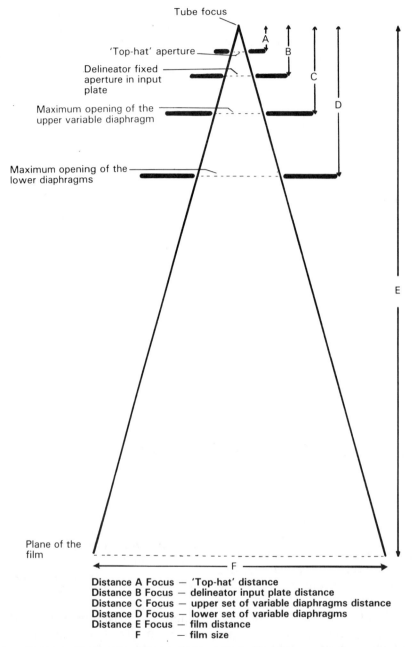

Tube focus

'Top-hat' aperture

Delineator fixed
aperture in input
plate

Maximum opening of the
upper variable diaphragm

Maximum opening of the
lower diaphragms

Plane of the
film

Distance A Focus — 'Top-hat' distance
Distance B Focus — delineator input plate distance
Distance C Focus — upper set of variable diaphragms distance
Distance D Focus — lower set of variable diaphragms
Distance E Focus — film distance
          F   — film size

Fig. 14.2 Location of the various apertures enabling dimensions of the apertures at different levels to be calculated so that the film field can be covered.

ated field size is fixed and the range of radiographic examination limited. For example, the simple skull unit is supplied with a set of diaphragm plates with different apertures designed to meet the requirements of the standard radiographic projections undertaken on the skull. Dental units also have fixed diaphragms. Occasionally fixed diaphragms are automatically introduced into the primary beam to limit the field so that it matches the

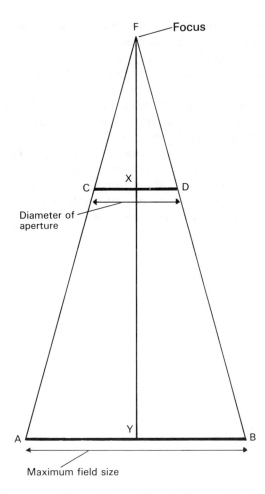

Fig. 14.3 Labelling of the similar triangles used in the calculation of the dimensions of the triangles FCD and FAB.

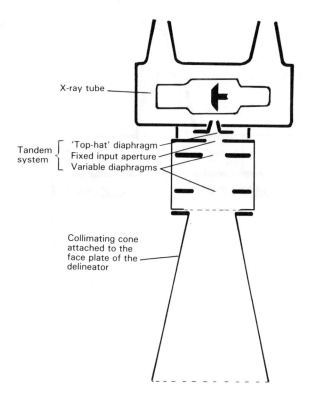

Fig. 14.4 Tandem system of collimation showing a cone added to the face plate of the delineator.

area being recorded. The image intensifier input phosphor is circular, and if the patient is to be protected from radiation which cannot be recorded, a circular diaphragm is required in addition to the usual rectilinear collimator normally provided. In some units, the additional circular diaphragm is linked to an interlock circuit which prevents fluoroscopy until the diaphragm is introduced.

(ii) The movable diaphragm — the Code of Practice for the protection of persons against Ionising Radiation demands that there is strict limitation of field size to the area necessary for the particular examination. To fulfil this requirement it is necessary to fit to all X-ray tubes a collimator with movable diaphragms,

unless there is a valid reason why it is not practical to fit such a unit.

Examination of Figure 14.4 shows the tandem system of collimation used on most modern units. The localising cone is never fitted to an undercouch tube but can generally be attached to most makes of units fitted to overcouch tubes. They are not essential but they do improve the quality of the image in regions of great thickness and density be adding to the elimination of scatter, and aesthetically by providing a clean cut-off of the radiation.

The diagram shown in Figure 14.5 shows two diaphragms: one is the diaphragm set up into the tube port, the other a diaphragm forming the input plate of the collimator. The size of these two diaphragms is calculated so that the maximum field size can be covered at the selected focus-to-film distance. Full details of a typical light-beam delineator will now be described showing how the movable diaphragms

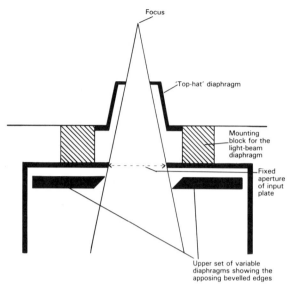

Fig. 14.5 Enlarged view to show the detail of the collimation provided around the tube port.

can be adjusted to restrict the field size. Figure 14.6 illustrates its principal features.

The light-beam delineator has a box-like housing of aluminium alloy lined with lead sheet on all its surfaces apart from the input and output face. The lead sheet is turned onto the borders of the output face to ensure that there is no gap in the lead shielding when the diaphragms are fully closed. The output face of the 'box' is covered with a thin radiolucent plastic sheet. This sheet protects the contents of the box but does not attenuate the useful primary beam. The centre of the plastic sheet is generally marked with a spot so that its shadow can be used to indicate the point through which the central ray will pass. There may be other lines which cast shadows on the field to be irradiated to aid beam alignment. These marks must not be radio-opaque. The output face may be fitted with slots to re-

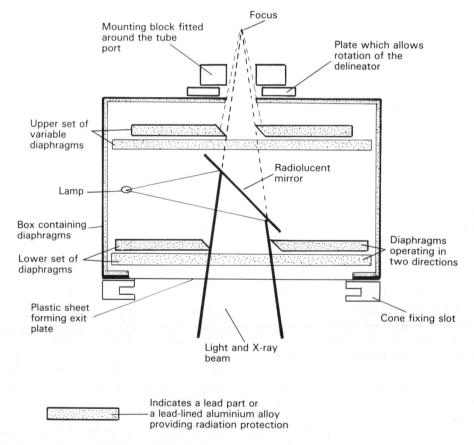

Fig. 14.6 Vertical section of a light-beam delineator.

ceive the base plate of a beam limiting cone. When the box is fitted to a tube on a support which has a motor driven vertical movement, a safety device must be fitted to the output face of the delineator box or localising cone if one is fitted to cut out the motor drive when the leading surface lightly touches an obstruction.

The top of the box is fitted to a fixing block which is secured to the mounting block attached to the X-ray tube housing around its port. There is generally an intermediate plate between the delineator and the tube mounting block which allows rotation of the axis of the delineator box around the tube port. This permits the operator to align the X-ray field with the part to be examined, reducing the field size and so the dose. Great care must be taken to ensure that there is no leakage of radiation from around the housing and between the delineator and tube housing. Fitted to the box or on a panel attached to it will be found the switches, controls and scales concerned with the operation of the unit and the brakes locking the tube support (see pp. 227–234).

The box contains one or more sets of lead diaphragms: if only one set is fitted, the unit is described as a single-leaf diaphragm or if more, a multi-leaf diaphragm. Figure 14.7 shows a double-leaf, which is a type very commonly fitted. The more sets of leaves, the more expensive but the more effective the cut-off of off-focus (extra focal) radiation will be. Examination of Figure 14.7 will show how this improvement arises. The multi-leaf type has a very complex mechanism within the box to operate the sets of diaphragms so that the diverging beam is collimated to cover the same field size.

The box also contains a lamp and a mirror set at 45° to the central ray of the X-ray beam. The mirror is made from a low attenuating material such as plastic or aluminium silvered on one side. This mirror is sited in the primary beam and by careful alignment at 45° to the beam of radiation and the beam of light from the lamp, the light reflected by the mirror illuminates an area which exactly coincides with the radiated field. To obtain this precise align-

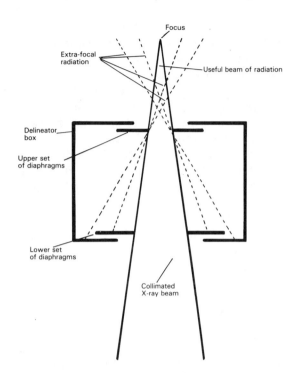

Fig. 14.7 Double-leaf diaphragm delineator more effectively eliminating off-focus (extra-focal) radiation.

ment all parts must be carefully sited and the filament configuration of the lamp of the correct form. The coincidence of the light and the radiation field must be checked frequently.

It is desirable that the illuminated area is marginally larger that the irradiated area and certainly never smaller. Any deviation from these limits should not be accepted, and an error of 10% or more must be corrected at once. There will be difficulty in aligning accurately both foci of a biangular tube as one focus being above the other will be directed to a different target area. Therefore a decision has to be made when setting up a delineator, either to accept a compromise with the radiation and illuminated fields slightly mismatched for both foci or, to have one focus, normally the fine focus, correctly aligned and the other out of register, but still within the permitted 10% error.

The lamp must provide an intense illumination so that the field margins can be seen in daylight. Such a high-powered lamp will become very hot after a short time and its life will be short due to rapid evaporisation of the filament. To extend the life of the lamp and reduce the amount of heat produced it is essential to provide an automatic cut-off for it after about 30 seconds. When the lamp has to be replaced, it is essential that a similar type is used so that the beam of light has the same configuration and the bulb correctly positioned, as failure to do so will produce malalignment with a lack of coincidence of radiation and light. The lamps selected require a 12 V supply which provides electrical safety for the operator and ensures easy acquisition of a suitable lamp as the voltage is that of a car headlight.

In working areas such as operating theatres where the ambient light is high an optical system sometimes replaces the light. The delineator box and diaphragms are similar but the lamp is replaced by a lens system which allows the operator to view the field. This system overcomes the problem of not being able to define the light illuminated field but has disadvantages: the operator must reach right over the patient to look through the lens system and will then see a reversed and inverted image which is not as easy to use for centring.

The lead leaf diaphragms are made from 3–5 mm lead sheet, thick enough to act as an effective barrier to the primary X-ray beam. They are mounted in pairs, one pair collimating the beam in one axis, the other pair the other axis. Each pair has an independent set of controls which allows the two pairs to be moved independently. In the double or multileaved systems the sets of leaves are connected through a system of gears and levers so that each set of diaphragms collimates to the same field size by forming an aperture appropriate to its distance from the focus. Because of the complexity of the gear and lever arrangement, the controls must be operated very carefully. To ensure the total closure of the radiation barrier when the diaphragm leaves are brought together their opposing faces are bevelled to 45° allowing them to overlap. This is a very important safety feature which can be lost if the soft lead faces are distorted by being banged together by the op-

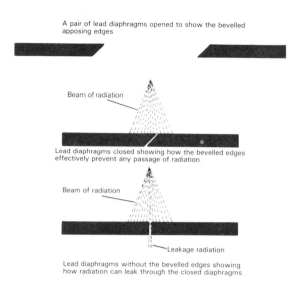

A pair of lead diaphragms opened to show the bevelled apposing edges

Beam of radiation

Lead diaphragms closed showing how the bevelled edges effectively prevent any passage of radiation

Beam of radiation

Leakage radiation

Lead diaphragms without the bevelled edges showing how radiation can leak through the closed diaphragms

Fig. 14.8 The advantage of lead diaphragms with bevelled edges compared with vertical borders.

erator, therefore when used, diaphragms should be moved slowly. Because of the importance for radiation safety the effectiveness of the closed diaphragms must be checked frequently (see Fig. 14.8). The layout of the diaphragm leaves is shown in Figure 14.9.

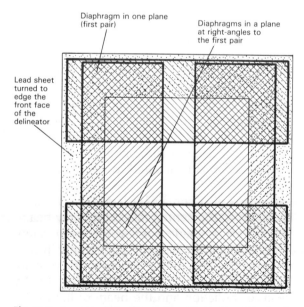

Diaphragm in one plane (first pair)

Diaphragms in a plane at right-angles to the first pair

Lead sheet turned to edge the front face of the delineator

Fig. 14.9 Layout of the two pairs of lead diaphragms moving at 90° to each other seen from below the delineator box. The lead sheet border of the lower plate is shown.

In some specialised units, when a circular field of fairly small diameter is most suitable for the area under examination an 'iris-leaf' circular diaphragm may be fitted to collimate the beam more effectively than would be possible with the more usual rectilinear light beam collimator.

Tests are necessary on a light-beam delineator to ensure:

a. the effectiveness of the beam collimation
b. the absence of leakage radiation from the housing or from the coupling between the delineator and tube housing
c. the alignment of the collimated radiation beam and the illuminated field, which ever focus is selected and whatever the direction of the primary beam
d. the alignment of the light indicated centre of the beam and the real centre of the X-ray beam
e. the accuracy of the indicators of field size displayed on the unit.

In addition to these tests regular and careful inspection must be made to check on the secure fixing of the unit onto the tube housing.

(iii) Beam limiting radiographic cones are tapered metal structures which may be fitted closely to the tube port or fitted on the outlet side of the light-beam delineator. The metal base of the cone cuts off the primary beam except for a central aperture which is cut to the correct size to suit the field size. The walls of the cone are made of steel or brass or sometimes of aluminium lined with lead sheet. Their shape is carefully calculated to follow the geometry of the beam as determined by the position of the focus and the central aperture in the base plate. In particular the exit diameter must be compatible with the input aperture.

Where cones are the principal means of collimation, it is essential to provide a number so that the smallest field size can be used. To encourage operators to change them frequently, they must be easy to fit on to the tube mounting, but at the same time, once fitted, they must be very secure, and this is usually done by a slot and a spring fitting which locks the cone base into its fixing plate. The location of the cone into the fixing slot ensures that the cone aperture is accurately aligned with the central ray of the X-ray beam. For easy selection of the most suitable cone, the diameter of the irradiated field must be scribed on the cone wall. This is usually indicated by marking the *cone factor* — the number of times the diameter will go into the focus-to-film distance. For example if the cone factor is 4 and the f.f.d. is 100 cm, the diameter of the field will be 25 cm. When the input and output diameters of a cone are calculated the following formula is used (see Fig. 14.10):

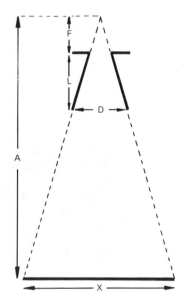

Fig. 14.10 Dimensions needed to calculate the cone factor.

$$X = \frac{A}{L + F} \times D$$

Where X is the field size
A the focus-to-film distance
L the length of the cone
F the focus-to-input of base plate
D the diameter of the exit of the cone.

If the cone is to be used on a motor driven tube support it must have a soft rubber edge fitted to its end and must also incorporate a safety device which will interrupt the downward motor drive if an obstruction is encountered.

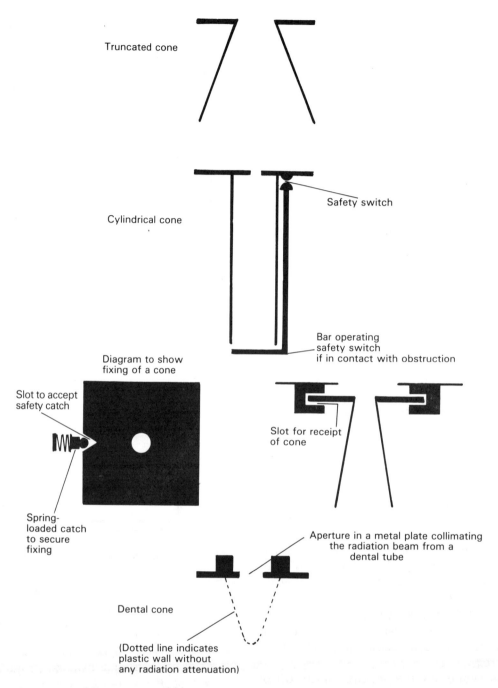

Truncated cone

Cylindrical cone

Safety switch

Bar operating
safety switch
if in contact with obstruction

Diagram to show
fixing of a cone

Slot to accept
safety catch

Slot for receipt
of cone

Spring-
loaded catch
to secure
fixing

Aperture in a metal plate collimating
the radiation beam from a
dental tube

Dental cone

(Dotted line indicates
plastic wall without
any radiation attenuation)

Fig. 14.11 Some types of X-ray cones available.

There are a variety of cones in use, including truncated, straight sided and telescopic shapes (Fig. 14.11). On dental units tapered cones are fitted which are merely centering devices, and by being several inches long prevent the use of too short a focus-to-film distance. These cones are made of plastic and have no lead lining so they do not collimate the beam of radiation. The collimation of these units is by the metal cone base plate only.

When a small cone is used the exposure must be increased to produce the same film density as it is necessary to replace the eliminated scatter. The exposure increase will also increase the radiation dose but this is acceptable as it is providing useful image information.

The advantages of a light-beam delineator with movable diaphragms compared with a fixed diaphragm or cone are:

1. clear indication of the field to be irradiated, and the calibrated scales allow the field size of the beam at the level of the cassette to be known.

2. Position of the central ray of the beam is clearly identified.

3. Any size of radiation field can be selected and the axis of the beam aligned to allow the smallest area to be used.

4. Gives greater accuracy in centering which will allow the use of a smaller field.

5. Focus-to-film distance can be varied with the new field size easily seen

6. Positioning is quicker when the position of the central ray is displayed

7. Radiographic examinations are performed more quickly as the field size can be varied by the use of simple controls rather than by using a number of different cones.

Disadvantages

1. Illuminated field displayed on the patient will be smaller than the irradiated field due to the divergence of the beam. This can be avoided by setting up the irradiated field size by means of the calibrated controls provided.

2. Shape of the collimated beam may not be the ideal shape, for instance, a specially shaped mammography cone will better suit the shape of the breast than the rectilinear field of the general purpose delineator.

3. Intensity of the illuminated area may not be sufficient to define the field borders.

(iv) The slot technique. If the irradiated area of tissue is very restricted little scatter is produced. This method of scatter reduction can be exploited by means of the slot technique (Fig. 14.12). A very narrow beam of radiation emerges through a rectangular slot diaphragm which is fixed to the tube port. This narrow beam is made to scan the length of the film during the exposure by rotation of the tube around its focal spot so that the beam is first directed along the peripheral beam of the conventional cone of radiation and then moved smoothly through the radial beams until it reaches the other peripheral beam where the exposure ceases. The cassette is placed in the conventional position but is overlaid by a diaphragm with a slot cut to just allow the narrow beam to pass through it. This diaphragm is moved during the exposure and its slot is always lined up with the narrow beam of X-rays so that the exposure reaches the cassette beneath. Although the slot scans the part during the exposure, the radiograph shows the normal projection.

The advantages of this technique are: (a) greatly reduced radiation dose because there is no need for an anti-scatter grid; (b) reduced geometric unsharpness because the reduced exposure factors allow the use of a finer focus.

The disadvantage is the comparatively long exposure time necessary for the scanning movement which limits its use to areas where motional unsharpness is not a problem.

Beam centering devices. These devices aid the positioning of the patient in relation to the X-ray beam. They provide the radiographer with a means of locating the central ray as it enters or leaves the patient. The devices do not in themselves reduce scatter although their use ensures a more accurate centering allowing a smaller field to be used. The most common types are as follows:

1. Simple mechanical devices (indicating the centre of the irradiated field)

a. *Metal pointers* are usually telescopic steel pointers which are fitted in place of a cone or assembled on a stirrup-shaped base which is fitted to the base of the cone. When the pointer is in position, it indicates the direction and location of the central ray. This centering device is not often used as it is inconvenient. It must be removed before the radiographic exposure and is very easily knocked out of alignment.

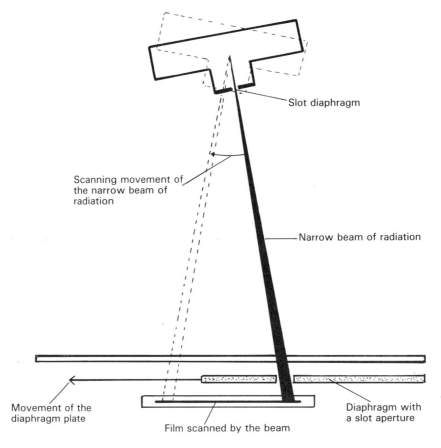

Slot diaphragm

Scanning movement of the narrow beam of radiation

Narrow beam of radiation

Movement of the diaphragm plate

Film scanned by the beam

Diaphragm with a slot aperture

Fig. 14.12 Principles of slot technique.

b. *Cones* are used for centering of some specialised units. The tapered cone fitted to the dental unit is the sole centering device provided on these units. Mammography units, with their specially shaped cones, aid centering although they do not actually indicate the centre of the beam.

2. Lights (indicating the centre of the entry field)

a. *Light-beam delineators* display the area to be irradiated and indicate the centre of the beam by a light obstructing centre spot or by bisecting opaque cross-lines. A detailed description has been given on pages 190–193.

b. *Externally sited lamps* (Fig. 14.13) do not normally outline the field but they do illuminate the axes of the field by two narrow beams of light directed from outside the

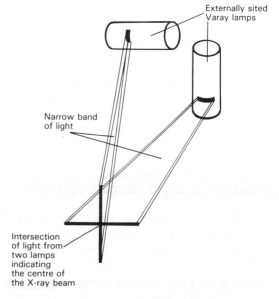

Externally sited Varay lamps

Narrow band of light

Intersection of light from two lamps indicating the centre of the X-ray beam

Fig. 14.13 Externally positioned lamps indicating the centre of the X-ray beam.

collimator housing which intersect at the centre of the irradiated field. There are two principal ways of producing the light beams:

(i) Varay lamps are fitted to the tube outside the radiation beam or in some cases fitted to the ceiling. The two lamps are mounted at 90 ° to each other, each lamp being housed in a cylindrical holder with the light emerging through a narrow slit on the face.

(ii) Remotely sited lamps, sometimes low-level laser lights, whose light beam is conveyed along fibre-optic pipes to two outlet points on the outside of the collimator, which direct the light to form two intersecting beams or occasionally to outline the borders of the film. This system has the advantage of removing the heat emitting lamps from the vicinity of the patient whilst still retaining an intense illumination, and the light emitting point is very compact. It is however much more expensive than the simple Varay lamps.

3. Mirror systems indicating the site of the central exit ray are unique to skull units and will be described with them in Chapter 16.

(ii) Reducing where possible the tissue thickness. Some tissue can be displaced from the irradiated area by external compression either mechanically with compression bands or cones or by positioning the patient so that their own body weight moves displaceable tissue out of the beam, e.g. the prone position for abdominal X-rays.

By reducing the thickness of the tissue to be traversed by the X-ray beam, the amount of scatter produced within the tissue is less, because the irradiated volume is less and the amount of primary radiation needed to expose the film adequately is less. These two factors will not only improve the image quality but will greatly reduce the radiation dose and because of the immobilising effect obtained when these devices are applied there will be less risk of patient movement requiring a repeat examination with its doubling effect on patient dose.

a. Compression bands are strips of nylon or cotton about 30 cm wide and 150 cm long. They are wound on to a controlled roller with the free end of the band fixed to a bar which can be hooked on to the far side of the X-ray table. The controlled roller has a ratchet mechanism and this is fitted securely to the near side of the table at any position along its length. With the free end of the band laid across the patient and hooked on to the far side of the table, the roller is turned to tighten the band across the patient. Once tightened the band is held in position by the ratchet locking device which will not release until the toothed ratchet is first released. This release system must be quick and easy to operate as firm compression is not comfortable for the patient and should be removed as quickly as possible after the examination is completed.

b. Compression cones are most commonly found in two sites:

(i) on the explorator (serial changer) used in fluoroscopy. The explorator carries a compression cone for use when areas such as the duodenum are to be examined. The compression cone is made of radiolucent plastic positioned over an aperture in a metal back plate. The cone is dome shaped. When pressed into the body it displaces some tissue and this reduces the thickness of tissue so reducing the amount of scatter produced and improving image contrast. The compression cone base plate has another use — it shields the unexposed parts of the film from radiation so allowing a series of exposures to be made on a single film. There must be a safety device to ensure that the compression on the patient cannot exceed a safe level and a quick release mechanism must be provided. In remote controlled units, the compression cone is motor driven but has a slipping clutch to prevent further compression when a preset value has been reached.

(ii) In mammography, where some levelling out of tissue thickness is desirable, it is possible to achieve some evening out by means of compression from a long cone. The cone must have a soft moulded leading edge to protect the skin of the breast. The same purpose may be achieved by fitting a plastic compression band which can be brought down on to the breast.

C. Careful selection of exposure factors. With a low energy beam, photo-electric absorption is the most important attenuating effect. It gives rise to total absorption of the incident photon so scattering does not occur. Therefore at low kV, below about 70 kVp, image contrast is increased by the absence of scatter from the film. However, the radiation dose is much greater because more of the photon energy is absorbed.

When the energy of the beam is increased above about 70 kV, the Compton effect becomes more dominant and scatter increases significantly. This gives rise to lower image contrast as the scattered photons add an overall unwanted density to the image. As the kV is further increased, fewer X-ray photons have to be used to produce the same image density, but if these higher energy photons are scattered they tend to continue in a much more forward direction than lower energy scattered photons and so are more likely to reach the film and increase the unwanted non-image forming density on the film.

To reduce the amount of scatter produced the kV should be kept low, but this is not advocated as it will increase the patient dose. Therefore because of the need to keep the radiation dose as low as reasonably achievable, the kVp should be as high as possible, consistent with the level of image contrast required, and taking into account all practical methods of preventing the scatter produced from reaching the film.

2. Reducing the amount of scatter reaching the film

Reduction in the amount of scatter reaching the film is obtained by means of the techniques described in (1) but even with the most careful use of these techniques scatter can only be reduced and never totally eliminated. Therefore the residual scatter must be absorbed before it reaches the film. This is achieved by:

A. the use of an anti-scatter grid interposed between the patient and the film;

B. arranging an air-gap between the patient and the film;

C. absorbing any back scatter produced behind the film.

A. By means of an anti-scatter X-ray grid. Anti-scatter X-ray grids improve the diagnostic quality of the radiograph by absorbing (trapping) the greater part of radiation scattered by the patient in the direction of the film. The absorption of scatter by a grid is possible because it is deflected from the path taken by the useful image forming radiation and can therefore be absorbed by a lead grid with its slats running in the same plane as the useful X-ray beam (see Fig. 14.14).

The basic principle of grid design is the provision of a series of slats formed of lead foil standing on edge separated from each other by strips of radiolucent materials which enables the useful radiation to pass through between the lead strips to reach the film below. Any radiation deflected from its original path is absorbed by the lead before reaching the film.

The efficiency of the grid is a measure of its ability to absorb scatter. However, the efficient removal of scatter involves some loss, by absorption, of useful radiation and this loss has to be overcome by increasing exposure factors. Therefore a balance has to be struck between the degree of scatter removal required to provide the information required for diagnosis and the justifiable increase in radiation dose that will be necessary. There are a number of factors which affect grid efficiency. These will be considered later.

The construction of X-ray grids. The purpose of a grid is to absorb the scattered radiation. It is formed from strips of lead. Lead is used because its high atomic number and its high density make it an ideal absorber of scatter. The strips, 500–2000+, are set on edge either parallel to each other or individually angled to the mean focal distance to form a focused grid as opposed to a parallel grid. Figure 14.15 shows the parallel and focused grid. Each

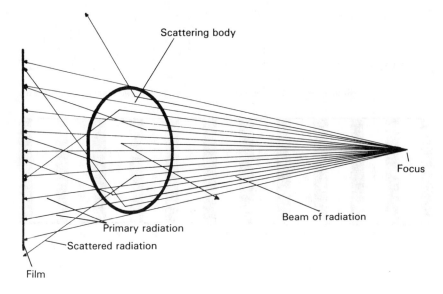

a. Scatter reaches film.

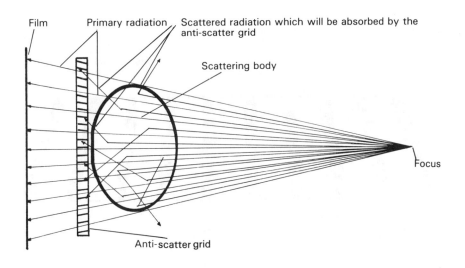

b. Scatter has been eliminated.

Fig. 14.14   Scattered radiation being eliminated by an anti-scatter grid.

strip is separated from its neighbour by an X-ray translucent interspace material. The whole is bonded together into a single flat structure and covered with plastic or aluminium to give the frail structure some strength and protection from moisture (see Fig. 14.16).

Ideally, the lead strips should be so thin that they cannot be seen with the naked eye when radiographs are viewed under normal conditions, but unfortunately there is a minimum thickness beyond which their absorption effectiveness is rapidly lost. Because radiologists require maximum absorption of scatter and minimal evidence of grid lines for image in-

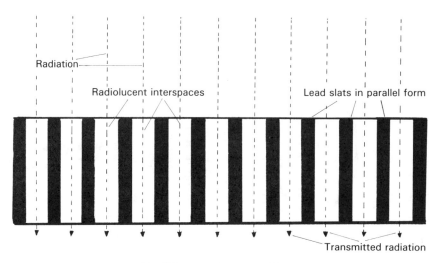

Radiation

Radiolucent interspaces

Lead slats in parallel form

Transmitted radiation

a. Parallel type anti-scatter grid

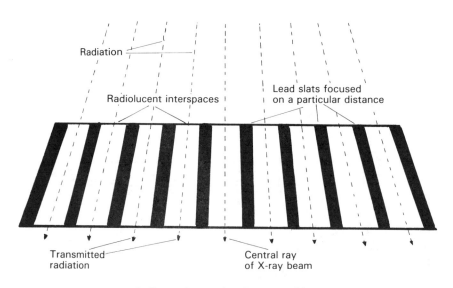

Radiation

Radiolucent interspaces

Lead slats focused on a particular distance

Transmitted radiation

Central ray of X-ray beam

b. Focused type of anti-scatter grid

Fig. 14.15 The position and alignment of the lead slats in the parallel and focused type of anti-scatter grids.

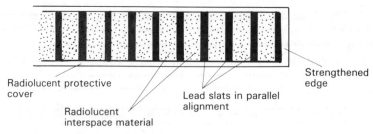

Radiolucent protective cover

Radiolucent interspace material

Lead slats in parallel alignment

Strengthened edge

Fig. 14.16 The construction of an anti-scatter grid, parallel type (in section).

terpretation, a compromise has to reached which will produce acceptable radiographs. The choice lies between 30 and 60 lines (lead strips) per centimetre.

The interspace material between the lead slats must offer little obstruction to the passage of useful radiation, and be truly radiolucent, therefore materials like paper, plastic or aluminium are used in grids today, although it is possible to purchase a carbon fibre interspaced grid where the technique justifies the extra cost of this new interspace material.

Plastic, paper, or possibly carbon fibre is chosen when the generator output is restricted, the exposure load high or where there is need for the radiation dose to be cut to a very low value. Aluminium is used because it forms a more robust grid. Its use necessitates more exposure because the aluminium attenuates the beam considerably more than the other materials, but it will absorb any soft radiation which may by its angle have passed through the interspace.

The cover of aluminium, plastic or carbon film enclosing the lead slats and the interspace slats should absorb as little radiation as possible, but should be thick enough to make the grid strong, durable and impervious to water. Thicker aluminium or steel surrounds the borders of the grid to protect the vulnerable corners from mechanical damage.

The slats normally run parallel to the long axis of the grid although the transverse type is available on special order. There are crossed grids (Fig. 14.17) where two linear grids are superimposed on each other with one grid having its slats (lines) at right angles to the other.

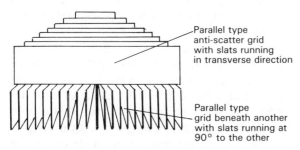

Fig. 14.17 Crossed linear parallel type grid shown diagramatically.

Parallel type anti-scatter grid with slats running in transverse direction

Parallel type grid beneath another with slats running at 90° to the other

Therefore grids are made in several forms: linear parallel, linear focused, crossed parallel or crossed focused.

Focused grids are designed for particular focus-to-grid distances. The distance is arranged to suit a focus-to-film distance of 100 cm or 180 cm and others are available for special techniques requiring different focus-to-film distances. These special grids are extremely expensive and difficult to obtain.

The grid ratio is the relationship between the height of the lead slats and the distance between them. It is one of the factors affecting the efficiency of the grid to eliminate scatter. If the height of the lead slat is 8 times that of the space between the slats, the ratio of the grid is 8:1, i.e.

$$\text{Grid ratio} = \frac{\text{height of lead slats}}{\text{distance between the slats}}$$

The greater the grid ratio, the more efficient the scatter absorption. Examination of Figure 14.18 shows two grids with ratios of 8:1 and 16:1. The 8:1 grid transmits more scatter than the 16:1 for its slats do not so effectively obstruct the passage of scatter which is only slightly deflected from the path of the primary beam. When high kV is used the scatter is much more forward directed than with lower kVs therefore it is important to use a grid with a high grid ratio to ensure a good clean up of scatter. If too low a ratio is chosen, the scatter having a small angle of deflection will be transmitted by the grid to the film.

It must however be remembered that when scatter is eliminated from the film, additional primary radiation must be applied to compensate for the absent scatter so that when a high ratio grid is used the exposure must be increased giving rise to an increased radiation dose and added loading on the tube. In practice the lowest grid ratio should be selected that will give the required level of scatter clean up to provide an image of diagnostic quality with an acceptable level of increased dose and tube loading.

Grid ratios in common use range from:

5:1   which is suitable for low voltage work where the quantity of scatter to be

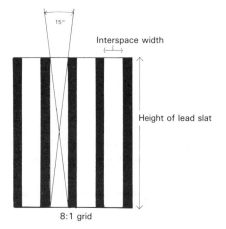

Angle through which scattered radiation can be transmitted

7.5°

16:1 grid

15°

8:1 grid

15°

Interspace width

Height of lead slat

8:1 grid

Fig. 14.18 The grid ratio, showing two 8:1 grids of quite different slat heights.

eliminated is small, where grid alignment is difficult and where it is not practical to increase the radiographic exposure.

8:1 suitable for middle range kV work.

16:1 suitable for high kV work where first class grid alignment is assured and the part being examined will be its nature produce much scatter.

12:1 an acceptable compromise between the 8:1 and 16:1, allowing a full range of general radiography to be undertaken without the problem of exchanging grids when different types of examinations are to be performed.

Grid efficiency is judged by its ability to remove scattered radiation with only minimal loss of useful primary radiation.

The factors which affect a grid's efficiency are:

grid ratio
thickness of lead slats
type of grid (linear or crossed)
nature of the interspace material.

Grids may reach an efficiency of about 80%. The efficiency value will vary when different kilovolts are used.

Grid factor of a grid is the amount of additional exposure that is needed to overcome the density loss due to the elimination of scatter and the absorption of primary radiation resulting from its use compared with the exposure without a grid. Therefore:

$$\text{Grid factor} = \frac{\text{exposure with the grid}}{\text{exposure without a grid}}$$

The factor will increase as the kV increases because there is more scatter produced and it is more forward directed. When this is eliminated, more density is lost and must be replaced by additional exposure if the image density is to be maintained. The amount of change is not great at normal diagnostic kilovoltages, e.g. an 8:1 grid used, where none was used before, will need an increase of 3.5 times the exposure at 70 kV and 4 times at 120 kV. The factor will be affected by changes in grid ratio and the nature of the grid. Therefore it is best to assess empirically the factor for a particular grid at a number of voltages.

Grid types: the focused and the non-focused (Fig. 14.15). They can be obtained in either a linear or crossed form.

The focused grid has its lead slats angled progressively in such a way that lines drawn through each lead slat will, if continued, intersect at a point a specific distance from the grid. The distance from the grid to the point of intersection is known as the focal distance of the grid. If the grid is well made and not of the highest ratio, this grid can be used over a narrow range of distances about the focal distance. The tolerances are specified by the manufacturer. When the slats are not progressively angled but are all perpendicular to the surface of the grid, the grid is a parallel or non-focused type.

The advantage of a focused grid is that the density of the radiograph is the same across the full width of the film, provided the grid is properly centered and correctly aligned to the X-ray beam. This is the result of the alignment of the lead slats with the radial X-ray beam. The parallel grid on the other hand cannot produce a uniform density across its width be-

cause the lead slats will only be aligned to the radial X-ray beam at its centre. They will become progressively more angled with respect to the X-ray beam as they are located further and further from the centre of the beam. The increasing angulation causes the radiation to be more attenuated with gradual loss in density from the centre to the edge of the film (see Fig. 14.19). The amount of radiation cut-off by a parallel grid over the outer third of the grid is normally acceptable as the area of interest is generally positioned over the centre of the grid and the thickness of the body is

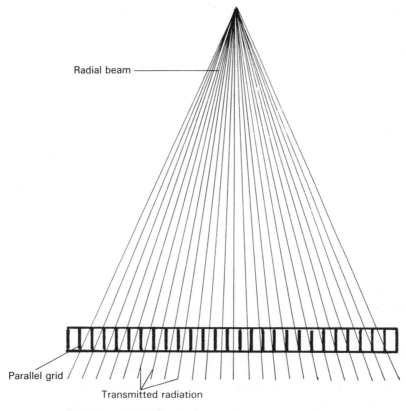

Radial beam

Parallel grid

Transmitted radiation

Note The cut-off of the primary radiation increasing towards the edge of the grid

Strip to show how the density of a film varies across its width due to the cut-off of primary radiation which increases from the centre to the edge

Fig. 14.19 The cut-off of radiation which arises with a parallel type grid as the slats become increasingly malaligned with the X-ray beam.

usually less in its outer third compared with the central third. The thinner region requires less radiation to provide the required density than the central part. Therefore as the absorption by cut-off is greatest in the area where the patient is thinnest the resultant image will have an even density across the whole film.

The parallel grid is preferred for some techniques for it is not so affected by differences in focus-to-film distance as the focused grid. If the field size is reasonably small, the cut-off in the outer part of the film can be tolerated. The shorter the focus-to-film distance, the greater the cut-off but when longer focus-to-film distances are used the angulation of the X-ray beam to the grid surface becomes greater. Therefore parallel grids can be used from about 90 cm to infinity.

A crossed grid, either parallel or focused, absorbs scatter more efficiently than a linear grid with a similar grid ratio; this is most marked at voltages below 100 kv. The increased efficiency of the crossed grid is due to absorption of scatter which will be transmitted by a linear grid since its direction is that of the interspace slats, but will be absorbed by the lead slats of the grid running at 90° to the first (see Fig. 14.17). This type of grid can only be used when the X-ray beam is perpendicular to the grid surface and even when this is arranged, great care must be taken with the alignment of the X-ray beam to the grid centre if cut-off is to be avoided. The removal of more scatter requires additional primary radiation to provide the same film density, therefore before a crossed grid is selected the increase in radiation dose must be considered and justified.

Grid lattice consideration. The grid lattice describes the layout of the lead slats. In order to prevent the image formed by the lead slats from interfering with the diagnostic value of the film it is important that:

1. The lead slat is as thin as possible so that it will be less visible on the film but still thick enough to provide absorption of the scattered radiation. As absorption of scatter is the function of the grid, the lead must be thick enough

to absorb the scatter even at the expense of some loss of information.

2. The lines formed by the slats are fine, and the degree of fineness is represented by the number of lines per centimetre. In general the greater the number of lines, the less obvious will they be to the observer. As the number of lines/cm increases the absorption of primary radiation increases if the thickness of the lead is unchanged since the interspace must become thinner (see Fig. 14.20). Therefore there is more lead in the grid which will necessitate additional exposure.

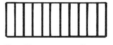 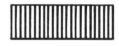

Few lines per centimetre   Many lines per centimetre

Lead slat of equal width in both grids, interspace much narrower in grid with many lines per centimetre

Fig. 14.20 Increased lines per centimetre resulting in narrower interspaces.

3. The most suitable type of grid — parallel or focused, linear or crossed — for the type of examinations to be undertaken is an essential factor which must be considered when a grid is specified.

4. Manufacture of grids is a difficult process which becomes more difficult as the number of lines increase. This is reflected in their price — a 60 line/cm will cost more than the 40 or 30 line/cm.

Grid identification. As it is important that the radiographer is aware of the grid specification so that it may be used correctly, the manufacturer of the grid labels it with the following information as well as indicating the direction of the grid lines:

1. type of grid: parallel or focused; linear or crossed; all metal (aluminium interspaces) or non-metal (plastic or fibre interspaces)
2. grid ratio
3. lines/cm
4. focal distance (on focused grids only)
5. tube side (on focused grids only)
6. serial number.

Grids in use. It is important when using a

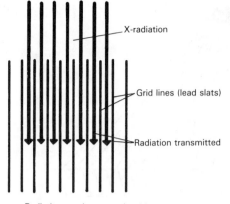

a. Radiation can be transmitted by a linear grid if the grid lines are aligned with the radiation

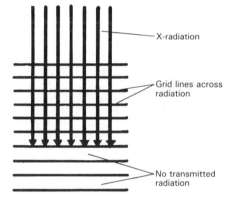

b. If the radiation is directed across the grid lines, no radiation will be transmitted

Fig. 14.21 The effect on transmitted radiation of aligning grid lines to the radiation and on placing grid lines across the radiation.

grid to be sure that it is precisely aligned to the X-ray beam to avoid radiation cut-off (Fig. 14.21). Therefore, when the X-ray beam has to be angled in relation to the grid, the grid lines must be aligned with the beam. When tomography is being performed, the X-ray beam is changing its direction during the exposure so the grid must adjust its position to maintain alignment with the X-ray beam throughout the exposure.

The effect of incorrect use:

1. Focused grids used upside down
   Focused grids can only be used when the angulation of the lead slats are directed towards the tube focus. The grid will be marked 'Tube-side' on the surface which must face the tube; if the grid is not used this way up, then, apart from a narrow strip in the centre of the grid, all the radiation is absorbed by the lead slats (Fig. 14.22).

2. Focused grids used outside the permitted focus-to-film distance
   Figure 14.23 shows how there is a progressive radiation cut-off as the edge of the film is approached. The degree of cut-off is increased as the grid ratio is increased. A cut-off of 40% is accepted at the margin of the grid.

3. Focused grid off-centre to the X-ray beam
   Figure 14.24 shows that the X-ray beam is not correctly aligned to the lead slats and this will cause radiation cut-off.

4. Off-level
   Figure 14.25 shows that with a focused or parallel grid, there will be cut-off when the grid is tilted in relation to the beam so that the beam strikes the grid at an angle. With a linear grid this effect will only occur when the beam is directed at an angle across the grid slats, and not in the other direction. Therefore, in practice, if a grid tilt is unavoidable or possible, the grid should be positioned so that the grid lines run in the same direction as the angled beam so that cut-off does not occur.

Care of grids. It is important to remember that grids are very fragile and can easily be damaged by rough or careless handling, and that any damage will degrade the X-ray image quite apart from the fact that damaged grids cannot be repaired and are costly to replace.

Therefore grids should: (1) be permanently protected by a thin covering of plastic, contained within an X-ray cassette or used on a rigid support. The patient's weight must never be applied to a grid without a strong underlying rigid support; (2) never be dropped or put down in a place where they may fall or have other equipment put on top of them; (3) be stored in a rack and never placed near heat.

Grid selection. The selection of the most

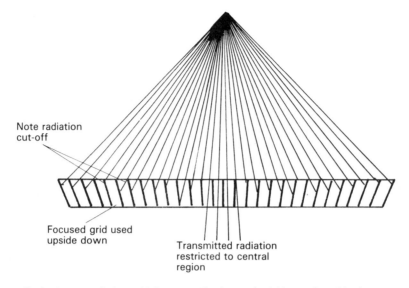

Note radiation
cut-off

Focused grid used
upside down

Transmitted radiation
restricted to central
region

Fig. 14.22 The cut-off of primary radiation which occurs if a focused grid is used upside down.

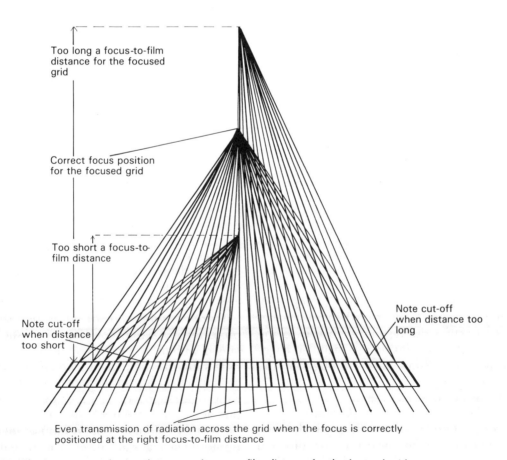

Too long a focus-to-film
distance for the focused
grid

Correct focus position
for the focused grid

Too short a focus-to-
film distance

Note cut-off
when distance too
long

Note cut-off
when distance
too short

Even transmission of radiation across the grid when the focus is correctly
positioned at the right focus-to-film distance

Fig. 14.23 The importance of using the correct focus-to- film distance for the focused grid.

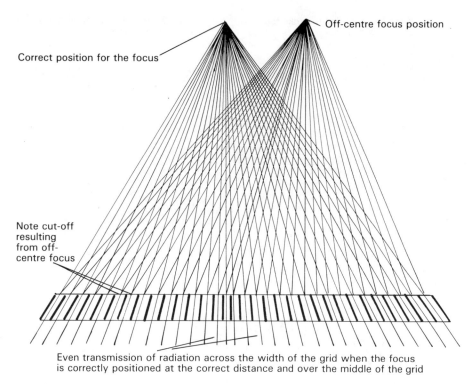

Off-centre focus position

Correct position for the focus

Note cut-off
resulting
from off-
centre focus

Even transmission of radiation across the width of the grid when the focus
is correctly positioned at the correct distance and over the middle of the grid

Fig. 14.24 The effect on transmitted radiation of off- centring the tube focus from the grid centre.

suitable grid for a particular examination or more commonly one suitable for a range of examinations necessitates consideration of the following:

1. quantity of scatter likely to be produced by the part of the body being examined
2. kilovoltage to be used
3. output of the generator or loading of the tube to permit the use of the increased exposure if a high ratio grid is being considered
4. radiation dose
5. technique to be used (any beam angulation)
6. focus-to-film distance
7. width of the grid.

Suggested grids:

30 lines/cm for general application and when used in a bucky. Ratios 6, 8, 10 and 12:1 depending on the kV and the generator output.

45 lines/cm for skull work, where great detail is required, the field is small and the scatter not too great in quantity Ratios 6 or 8:1 are suitable.

45 lines/cm is the best grid for stationary grid work where the grid lattice is hardly visible at the normal viewing distance

60 lines/cm is the grid which can be used where very fine detail is to be displayed and more obvious grid lines are not acceptable.

The selection of grid ratio depends upon the kV to be used; for high kV work above 120, a 16:1 is desirable. In the normal range of kV (up to 100) 6, 8 or 12:1 is suitable, the higher ratio being most suitable for areas where there is great scattering and the lower one where the generator output is limited and grid alignment may well be difficult, e.g. ward radiography.

Grid tests. Grids must be tested regularly to determine that they are without defect and do not degrade the image to unacceptable limits. With use they may become distorted and so cause greater cut-off at their borders or may

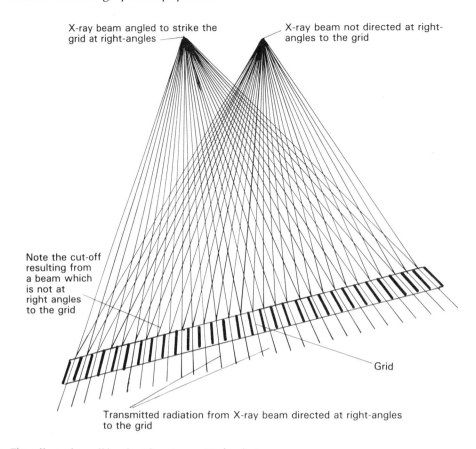

X-ray beam angled to strike the grid at right-angles

X-ray beam not directed at right-angles to the grid

Note the cut-off resulting from a beam which is not at right angles to the grid

Grid

Transmitted radiation from X-ray beam directed at right-angles to the grid

Fig. 14.25 The effect of an off-level grid on transmitted radiation.

show a very obvious line where they are severely damaged by bending.

The radiographer is recommended to determine the grid factor at various commonly used kilovoltages so that correct allowance can be made in the exposure when they are selected.

It is also recommended that all students malalign the grids, use them at different distances and invert a focused grid so that the characteristic appearances of grid faults can be readily recognised. Tests on grids should be undertaken with a phantom (a pile of wood boards) to simulate a patient so that the tests can be performed with normal exposure factors. The use of low kV will produce artifacts which are not of practical significance.

Grid movement. The linear anti-scatter grid can be used as a stationary or moving device.

The stationary grid will cast an image of its lead slats on the film and so may make in-

terpretation of the image more difficult. If the grid is moved during the exposure there will be no image of the slats visible on the film.

Therefore the advantage of the moving grid is improved image quality and better scatter removal for thicker lead slats can be used as they will not appear on the film.

The disadvantages of a moving grid are associated with the provision of movement, including an increased object-to-film distance because of the need to provide space for the movement to take place without risk of jamming, the inability to take the unit from its site under the patient support table, the increased cost of the unit and the possibility of grid lines remaining because of the stroboscopic effect.

The action of the grid. When the grid is moved during the exposure the grid lines are blurred by movement, but the absorption of scatter is unchanged, therefore image contrast is improved by elimination of the distracting grid lines which break up the image. The exposure will need to be increased when the grid is moved for all of the film will at some time during the exposure fail to receive primary radiation because this will have been absorbed by the lead slat lying between it and the patient. The stationary grid on the other hand will give strips of film under the interspace material which will never be obscured by lead, therefore this part will have less attenuation than any part of the film with a moving grid above it.

The grid, generally focused, is mounted in a frame which is made to move across the X-ray beam in a direction at right angles to the grid lines. The grid in its frame and the movement mechanism are known as the Potter-Bucky diaphragm, after the inventors.

Features common to all types of bucky assemblies (moving grid mechanisms)
1. The grid movement must start before the exposure commences and continue until after the exposure is completed.
2. The speed and range of grid movement during the exposure must be sufficiently large to blur out the grid lines.
3. The range of grid movement from the central position must not be large or the central ray of the X-ray beam will be directed too far from the centre of the grid. This will cause radiation cut-off. The range of movement is generally not more than 5 cm, 2.5 cm either side of the centre.
4. The movement must be smooth and continuous throughout the exposure.
5. The mechanism providing the grid movement must be simple.
6. The whole assembly must be as thin as possible so that the object-to-film distance is not too large.
7. A bucky assembly is comprised of:
   a. a frame to hold the grid, which in some units is accessible to the operator so that the grid of a different ratio can be inserted.
   b. an anti-scatter grid, commonly 43

× 43 cm so that it will cover the 43 × 35 cm film when the long axis is placed along the patient table or across it
   c. the mechanism for moving the grid
   d. a steel cassette tray is generally part of the assembly. It is positioned as close as is practical under the grid. The bucky tray can be removed to allow other devices such as a multisection tomographic cassette to be inserted in its place.

The whole assembly is mounted on bearings which run in a track on the underside of the X-ray patient table. This track allows the assembly to be moved along the length of the table, so that the grid and the film can be positioned under any part of the recumbent patient. This assembly is heavy and must have very positive locks and be counterweighted so that the bucky will hold its position even when the table is tilted.

The type of grid movement selected is controlled by the type of work to be performed, the exposure time, the space available to accommodate the mechanism and the importance of complete blurring of all grid lines. The choice lies between:

1. The simple oscillating movement
2. The reciprocating movement
3. The vibrating or trill movement
4. The single stroke movement — this is not installed in any units purchased today but may well be found in old units and as it cannot be used satisfactorily without appreciation of its method of operation, it is explained in the text.

   1. The simple oscillating movement
The grid oscillates forwards and backwards about its central rest position. The oscillating movement is produced by a simple electric motor. The motor causes a disc which is mounted on a spindle to rotate at a constant speed, a rod-like arm is attached to a point on the outer border of the disc. The other end of the arm is attached to the grid. Each time the disc

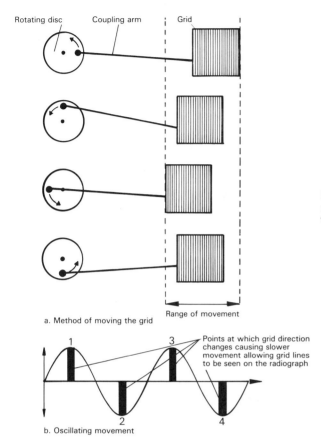

a. Method of moving the grid

b. Oscillating movement

Fig. 14.26 Simple oscillating grid movement.

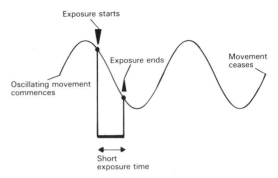

Fig. 14.27 Grid movement showing the position of maximum speed where a short exposure could be made with effective blurring of grid lines.

turns, the arm pushes or pulls the grid forwards and backwards in a track fixed at the top and bottom of the grid assembly (see Fig. 14.26a). The movement is sinusoidal.

Examination of the trace of the grid movement shows that at Points 1, 2, 3 and 4, where the grid is changing direction, the rate of movement is at a minimum and may be slow enough to allow an image of the grid lines to become evident, because the grid is virtually a stationary grid for part of the exposure and during this time the grid lines are produced on the film. This effect is more likely to occur when a 2-pulse generator is used since the electric motor speed is tied to the Ac supply making a stroboscopic effect possible. If the frequency of grid oscillating cycle peaks at the time as the radiation peak

voltage the grid line image will be more obvious. The stroboscopic effect will be explained more fully after the single-stroke bucky has been described.

By careful setting of the exposure contacts in relation to the grid's position, it is possible to arrange that short exposures take place when the grid is moving at its greatest speed. Figure 14.27 indicates the point at which a short exposure will start.

2. *The two-speed reciprocating movement*
A grid operated by a reciprocating mechanism moves rapidly in one direction and returns more slowly to its start position. The movement is brought about by a solenoid and a strong spring set on either side of the grid. The solenoid when energised produces a strong attractive force which draws the grid very rapidly towards itself. The spring attached to the other side of the grid is under high tension when it is fully stretched by the movement of the grid towards the solenoid so when the solenoid is de-energised the spring pulls the grid back to the start position. Therefore if the solenoid is regularly energised and de-energised, the grid will move forwards and backwards at regular intervals of time. With the two-speed reciprocating movement, the time taken to move forward is shorter than the time to return and because of the tension of the spring and rapid de-energisation the change of

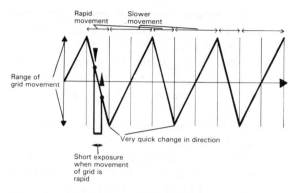

Fig. 14.28 Two-speed reciprocating movement.

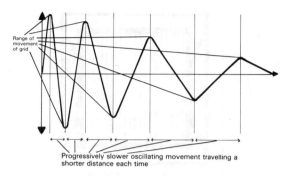

Fig. 14.29 The trill (vibrating) movement.

direction is very rapid leaving no time for grid lines to be imaged. Examination of Figure 14.28 shows the trace of movement of the grid operated by a two-speed reciprocating mechanism.

The movement repetition rate has to be chosen to suit the shortest exposure time which may be required to ensure that even with this time the grid is moving fast enough to blur out the image of the grid lines. When selecting a reciprocating form of grid movement the shortest exposure time that may be used with the radiographic techniques to be undertaken on the equipment must be determined so that the correct motor can be installed which will drive the grid at a speed to satisfy the demands of the very short exposure. For example, radiography of small children using rare-earth screens to reduce radiation dose will almost certainly necessitate a faster than average grid movement.

The two-speed reciprocating movement is certainly more efficient than the simple oscillating movement, but it is more costly to produce and requires a more complicated mechanism to operate it which is more bulky than the simple oscillating mechanism.

3. *The trill (vibrating) movement*
The trill movement is an oscillatory movement which differs from the simple oscillatory movement described previously: its

repetition rate is not regular, it gets progressively slower and the magnitude of the movement diminishes with time. A trace of the movement is shown in Figure 14.29 illustrating the variation in speed and magnitude.

This is an ideal grid movement as it is cheap and easy to produce, allows a wide range of exposure times to be used without risk of grid lines on the film and the mechanism is compact and simple. Short exposure times are made when the grid is moving quickly and there is no risk of stroboscopic effects as there is no exact repetition in time of grid movement during the whole period of its movement. The grid movement takes up to 15 seconds to die away, so allowing for very long exposure times as well as the very short.

The grid frame is attached to two pairs of flat springs as shown in Figure 14.30. The grid is drawn off-centre before the exposure commences by energising a solenoid which attracts the grid in its frame because of a soft iron disc attached to the frame. The movement of the frame places one pair of springs under tension and the other pair under compression. When the exposure sequence commences the solenoid is de-energised so that the grid in its frame oscillates between the two pairs of springs. At first the springs have energy causing the oscillations to be large and rapidly recurring, but progressively the energy stored in the springs reduces caus-

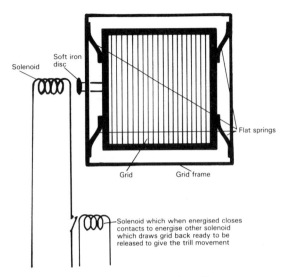

Fig. 14.30 Mechanism producing the trill movement.

ing the movement to become less and much slower. The whole sequence of energising the solenoid, drawing back the grid and de-energising the solenoid precedes every exposure even if some residual movement of the grid remains.

4. *Single stroke movement*
Although this method of moving the grid is obsolete, it is important to understand the operation since the radiographer must set the controls properly if the full radiographic exposure is to be delivered and no grid lines are to be visible. All the other forms of grid movement merely require the radiographer to select them.

In a single stroke movement, the grid moves in one direction only, travelling at a constant speed which has to be selected by the radiographer to match the exposure time. The grid is manually drawn back to the start position before every exposure and then is released electrically just before the exposure starts. Throughout the exposure the movement must continue; if the movement is complete before the exposure time is over, the radiation is prematurely terminated by the unit. The movement is about 5 cm, 2.5 cm on either side of the central position, therefore if the exposure time is long, the speed of grid travel has to be much slower than that needed for a short exposure. Figure 14.31 shows the relation of grid movement to exposure time.

The control of movement time is normally a small circular dial with a range of times scribed upon it, and the operator selects a time on this dial which is slightly in excess of the exposure time they have selected. It is essential to choose the correct time for too fast a grid movement will cut the exposure short and too slow a movement will result in a film with the image of grid lines upon it. With this regular movement there is considerable risk of stroboscopic effect. The movement is controlled by an oil dashpot mechanism which is bulky and liable to malfunction. Not surprisingly this system with all its in-

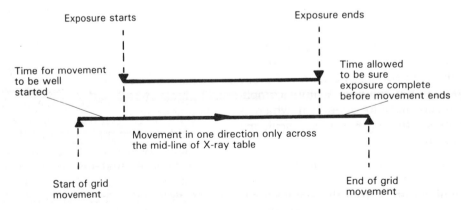

Fig. 14.31 Single-stroke movement — relation of the exposure of the grid movement.

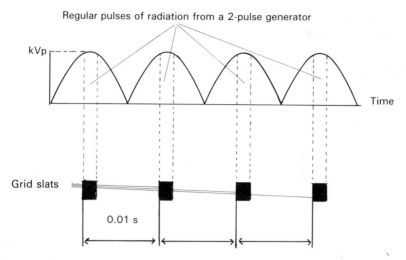

Fig. 14.32   Stroboscopic effect.

herent problems is no longer produced so the detail of its mechanism has not been included in this text.

The stroboscopic effect. A stroboscopic effect will arise when two sequences of periodic occurences coincide. In this radiographic application the two sequences are the pulses of radiation and the movement of the grid slat. Figure 14.32 shows the regular pulses of radiation generated by a 2-pulse generator and below it the grid slat moving over the film regularly covering, and uncovering the film beneath it. If the speed of the grid movement causes a lead slat to cover the same strip of film every time the radiation pulse is generated, the coincidence of these two actions will imprint the grid's image on the film as if the grid was stationary although it is in fact moving throughout the exposure. This effect is most likely to arise with a simple oscillating grid where the motor moving the grid and the generator producing the radiation are supplied from the 50 Hz alternating electrical mains supply. A single stroke grid movement may show this effect when by chance the grid movement coincides with the radiation pulses and this problem is easily overcome by a slight adjustment in grid speed.

B. By means of an air-gap. In areas, such as the chest, where the amount of scatter pro-

duced is not great, it is possible to produce a radiograph with much less scatter present than normal by introducing an air-gap between the patient and the film. This technique avoids the necessity for an anti-scatter grid so obviating the need for additional radiation dose and gives an image with lower contrast than with a grid.

An air-gap of at least 15 cm is needed if scatter elimination is to be effective. This gap will greatly increase the object-film distance causing an increase in image unsharpness and enlargement of the image if the technique is not modified to restore these factors to their normal value. The modification required is an increase in focus-film distance which will make the ratio of object-film distance to focus-film distance similar in both cases (see Fig. 14.33). This will overcome the image enlargement and also give the same geometric unsharpness. If magnification is desirable or acceptable, the geometric unsharpness can be reduced by using a smaller effective focus. This alternative is the basis of macroradiography.

The method of scatter elimination. Figure 14.34 shows that the scatter produced in the body being deflected from the normal path of the beam fails to reach the film and if not absorbed would fall well outside the area under examination. This is the sole method by which an air-gap eliminates scatter from the useful

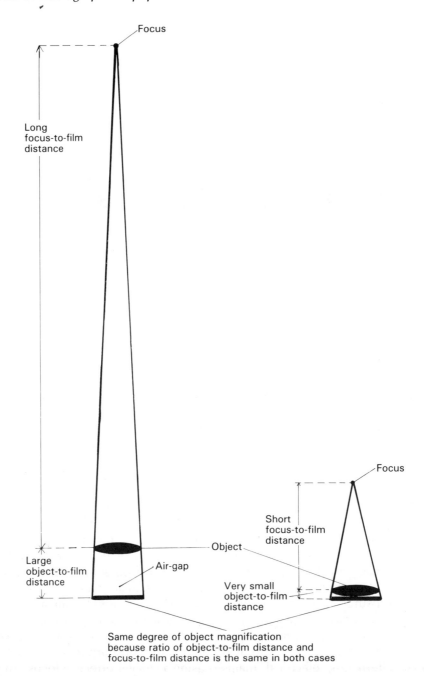

Fig. 14.33 Air-gap technique.

field — the air within the gap plays **no** part in the elimination process.

The provision of an air-gap. The air-gap is provided by interposing a suitably sized box between the patient and the film. The box has a non-opaque face on which the patient rests; the exit face of the box is normally open. The four sides are lead lined to absorb the scatter so providing radiation protection for the personnel in the room and ensuring that the area of interest in the patient is the only area receiving radiation (Fig. 14.35).

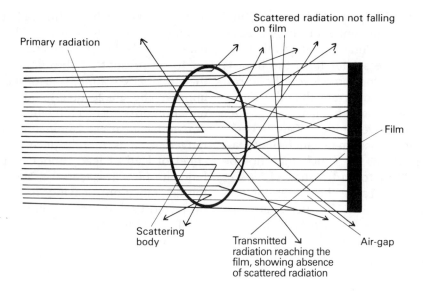

Fig. 14.34 The principle of air-gap technique in the reduction of scattered radiation reaching the film.

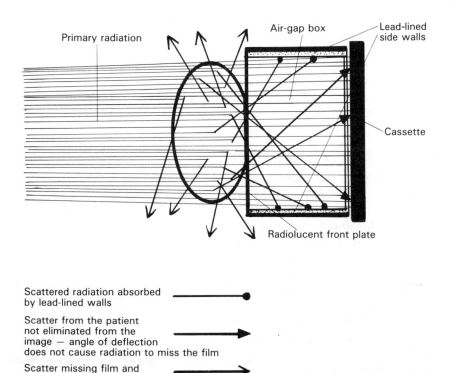

Fig. 14.35 Air-gap provided by a box with lead-lined walls.

Applications for air-gap technique. Chest radiography — in a patient with heavy breasts which produce considerable scatter this technique eliminates the scatter from the breasts whilst still retaining the same level of contrast in the apices. It is important that the image does not have an enlargement factor greater than with a normal technique. This necessitates a very long focus-film distance of at least twice the normal 180 cm which may not be possible in an X-ray room because of its size and/or layout, or because the generator output is too low to allow the increased mAs needed to expose the film satisfactorily to be delivered in an exposure time which will 'freeze' the patient movement.

Macro-radiography — in this technique the object-film distance is intentionally increased to produce an enlarged image, therefore the opportunity to reduce radiation dose by the elimination of an anti-scatter grid should be taken. This technique reduces the exposure needed and so permits the use of a micro-focus.

C. A low attenuating filter between patient and film. A wafer-thin copper filter can be placed between the patient and the film to absorb some of the scatter before it reaches the film since the scattered X-ray photon has lower energy than the useful primary beam and will be more readily absorbed than the primary photon. The film will show improved image contrast but it is important that the filter is very thin or it will itself produce scatter and absorb too much of the useful radiation.

This method of scatter reduction is not often used but may be useful for bed-side radiography when an anti-scatter grid is not available and the kilovoltage is low, or where it is difficult to align a grid correctly. The aluminium faced cassette will eliminate some scatter and so improve the image contrast compared with the plastic fronted cassette, but its increased absorption of useful radiation has caused the low attenuating plastic fronted cassette to be in general use today.

D. Back-scatter absorption. Some primary radiation will pass through the film and unless it is absorbed it will be scattered by interaction with objects, such as the wall, behind it. A proportion of this scatter will be scattered back towards the film causing additional scatter to be present on the film. It is important that this back-scatter is absorbed not only to improve the image quality but to reduce the radiation dose received by the patient or other personnel nearby. Elimination is easily arranged — it is merely necessary to place a sheet of lead or lead rubber immediately behind the film. The lead will absorb any transmitted radiation, leaving no scatter to be projected back on to the film.

All X-ray cassettes should be checked for the presence of a back-scatter absorbing layer and if one is not present, as in some cassettes designed for use with units employing certain types of automatic exposure control, an absorbing sheet must be placed behind the cassette and the automatic exposure monitoring chamber. If direct (non-screen) radiography is to be undertaken a back-scatter absorbing

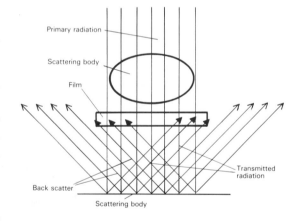

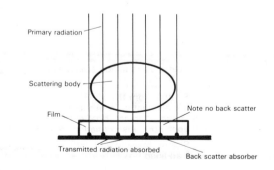

Fig. 14.36 The effect of back scatter absorbers.

layer must always be used behind the film. Figure 14.36 illustrates the distribution of this scatter, and also indicates how important the absorber is to the general control of scatter.

3. Reduction in the effect of the scatter

When the density on a film is produced by the effect of X-radiation alone, primary and scattered radiation blacken the film irrespective of the photon energy so that the image is degraded by the non-image forming scatter. But when intensifying screens are used, the blackening is largely the result of the light emitted by the phosphor and this does require a certain level of photon energy to cause the excitation. If the photon energy is below this level then it takes no place in image formation. Therefore the image has greater contrast because the non-image forming scatter has not contributed to the film blackening and so the use of intensifying screens has limited the effect of any scatter remaining after all other methods of control have been applied.

Rare-earth phosphors are particularly effective since the binding energy of their electrons is greater demanding a higher energy photon to cause excitation.

15
Radiographic tables, cassette/film holders and tube supports

RADIOGRAPHIC TABLES

There are many types of radiographic table available today, ranging from the simple very basic patient support table suitable for simple general radiography to the very sophisticated units designed to perform particular functions.

The basic table

The basic table will be considered in three parts: the table top, the sub-frame and the table base.

The table top

The top is formed from a sheet of flat or dished radiolucent plastic material of about 75 cm wide and 225 cm long, thick enough to support the patient's weight but keeping the attenuation it offers the X-ray beam to a minimum. Carbon fibre which is even more radiolucent may be used instead of plastic where the patient's dose must be kept very low, or where the lower radiographic exposure required when this material is used is necessary to reduce the tube loading. However, carbon fibre is very expensive and so is not used unless the extra cost can be justified by its advantages.

In addition to the low attentuation the table top must be easy to clean and not easily scratched or damaged. The sides of the top are strenghthened by metal side rails which also provide attachment for accessories such as displacement bands, handgrips, lateral cassette holders and in some cases the pivot unit for tomography.

In very simple models, the table top is often fixed to its base allowing no movement but more commonly the table top can be moved both transversely and longitudinally on its base. The table with this double movement is described as a 'floating top' table (Fig. 15.1). Table top movement allows the patient to be positioned without moving him/her on the table. Its advantages include:

1. The ability to undertake multiple examinations of the very sick or badly injured patient with minimum disturbance.
2. Quicker, easier and more accurate positioning.

Its disadvantages are:

1. An increased table top-to-film distance which cannot be avoided if movement is to be possible (see the description of the table runners on page 219, and Figure 15.2).
2. Increased image magnification and unsharpness unless compensation for these effects is made by increasing the f.f.d.
3. The need to provide very positive locks to secure the table top.
4. Difficulty in centering the part of the patient to be examined accurately under the X-ray beam.

The table movement must be smooth and

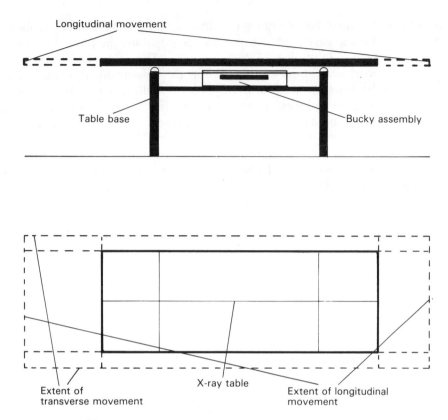

Fig. 15.1 Floating top X-ray table.

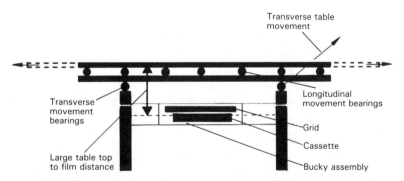

Fig. 15.2 Enlarged view of a floating top X-ray table to show clearly how the provision of longitudinal and transverse table top movement causes a large table to top to film distance.

the range of movement provided sufficient to enable all parts of the patient to be examined without disturbance. Electromagnetic brakes are generally provided which are operated either by the radiographer's hand or foot. In simple tables the movement is manually operated and so must be engineered to make it light and easy to move the patient. Movement is provided by means of roller bearings running in a channel. For longitudinal movement the channels are secured along both sides of the base support and across the width of the base for lateral movement. The channels for one direction of movement must be set on top of the other, and it is this unavoidable design feature which causes the increased table top to film distance in this type of table (Fig. 15.2).

As previously mentioned, the effect of this increased distance can be compensated for by an increased f.f.d. or may be reduced to acceptable levels by dishing the table top. A dished table top does however present difficulty when a horizontal beam is required. Some manufacturers have designed tables which allow the cassette in its tray to be raised up under the table once the movement has been completed. It is generally felt that an increased f.f.d., even if it is very limited, and the use of a smaller focal spot are the most satisfactory way of overcoming the difficulty, but the magnitude of the problem must be assessed when considering a particular unit.

Some manufacturers attach their table top to its base with a locking system which can be released to allow the table top to be removed from its base and attached to a set of wheels converting it into a transport trolley. This is a desirable feature in accident departments where patient movement must be restricted to an absolute minimum. But in selecting this type it must be accepted that two porters are needed to transport the patient on the large and heavy trolley.

The longitudinal movement can be used to change the position of the patient in relation to the recording unit. This enables the patient to be examined by closed circuit TV (CCTV) to site a catheter and then transferred to a position over the film changer unit to record the series of images. Alternatively, the table may be driven autonomatically to predetermined positions to enable the flow of contrast agent in the peripheral blood vessels to be followed and recorded. These tables are called *catheter tables*. Their basic design is the same as the basic table, and the modifications needed to provide for the specialist function are an extended longitudinal movement and the more common use of carbon fibre for the table top.

When there is automatic table movement, safety devices must be provided to protect the patient and the equipment from damage resulting from parts moving in relation to each other and to ensure that no movement can take place whilst the patient is being placed on the table. The safety devices may be mechanically or electrically operated. Electrical devices normally operate by means of a micro switch. The micro switch operating lever is compressed by the moving table and this action opens or closes contacts within the switch, breaking or making the continuity of the safety circuit as the circuit demands. It is important that the operator is aware of the presence and location of the devices so that a source of malfunction may be eliminated if the table movement fails to operate as expected.

The sub frame

The sub frame, interposed between the table top and table base, supports the equipment which is used to record the image. The most commonly found piece of equipment supported on the sub frame is the bucky assembly. This is mounted on nylon wheels which run in channels along the length of the sub frame. The sub frame should be as long as possible to give the greatest range of movement of the bucky and the cassette tray beneath the patient. As moving parts and electrical connections have to be housed on the frame, for safety and to prevent dirt or debris interfering with the operation of the equipment, it is usual to find a plastic cover on the sub frame and a pair of support rollers attached to each end of the bucky assembly. The rollers support the width of the table top to prevent any sagging of the top interfering with the free and even movement of the grid. Electro-mechanical locks are provided to prevent movement of the assembly during the exposure.

The table base

There are three types of base available which allow for the various types of radiographic techniques that have to be performed: the flat bucky table, the tilting table and the special table base.

The plain flat bucky base is a simple support

for the table top and sub frame and can be provided by four legs supporting the corners of the sub frame. It is used in general work where it is not necessary to examine the patient in any position other than the horizontal.

The base must be rigid and strong and is normally securely bolted to the floor, unless the table is to be used for patient transport as well as radiography. The height of the table from the floor is the same as a standard patient trolley and cannot normally be altered although some tables have been designed to allow the table top to be lowered to a level which makes it easier for the patient to get on and off the table and then be raised to a comfortable working height. This type of table should be considered where there is a high proportion of elderly or disabled patients to be examined.

The tilting table

This can be used for all of the functions performed by the flat table but with the tilting facility has its prime use in fluoroscopy.

It has a table top and sub frame similar to that provided for the plain flat table mounted on a base which allows the top to be tilted from the horizontal. Tables are available with different degrees of movement, the greatest being the 90°/90° table which rises from the horizontal to the vertical position in either direction, to the more simple model which provides a 90° tilt in one direction and a restricted tilt of 10–60° in the other direction, termed the adverse direction. Figure 15.3 illustrates the range of movement.

The more simple form is normally adequate for the examination of the alimentary tract; the 90°/90° tilt is ideal for myelography, especially the examination of the cervical region. Therefore careful consideration should be given to the type of table necessary for the work to be undertaken, as the price of the 90°/90° table is very much more than the table with limited movement. This increase in price is the result of the special movement necessary to raise the table to the vertical position in both directions using one tilting mechanism. This is a compli-

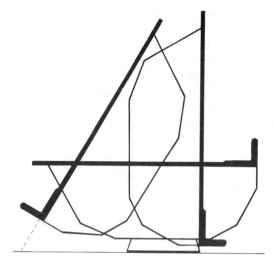

Fig. 15.3 View of a tilting table showing the table in the vertical, horizontal and tilted position.

cated mechanical problem which requires translation as well as elevation (a movement similar in action to that of the fair ground swinging boat).

The table movement is driven by a high-powered electric motor which drives a series of gears and chains to move the cogs secured to the table top. The controls for the table movement are sited with other controls on the table's serial changer, although they may be duplicated on a remote control unit. Because of the complexity of the combined movement that is possible on the table, by the top and by the equipment attached to the table, it is essential that many additional safety interlock circuits are provided to prevent damage to the patient or the equipment occurring as a result of the combined movements.

The elaborate movements may be monitored and more closely controlled by means of a microprocessor which can predict the effect of the various movements. The electromagnetic brakes must provide a very positive action. The weight of the table to be tilted is very great, but this is moved smoothly and easily by the motor aided by a system of counter-weights. That is the weight to be lifted is matched by an equal weight, which is attached to it by a system of wires and cables positioned diagonally opposite to it. As one weight is raised or lowered, the other weight, the counter-weight, moves to balance it in its new position.

The height of the table is kept as low as possible but it is not possible to get it very low as the lifting mechanism, and often an under-couch unit, have to be stored beneath it. Then of course its height must be similar to a trolley top level and at a convenient working height. This height requires the provision of an integral step for the use of the patient. Other accessories are provided to support the patient as the table tilts. These include hand grips, shoulder supports and patient harness for securing them to the table.

The tilting table as a fluoroscopy table

When a tilting table is used for fluoroscopy, the table sub frame supports the serial changer and the undercouch X-ray tube as well as the bucky assembly.

The X-ray tube and serial changer are linked together in a fixed relationship. The combined unit of serial changer and tube are counter-weighted and should be balanced so that the unit is light enough to move despite its weight and should retain its position when the table is tilted and the brakes are off. This is difficult with a serial changer carrying various sizes of cassette of different weights. In modern units

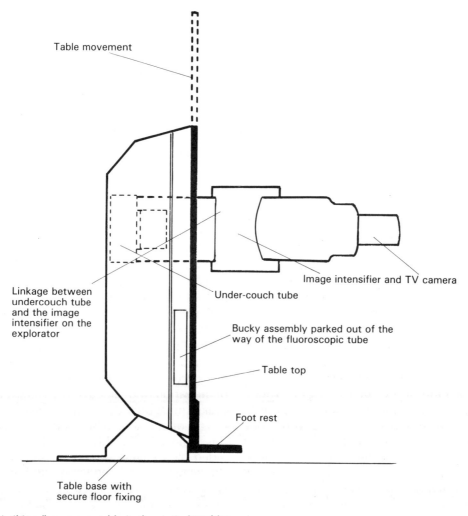

Table movement

Linkage between undercouch tube and the image intensifier on the explorator

Under-couch tube

Image intensifier and TV camera

Bucky assembly parked out of the way of the fluoroscopic tube

Table top

Foot rest

Table base with secure floor fixing

Fig. 15.4 A tilting fluoroscopy table in the vertical position.

the movement is either power-assisted or motor driven to enable the operators to move the carriage easily as they examine the patient. Figure 15.4 indicates the relationship of the undercouch tube to the serial changer with the table in the upright position. Figure 15.5 illustrates more fully the link between the tube and serial changer, showing the collimator attached to the tube and the serial changer carrying the image intensifier. The link between the parts is described as the tower. The table top-to-tube distance is usually fixed between 40–50 cm.

The serial changer and image intensifier carriage. The serial changer, sometimes described as the explorator, is designed to provide a means of rapidly recording radiographic and fluoroscopic images during a fluoroscopic examination allowing the operator to change quickly the position of the unit to record the area of interest. The operator either moves the unit without assistance, or is assisted by a motor or by controlling a motor which drives all movements. The serial changer moves smoothly over a large area of the table top by means of a combination of longitudinal and lateral movement. The movement is halted as soon as the movement controls are released. The unit must move in towards the table top and out from it as required — this movement allows the patient-to-recording plane to be kept to a minimum.

The electric motors driving the movements are housed beneath the table top, and once

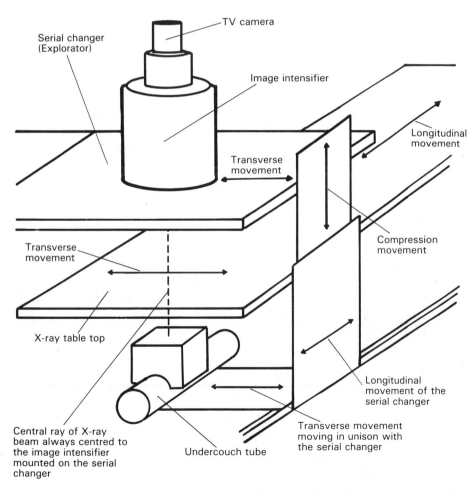

Fig. 15.5 Linkage of the undercouch X-ray tube with the serial changer (the explorator).

the unit is positioned further movement is prevented by electro-magnetic brakes. Many safety devices are included in the serial changer movement controls to ensure that immediately the unit meets an obstruction it stops at once, or in the case of the compression movement when a pre-selected pressure is applied to the unit by the patient's body. In some modern units the safety devices are co-ordinated by a microprocessor, others rely on pressure and a slipping clutch to prevent the movement continuing when it is unsafe to do so.

The unit controls (Fig. 15.6) are grouped conveniently on the side of the unit enabling the operator to move the unit, lock the movements, screen or radiograph as required, tilt the table to any position between the horizontal and the vertical and still remain protected from all primary and most scattered radiation. All these controls may be duplicated on a separate unit allowing the unit to be operated remotely, which affords the operator greater

radiation protection. When the unit is operated remotely it is essential to provide a more powerful motor to ensure that it is able to move without manual assistance.

A compression cone mounted on a metal plate with a central aperture is provided to allow compression to be applied over the duodenal area. The metal plate carrying the cone prevents scattered radiation reaching the film around the small field so that a series of exposures can be made in rapid succession on a single film. This plate with its cone is introduced into the radiation field manually or by the operation of a small motor whose controls are placed close to the operator.

All serial changers are provided with diaphragms which allow a film to be divided into a number of sections, either vertically or transversely by selection of the appropriate programme. Figure 15.6 shows the layout of a typical serial charger.

A moving grid is generally provided, although in some units the grid is stationary.

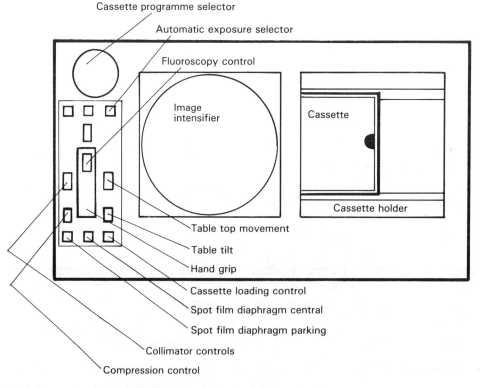

Fig. 15.6 Serial changer (explorator) with a simple control panel.

However, if this is the case, a fine line grid must be provided.

Full size films can be taken by providing a cassette transport system which operates on rails and which allow the cassette to be moved in front of the input face of the image intensifier. The cassette carriage is designed to allow a selection of sizes of cassette to be used. The fitting of cassettes into the carriage, which forms part of the transport system, must be easy and quick and whilst in the waiting position must be protected from any scattered radiation. This is normally done by the fitting of a radio-opaque plate on the carriage behind the cassette waiting position.

When the operator selects radiography, the cassette carriage moves across to the exposure position and the movement of the carriage often initiates the grid movement and brings the unit into the prepare stage. In some units, once the prepare phase is over, the positioning of the cassette in its correct position operates the exposure switch. This facility is useful for a rapid sequence of exposures since the series can be made without the delay which would arise if the unit was allowed to go out of the prepare position. The sequence of events when radiography is selected is as follows:

1. Fluoroscopy is switched off as the carriage starts to move.
2. The X-ray tube anode is accelerated to the required speed and the tube filament boosted to the heat required for the selected mA.
3. The cassette carriage with its contained cassette is brought into the exposure field and held in position.
4. The grid is set in motion.
5. The exposure is made.

After the exposure is over the cassette carriage leaves the field and the sequence of events set out above takes place in reverse order.

Provision for the fixing of accessories. Slotted metal side rails are fitted to the table sides to allow a variety of accessories to be fitted at any position along the length of the table. Once they are in position they are locked in this position so that they can withstand the strain applied to them when the patient or the table is moved. There are many accessories available which fit into the side rails, including: a patient step (a foot rest), a lateral cassette holder, shoulder rests, a compression band, hand grips and, on some units, patient cradles. Units may provide facilities for lateral fluoroscopy by means of a second image intensifier TV unit fitted to the edge of the table with a second X-ray tube centred to it. A linear tomographic attachment may be fitted to some units.

Radiation protection. It is important to protect all the staff from scattered radiation and to ensure that it is not possible for anyone other than the patient to receive primary radiation from the undercouch tube. This protection is provided by:

1. Metal covers on the sides of the table and a metal flap to cover the space between the table top and the sub-frame during fluoroscopy. This space is needed to give access to the bucky tray. Lead impregnated plastic or rubber aprons and flaps are fitted to the serial changer to attenuate scatter from the patient.
2. The field size of the primary beam is restricted by a diaphragm in the tube port to the smallest size that will cover the largest area to be recorded by the system. In addition to this, a variable collimator is fitted to reduce the field size to cover the area of interest; the diaphragms of the collimator are adjusted by hand or automatically in response to instructions from sensors monitoring the cassette size and are closed down as the focus-to-film distance increases so that the radiation beam never extends beyond the cassette margins. When automatic collimation is provided, it must always be possible to over-ride it so that the field size can be reduced to an even smaller area if the information to be recorded can be covered by a smaller field. As a safeguard against accidental irradiation by primary radiation when the serial changer is parked clear of the table to allow the overcouch tube to be used without obstruction, the diaphragms are automatically closed.
3. Fluoroscopy units must incorporate a

timer which records the length of the fluoro-scopic examination and indicates the end of a preselected time by an audible alarm. If this is ignored and screening is continued, the fluoroscopy exposure will be terminated preventing any further X-ray generation until the timer has been manually reset by the operator.

4. The screening switch operated by the radiologist is designed to be a hold-on switch which, if released, stops irradiation and prevents accidental fluoroscopy.

5. In common with other X-ray tubes, the tube used for fluoroscopic examinations must be fitted with additional aluminium filtration to provide the total filtration required by the Code of Practice.

6. Recently, remotely controlled fluoroscopic units have been introduced, and these allow the operator to remain behind a protective screen whilst performing the examination on the patient. This system has the disadvantage of isolating the patient from the operator making their care more difficult and the examination probably more worrying for them and has poorer scatter control (Fig. 16.2), but there are advantages which will be described in Chapter 16. It is important that radiation surveys are performed around the X-ray table in the horizontal and vertical position to identify the areas of high and low levels of scatter.

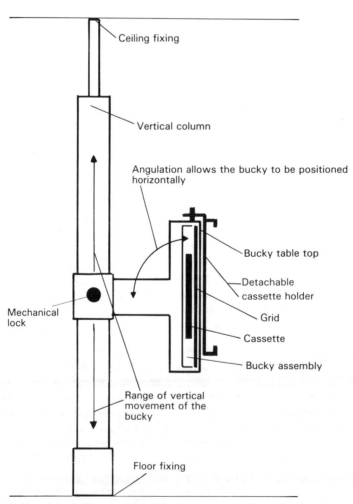

Fig. 15.7   Upright bucky with a detachable cassette holder for chest radiography.

THE VERTICAL BUCKY AND CHEST STAND

The bucky assembly described previously is mounted under a square patient support table. The whole unit is fitted on a vertical column through a mounting block which allows the table to be raised and lowered to align it to the X-ray beam. The table is hinged so that it can be positioned horizontally or vertically, or any position between. The mounting block also allows rotation enabling the table to be turned to align the grid to the X-ray beam.

The table, bucky assembly and its mounting are counter-balanced and all the movements are provided with scales and secure locks. A cassette holder is attached to the table face and with the table vertical converts it to a chest unit. (Fig. 15.7).

An integrated bucky and tube unit

Figure 15.8 shows the layout of this unit, in which the X-ray tube and bucky are mounted on the same arm. The arm is fixed to a vertical column allowing the integrated table and tube to be raised and lowered, and turned through almost 360°.

This unit has great versatility. It is a very useful unit for all extremity work, and can be used for chest radiography, if a slightly shorter focus-to-film distance can be accepted. Almost all general work can be performed if a patient trolley is placed over the unit table. This type of unit is recommended for a basic radiological service because it is simple to use with its fixed focus-to-film distance and its tube always centred to the mid-point of the table.

UNDERTABLE CASSETTELESS FILM UNITS

There are specialised tables in which the cassette tray is eliminated and a light-tight film transport system substituted. The films are transferred from a storage magazine to the exposure position beneath the anti-scatter grid where they are clamped between the intensifying screens to ensure good film/screen contact. Once exposed the film is removed to a take-up magazine for transfer to the darkroom or conveyed along an extended path direct to the processor unit.

These units are very expensive but can be justified where there are many examinations using a series of large films normally exposed in the bucky tray, e.g. urography. They have advantages over an ordinary table because they eliminate the manual labour of cassette handling. Individual cassettes with their intensifying screens are not required and the system being enclosed eliminates the risk of screen damage so there are fewer artifacts on the films. There are many other useful features included on these units which can be found in the manufacturer's literature.

AUTOMATED CASSETTELESS CHEST UNIT

The cassetteless chest unit is useful in the few departments where the volume of chest radiography justifies the cost of the unit. It has advantages over ordinary full size cassette radiography. Its use reduces the manual work of the radiographer by eliminating the handling of many heavy X-ray cassettes. It increases the number of patients who can be examined and allows the radiographer to remain with the patient while the film is processed. The enclosed film path protects the intensifying screens from damage or dust.

This system is used as an alternative to photofluorography as it requires less radiation to expose the film adequately and this reduces the patient dose, a great advantage, but of course the cost of film is much greater.

Figure 15.10 shows the layout of the unit and illustrates the path taken by the film.

X-RAY TUBE SUPPORTS

The X-ray tube requires a support which will allow it, by longitudinal and transverse movements, to be positioned anywhere over a reasonable floor area and to be varied in height, allowing at least 100 cm focus-to-table top distance.

The support must be:

1. able to carry the considerable weight of

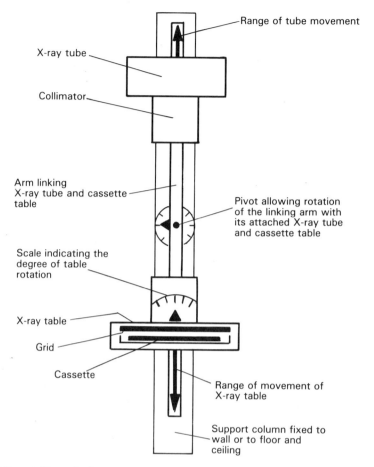

Fig. 15.8 Integrated X-ray table and tube unit.

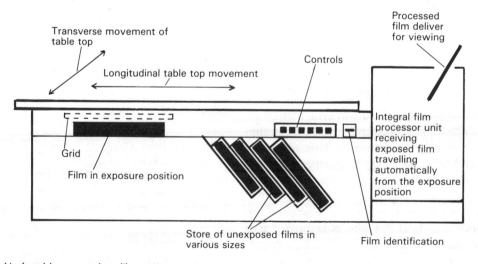

Fig. 15.9 Undertable cassetteless film unit.

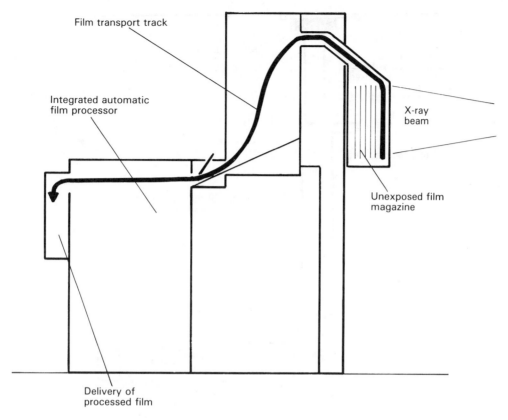

Fig. 15.10 Automatic cassetteless chest X-ray unit with a film magazine.

the X-ray tube and have locks which will secure the tube in any position.

2. counterpoised to reduce the weight which has to be moved manually or by a motor.

3. designed to ensure that in the event of mechanical or electrical failure the unit will remain securely supported.

4. provided with movements which allow precise angulation of the X-ray beam around the tube attachment point and clearly indicate the amount of angulation and rotation.

5. provided with easily accessible controls for the release of locks and sometimes providing motor power to allow the unit to be moved easily from one position to another.

Three types of support are available

1. *Floor/ceiling support* — floor mounted, running in a floor track travelling in one direction only.

2. *Ceiling mounted* — carried on ceiling beams, covering a rectangular floor area with a larger transverse axis than is possible with a floor/ceiling support.

3. *Table mounted* forming an integral part of the X-ray unit. The unit is normally designed for a particular purpose such as a remotely controlled fluoroscopy unit, a tomographic table or a skull table. However, this principle is recommended for the simple inexpensive basic radiological unit for use in developing countries.

A description of the first two types is given here, while the third type will be included with the description of the complete unit.

1. Floor/ceiling tube support

The tube support is formed from a vertical column with a counter-poised cross-arm on which the X-ray tube is mounted (see

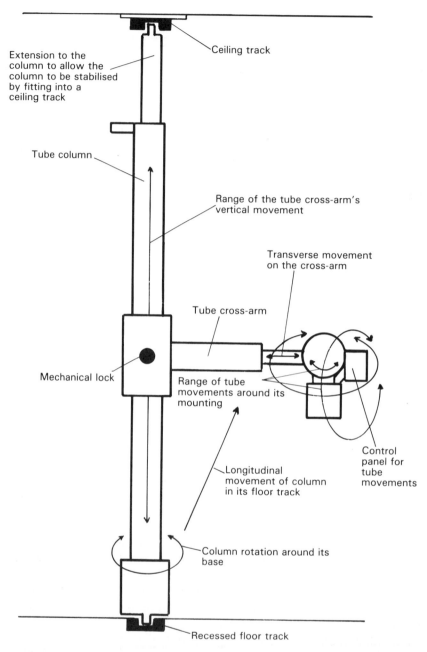

Extension to the column to allow the column to be stabilised by fitting into a ceiling track

Ceiling track

Tube column

Range of the tube cross-arm's vertical movement

Transverse movement on the cross-arm

Tube cross-arm

Mechanical lock

Range of tube movements around its mounting

Control panel for tube movements

Longitudinal movement of column in its floor track

Column rotation around its base

Recessed floor track

Fig. 15.11 Floor-to-ceiling tube support.

Fig. 15.11): The column travels in a floor track which is recessed into the floor, and for added stability the column is extended upwards to allow it to run in a ceiling track. Should a ceiling support not be possible a wider base running in two widely separated floor tracks will provide stability. The floor tracks may occasionally be mounted on the floor surface instead of being recessed, but this is not an ideal arrangement as it forms an obstruction to a free passage around the table.

An electric motor may be attached to the

column base to provide linear longitudinal movement required for simple tomography.

The column runs the length of the track allowing the X-ray tube to be positioned anywhere along the track which generally extends well beyond the head and the foot of the table, its length only limited by the layout and size of the room. The cross-arm allows the tube to be moved vertically and to a limited extent allows transverse movement across the table. The vertical column can be rotated at its base so that the cross-arm can be positioned around the vertical column. The X-ray tube can be rotated on the cross-arm about its long and short axes. It is usual to find the normal operating position of the tube self-locating. All movements are counter-poised to reduce the effort needed to produce the required movement and once this position is reached, further movement is prevented by locks.

The locks are usually electro-mechanical. A number of scales are provided to register the position of the tube:

a. on the column to give the focus-to-table top distance and the focus-to-bucky distance

b. on the cross-arm to indicate the central position of the tube and the distance from the centre in both directions

c. to indicate the degree of angulation or rotation around the X-ray tube or the column.

Other features found on most tube columns include:

a. a control unit fitted on the tube mounting to allow the locks securing all movements of the tube column and cross-arm to be operated from a central convenient point. These controls are often incorporated with the controls of the X-ray beam delineator.

b. a fixing point for the attachment of a tomographic coupling rod linking the X-ray tube and the bucky tray.

In some modern sophisticated units there are electrical sensors mounted on the tube column to record the selected focus-to-film distance and transmit this information to a micro-processor which adjusts the X-ray beam

to a field size which will just cover the area of the selected cassette within the bucky tray.

Controls and indicators found mounted alongside the tube

1. Vertical tube movement brake.
2. Longitudinal and transverse tube movement brakes.
3. Rotation locks.
4. Delineator light switch.
5. Delineator diaphragm controls and scales.
6. Pair of indicator lamps to display visually which tube is energised, if more than one overcouch tube is supplied from the same generator.

2. Ceiling mounted tube support

The ceiling mounted tube support allows the X-ray tube to travel over a very large floor area. It is suspended from the ceiling on two sets of tracks (Fig. 15.12). One set of tracks runs parallel to the long axis of the X-ray table and the other across it. The longitudinal tracks are secured to boards fixed to the ceiling or to steel girders fitted close to the ceiling supported by the room walls, and in either case the fixing must carry the combined weight of the tracks, the tube and its support. The transverse tracks run across the longitudinal tracks and from them is suspended the tube support carriage with its telescopic column so that it is free to move along the track. In this way the X-ray tube can be located at the required height over a very large floor area. To obtain a 100 cm focus-to-film distance, it is necessary for the finished floor-to-ceiling height to be 3.25 m. This ceiling height allows for the space taken by the longitudinal and transverse tracks and the telescopic tube support (Fig. 15.13). If a particularly large floor area is to be covered an additional longitudinal track will be required.

The high tension cables for the tube are carried by the support and looped along the track to drop down over the generator tank. The supports for the cables must run freely along the track to avoid any strain being

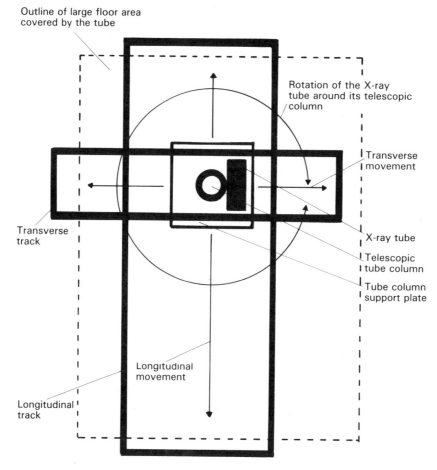

Outline of large floor area
covered by the tube

Rotation of the X-ray
tube around its telescopic
column

Transverse
movement

Transverse
track

X-ray tube

Telescopic
tube column

Tube column
support plate

Longitudinal
movement

Longitudinal
track

Fig. 15.12 Layout of the ceiling tracks of a ceiling mounted tube support.

applied to the cables when the tube is moved to another position.

The tube support allows the tube to be rotated around three axes: longitudinal, transverse, and around the telescopic column. The controls for the various movements are grouped in a control unit attached to the tube mounting. Counter-balance is provided for the tube so that it will retain its position even when the electrical supply to the brakes is switched off. The longitudinal movement may be powered by a servo-motor, and this aids the operator in general work and allows linear tomography to be performed by coupling the motor driven tube to the bucky tray through a fulcrum fitted to the table top.

Advantages of a ceiling mounted tube support over a floor/ceiling tube support

1. Floor around the table is free of floor track and tube column
2. One tube can serve more than one table
3. Freer use of a horizontal beam, for example, it can be used from both sides of the table
4. Longer focal film distances can be obtained particularly with horizontal beam work directed at the table because of the increased range of movement
5. Allows easier alignment to accessory equipment such as the vertical bucky stand
6. Movement along the ceiling tracks is smoother and freer than a tube column run-

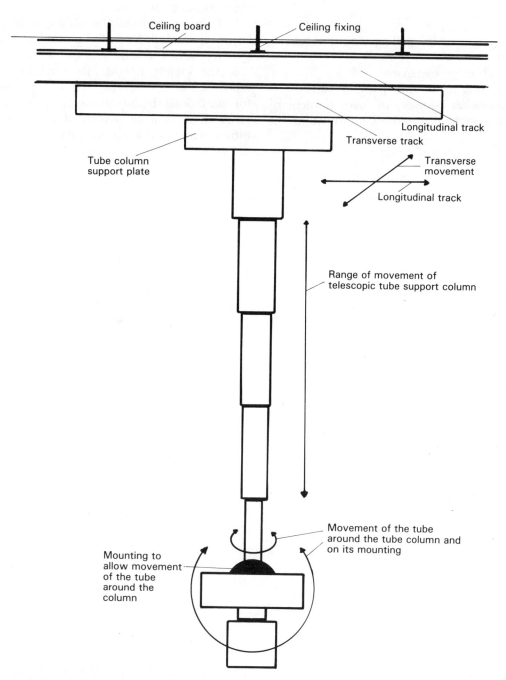

Fig. 15.13 Ceiling supported tube column.

ning in a floor track which may be damaged or dirty.

Disadvantages of the ceiling mounted tube support
1. Much more expensive.
2. Centring to the bucky less positive.
3. Somewhat slower to use particularly when the table is required for most of the work.

4. Focus-to-table distance is not so easily read and often is not accurate as the tape measure tends to drift.
5. Reinforcement of the ceiling or the provision of steel girders will be needed to carry the weight of the tube support.
6. The ceiling height may limit the maximum f.f.d. and affect the lowest level available for horizontal beam radiography, since the range of vertical movement of the telescopic tube column is fixed in manufacture.

16

Specialised fixed units and accessories

In the last chapter the design and function of simple radiographic tables, simple cassetteless systems and tube supports have been described. In this section a brief description is given of the modifications made to general equipment to fulfil the needs of specialised techniques better. It is obviously not practical to include details of all such units nor to explain their particular features as they are so numerous and new designs with improved facilities are constantly becoming available. Readers requiring detailed information on a particular unit are recommended to examine the manufacturers data sheets published for the unit.

1. REMOTELY OPERATED RADIOGRAPHIC/FLUOROSCOPIC TABLE WITH AN INTEGRAL TUBE SUPPORT

In this form of unit, the integral tube support links an over-table tube to an under-table image intensifier or bucky tray (see Fig. 16.1). It is designed to be operated remotely and should be used in this way as the scattered radiation produced by the X-ray beam of an over-table tube is largely directed upwards giving a higher radiation dose to the eyes and thyroid gland of the operator standing beside the patient. Figure 16.2 illustrates the distribution of scattered radiation around a unit with an under-table tube and an over-table tube.

The over-table tube on its support can be raised or lowered to vary the focus-to-film/image intensifier distance and will even at its shortest distance have a longer focus-to-intensifier distance than a unit with an under-table tube.

Advantages of the unit with an integral tube support

1. Less tiring for the operator through the power-driven movement essential in a remotely operated unit.

2. Less radiation dose if the unit is operated remotely from a control unit behind a radiation protective screen.

3. Longer and variable focus-to-film distance can be used for fluoroscopy to give improved image quality as a result of the improved beam geometry.

4. The absence of the bulky over-table image intensifier support gives a better view of the patient who is no longer bothered by equipment suspended close above him.

5. A single tube can provide fluoroscopic and radiographic requirements.

Disadvantages

1. The provision of remote control makes the unit much more costly.

2. Some limitation in the techniques possible with the tube securely linked to the table.

3. Increased radiation dose if table-side pro-

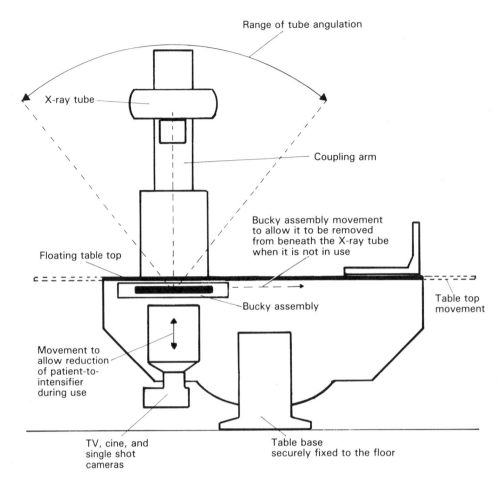

Fig. 16.1 Radiography/fluoroscopy table with an integral tube support.

cedures are undertaken with fluoroscopic control.

4. Remote operation requires greater patient co-operation, and if this is not possible, an electrically operated patient cradle will be required to position the patient.

5. Longer examination times, partly due to the separation of the patient and operator during fluoroscopy and the need to move the image intensifier or bucky tray to allow the alternative unit to be centred to the X-ray beam

Even more complicated fluoroscopic units can be obtained which allow a greater range of movement, permitting bi-plane fluoroscopy and tomography but these units are extremely expensive and can only be justified if there is a very frequent need for their special facilities.

2. SKULL UNITS

The design of specialised skull units has simplified general skull radiography and neuro-radiological techniques by providing:

1. A quicker and easier positioning of the patient, tube and cassette
2. Greater accuracy and easier reproducibility of radiographic projections
3. Special features which are built in rather than attached when needed.

The basic principles of the design

There are two systems in use: the Lysholm and the Dulac system. The Lysholm, a simpler system, is the most commonly used system in the less expensive units suitable for general skull

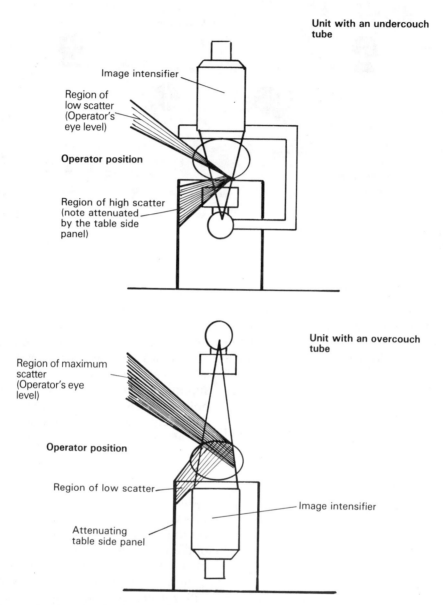

Unit with an undercouch tube

Image intensifier

Region of low scatter (Operator's eye level)

Operator position

Region of high scatter (note attenuated by the table side panel)

Unit with an overcouch tube

Region of maximum scatter (Operator's eye level)

Operator position

Region of low scatter

Image intensifier

Attenuating table side panel

Fig. 16.2 Difference between the distribution of scattered radiation in a unit with an undercouch and an overcouch X-ray tube.

radiography and simple specialised techniques.

The Lysholm system

The distinguishing feature of this system is the position of the centre of rotation of the film holder and the X-ray tube. This is on the same plane as the film (see Fig. 16.3a). The focus-to-film distance is fixed, usually 100 cm.

The Dulac system

The Dulac system is often known as the isocentric system. The X-ray tube and film holder rotate about a fixed point in space; the point chosen to be the centre is the centre of the area of the head to be examined (see Fig. 16.3b). As the centre of rotation is at a point in the patient's head, it is possible to increase or decrease the focus-to-film distance

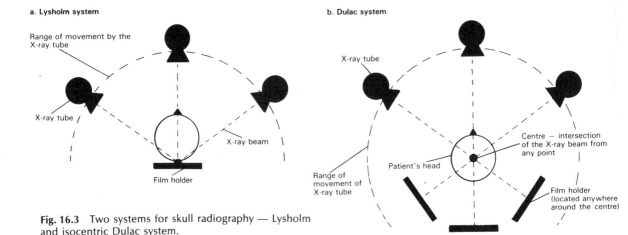

a. Lysholm system

Range of movement by the
X-ray tube

X-ray tube

X-ray beam

Film holder

b. Dulac system

X-ray tube

Centre — intersection
of the X-ray beam from
any point

Patient's head

Range of
movement of
X-ray tube

Film holder
(located anywhere
around the centre)

Fig. 16.3 Two systems for skull radiography — Lysholm and isocentric Dulac system.

and therefore the patient-to-film distance, without altering the position of the patient making techniques such as macro-radiography possible. If the film is placed in the axis of rotation of the X-ray tube and fixed whilst the tube support is allowed to rotate, Lysholm techniques can be used.

Advantages of the Dulac system

1. The patient's head can be positioned and well supported whilst the tube and film are rotated around it.

2. An image intensifier and TV camera, a cine camera, a rapid film changer, full size or 100 mm or a tomographic attachment can be added.

Disadvantages

1. Price.
2. Size.

Lysholm skull unit

The unit consists of a rigid vertical column on which is mounted a freely sliding carriage, accurately counter-balanced to facilitate movement and locking in an accurately set position. The column is given added stability by an extension column either to the ceiling or to the wall behind the unit, and if this is not practical, an extended base-plate must be fitted to reach out under the the object table. The sliding carriage has a pivot about which a C-shaped arm supporting the X-ray tube can rotate. This pivot point is also the centre of rotation for the object table.

The object table has a transparent perspex top with two fixed rails for the attachment of accessories such as an immobilising band or lateral cassette holder. Under the table is a support frame for the bucky and cassette holder which can be rotated to permit the alignment of an angled X-ray beam. The largest cassette which can be used is a 24 × 30 cm. This small field permits the use of a steep angle tube.

The X-ray tube is mounted at a fixed focus-to-film distance, and is attached to its support by a worm gear which allows angulation of the central ray to a point away from the centre of the table. The beam is collimated by a series of simple diaphragms with various sizes of aperture, by cones or by a light beam delineator with rectilinear or iris diaphragms.

There are two devices to aid positioning. The delineator or varay lights which locate the centre of the incident beam, and a mirror system positioned beneath the transparent table top to allow the operator to see where the exit beam will emerge from the patient (see Fig. 16.4b).

The rotation around the carriage on the vertical column allows the X-ray beam to be directed vertically or horizontally.

Accessories can be fitted to allow the cassette to be supported vertically and to allow a series of angiography films to be taken using a vertical or horizontal X-ray beam. In some units it is possible to attach a motor driven tomographic attachment and to use it with the patient in the recumbent or erect position.

Scales are provided at all points on the unit where movement can take place, this enables projections to be precisely performed.

Dulac system

A Dulac system is normally formed from a C-arm or a U-arm mounted on a telescopic vertical column which is generally suspended from the ceiling by a plate which allows the column to rotate around its base. The C-arm is attached to the column by a mounting so

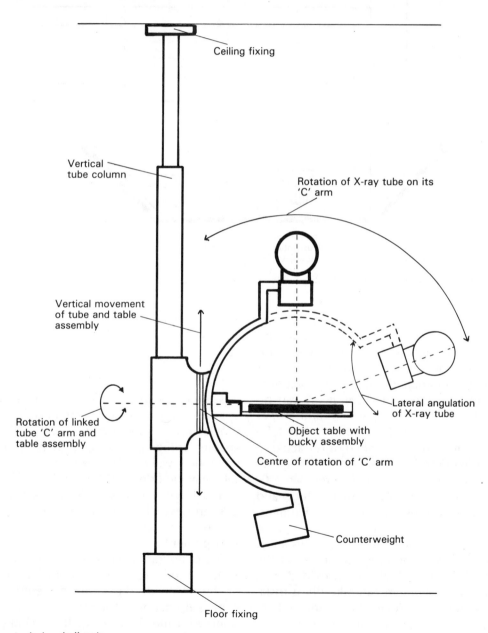

Ceiling fixing

Vertical tube column

Rotation of X-ray tube on its 'C' arm

Vertical movement of tube and table assembly

Lateral angulation of X-ray tube

Rotation of linked tube 'C' arm and table assembly

Object table with bucky assembly

Centre of rotation of 'C' arm

Counterweight

Floor fixing

Fig. 16.4a Lysholm skull unit.

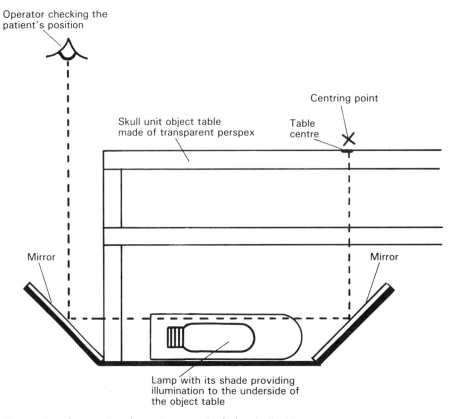

Operator checking the
patient's position

Centring point

Skull unit object table
made of transparent perspex

Table
centre

Mirror

Mirror

Lamp with its shade providing
illumination to the underside of
the object table

Fig. 16.4b Mirror system for centring the patient on a Lysholm skull table.

that the arm can rotate around its attachment (Fig. 16.5). The X-ray tube is fixed to one end of the arm and the cassette holder, image intensifier or film changer fixed to the other end. By a combination of all the rotational movements provided, the central ray can be directed to any point on a sphere and always directed to its centre. The length of the telescopic column can be extended or retracted to allow the isocentre to be adjusted in height.

The cassette being attached to the same C-arm follows the movements of the tube and can be raised and lowered on the attachment, retaining its alignment with the tube, to reduce or increase the object-to-film distance. The part for examination is positioned at the centre of the sphere. Scales are provided at all places where movement can take place to facilitate positioning. Collimation and light indication of the X-ray beam are provided.

Again as with any ceiling suspended unit the finished ceiling height must be at least 3 metres.

3. ANGIOGRAPHIC UNITS

It is the purpose of angiography to record the opacified blood vessels. This necessitates the provision of a radiographic system which will enable radiographic images to be taken at a rate which will display the region's blood vessels opacified despite the rapid passage of the contrast agent and yet still manitain a degree of sharpness which will allow very fine vessels to be seen and in some instances permit enlargement.

The radiographic images can be recorded directly on full size films by photo-fluorography, or by TV with digital image enhancement with subtraction. The last option is only selected if the demand for the technique can justify the great expense of these facilities.

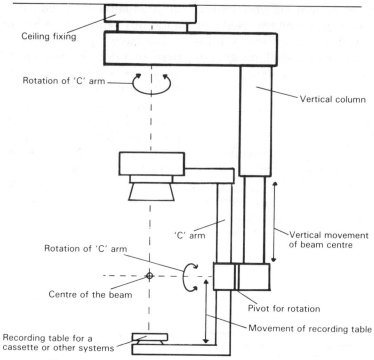

Fig. 16.5a Lateral view of a ceiling supported 'C' arm

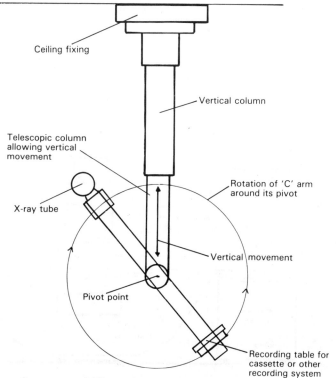

Fig. 16.5b Front view of a ceiling mounted 'C' arm. isocentric system.

In this section the patient support tables, tube supports and film changers used for these techniques will be described. Photofluorography and TV with digital image enhancement are described on pages 179–182 and 176.

Patient support tables

The patient tables for these examinations support the patient above the recording equipment and apart from cerebral angiography, allows the patient to be moved to keep the part for examination over the recording field. The table top must have very low attenuation and yet support the patient's weight. Carbon fibre may be added to the plastic forming the table top to give strength to the structure whilst reducing its attenuation. Any reduction in attenuation will reduce the patient's radiation dose and the loading on the tube.

The table top may be mounted on a simple base or on a fluoroscopy table by a system which gives a very large longitudinal range of movement with an extension beyond the base to allow a film changer to be positioned beneath the table (see Fig. 16.6). With very simple units, it may be necessary to provide a trestle support for the extended end to give stability. The range of table movement allows the patient to be positioned first over the image intensifier for the introduction of the catheter and then moved over the film changer. If peripheral vessels are to be examined, it may be necessary to move the patient during the examination to follow the contrast agent as it travels along the vessel. This movement may be manual but more commonly is motor

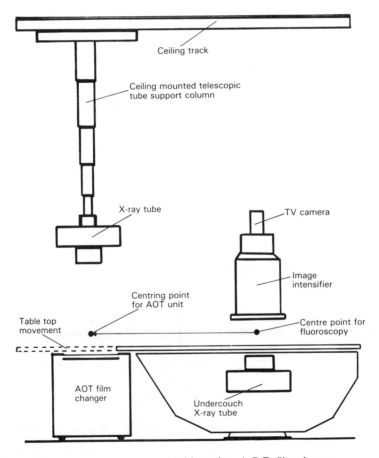

Fig. 16.6 Angiographic unit formed from a fluoroscopy table and an A.O.T. film changer.

driven by a motor which is operated by a pre-set programmer unit which controls all aspects of the examination once the initiating switch is operated. Exposure factors are automatically controlled taking into account the changes of part thickness and density that are encountered during the movement along a limb.

The patient table may be suspended from a support, attached to ceiling tracks, which clears the floor of obstructions and gives free access to C-arm units. Greater longitudinal and transverse movement is possible and the table top height can be adjusted to an ideal working height for the operator because the column supporting the table is telescopic. This form of support is frequently used in installations dedicated to angio-cardiography where

the cost of such systems can be justified by their workload (Fig. 16.7).

Tube supports

The X-ray tube used in angiography may be supported in the conventional way from a ceiling mounted tube support or mounted on a C-arm, as described. The C-arm is better for angio-cardiography than the simple tube support because its variable geometry allows the X-ray beam to be aligned to the ideal plane to display the heart in the optimum projection. Of course, if an oblique angle is used it is necessary to angle the recording equipment to allow the central ray of the X-ray beam to remain perpendicular to its surface. This is sim-

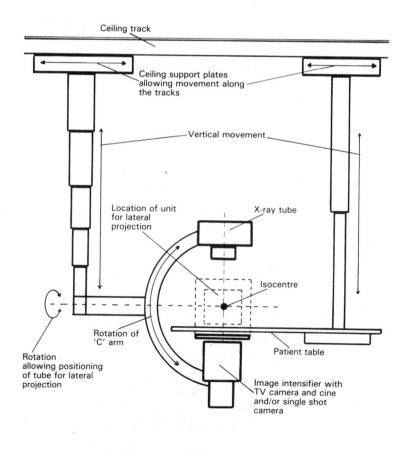

Fig. 16.7 Angiographic unit formed from a ceiling suspended 'C' carrying the X-ray tube and the image intensifier with cameras.

ple with a C-arm for the recording unit(s) can be mounted on the other end of the C-arm.

The recording unit may be an image intensifier with closed circuit TV, perhaps including digital image enhancement, or an image intensifier with photofluorography, single shot and/or cine photography or a small full-size film changer. The last option requires a special mounting block on the C-arm to allow the image intensifier or the film changer to be aligned to the X-ray beam. Figure 16.8 shows the two units on the C-arm at 90° to each other so that a simple rotation of 90° by the mounting block will present the alternative unit. The addition of a second C-arm on a separate support allows bi-plane techniques to be performed.

Film changers

The film changers to be described are those taking a series of full size radiographs; small format single shot and cine cameras was discussed on pages 179–182.

There are two methods of exposing a series of radiographic images. The first uses conventional cassettes, the second delivers just films in rapid succession into the X-ray beam.

Cassette changers are used when a relatively slow rate of repetition and a limited number of images will supply the information required.

For cerebral angiography

Figure 16.9 illustrates the system. Three or five cassettes are exposed in each position. The unit containing the cassettes is mounted on a skull table, and the series of cassettes are changed by hand. Each cassette is held in a steel tray to absorb any radiation transmitted through the cassette above it. Each tray has a handle to facilitate its rapid withdrawal from

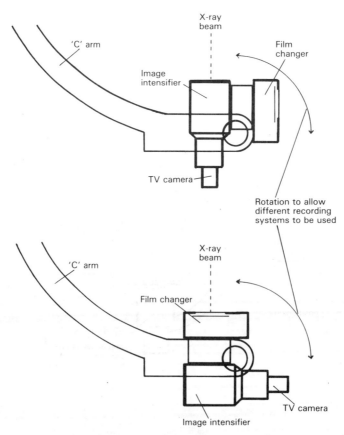

Fig. 16.8 Special mounting on one end of a 'C' arm to allow different recording systems to be selected.

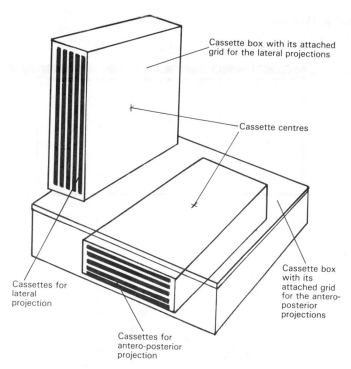

Cassette box with its attached grid for the lateral projections

Cassette centres

Cassette box with its attached grid for the antero-posterior projections

Cassettes for lateral projection

Cassettes for antero-posterior projection

Fig. 16.9 Cassette changer for use with a skull unit.

the changer after it has been exposed. As the tray containing the exposed cassette is pulled from the unit a strong spring pushes the remaining cassettes up so that the top cassette is close behind the grid ready for the next exposure.

This system is adequate for general departments but does require considerable practice for a high repetition rate to be achieved.

For angiography of the limbs
Figure 16.10 shows a 6-sided drum which holds a 30 × 120 cm cassette on each surface. The drum rises before each exposure to be close beneath the patient table with its stationary grid. After a cassette is exposed, the drum lowers and rotates to present another cassette for exposure.

The long film allows the blood vessels of upper or lower limb to be displayed from their origin to their end on a single cassette. Wedge shaped aluminium filters are fitted to the X-ray tube to attenuate the beam so that the image

of the thicker region and the thinner region are satisfactorily displayed by a single exposure. The focus-to-film distance must be very long to cover the long cassette and collimation carefully set to suit the area under examination and to ensure that the cassettes awaiting exposure or after exposure are not fogged.

Advantages claimed for this system are:

1. less dose to the patient.
2. the patient does not require repositioning during the examination to cover the length of the limb.
3. the vessels are displayed whatever the rate of blood flow as each film covers the entire length of the vessel.
4. exposure control is simplified as the same factors can be used for all parts of the limb.

Film changers
There are two types of cut film changer most commonly used with different ways of storing

Side view of unit

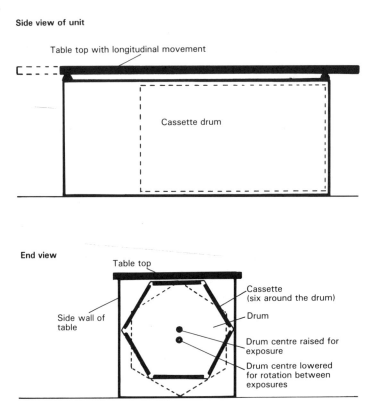

Fig. 16.10 Unit for the angiographic examination of the full length of the limbs.

the films before exposure (Figs 16.11 and 16.12). In one unit they are assembled vertically in a cassette where each film is held in a separate section, while in the other the films are in a pack. Manufacturer's data sheets provide full details of the units so in this text only the general operating principles and the features common to both are described.

The operating parts are contained in a light tight housing which is lead-lined to prevent X-radiation entering through the casing except through the area aligned to the X-ray beam. A storage magazine contains the unexposed films. This magazine is withdrawn from the unit for loading with film and then returned to the unit where it is opened in the dark ready for the films to be extracted for exposure. A collecting magazine is positioned in the unit to receive the films after exposure. This magazine can be closed within the unit so that exposed films can be removed without risk of light fogging the films.

The films are drawn one at a time from the stock of about 20 unexposed films in the storage magazine. They are then carried by a transport system to the exposure area where they pause to receive the X-ray exposure before moving on to the collecting magazine.

When the film is in the exposure area it lies between a pair of intensifying screens which compress it tightly to give good film screen contact. The top screen is secured to a good firm backing of radiolucent material, often carbon fibre. The back screen is mounted on a metal plate which is raised to clamp the film in position as soon as it is aligned in the exposure area. A stationary grid is fitted over the exposure area.

It can be seen that the co-ordination of all the actions needed to position and expose a series of some 20 films at a rate of 3 exposures a second requires the siting of many sensing, operating and safety interlock devices within the unit and the provision of a micro-processor

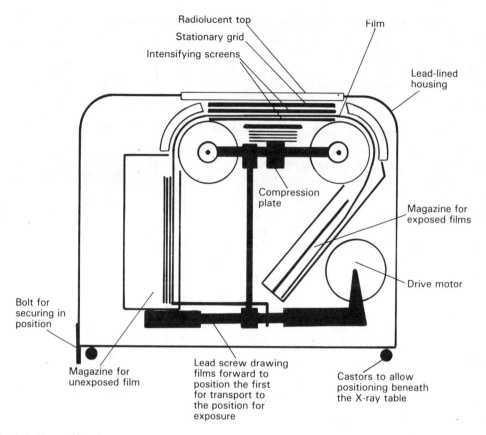

Fig. 16.11 A.O. T. cut film changer.

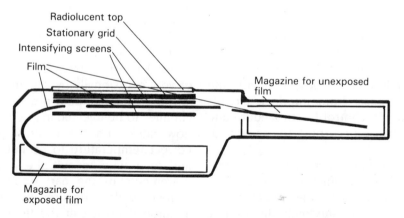

Fig. 16.12 Film changer of compact design suitable for attachment to a 'C' arm unit.

or programmer to handle their signals and actions.

The operator's handbook should be read very carefully as these units are very complex and any lack of care or understanding may re-sult in equipment malfunction. The examinations undertaken with this equipment are not without risk, deliver a high radiation dose and are very costly in time and materials so it is important that the equipment is operated correctly. All manufacturers provide clear setting up procedures and have guides to the location and correction of faults which can be dealt with by the operator.

Cut film changers are made to accept either 35 × 35 cm or 24 × 30 cm films. In General departments a single unit is usually sufficient although bi-plane units are available. The larger changers are normally floor mounted and when in use are securely locked into position to prevent any movement through their vigorous action.

The height of the unit is not variable but some units are mounted on a base which gives a limited amount of movement. The smaller units may be floor mounted but because they are much lighter and more compact they can be mounted on a C-arm. This allows them to be used in the ideal position for the radiographic projection and for the convenience of the operator. Figure 16.13 shows two large units in bi-plane position.

The programmer unit. A programmer unit houses what could be described as a linear programme, and this ensures the correct operating sequence of all the units taking a part in the procedure. The operator introduces information on the number and timing of the series of exposures and the moment when the contrast agent is to be injected. The unit integrates the film transport with the exposure sequence so ensuring that a film is in the correct position every time an exposure is to be made. In addition to all these demands the unit receives signals from interlock circuits and sensors which control the procedure and prevent any harm occurring to patient or equipment.

The older form of programmers are complicated electronic units which require controls and switches to be set by the operator. The modern units operate automatically from a punch card programme which is placed in the unit. This card supplies information to a microprocessor which controls and monitors the procedure. A number of different punch card programmes are kept, one for each of the procedures that may be undertaken.

Contrast injectors. In angiography, contrast

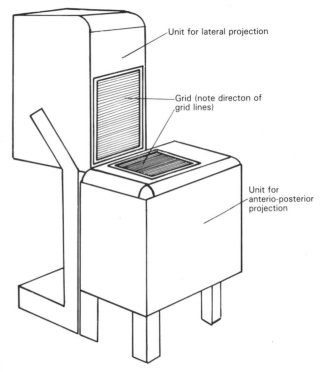

Fig. 16.13   Bi-plane A.O.T. film changer.

agents are introduced into the vascular system through a cannula or a catheter. Although there are a few occasions when the contrast can be injected manually, the majority of injections require a power driven syringe to deliver the quantity of contrast needed in a short time. The drive power is supplied electrically or very occasionally by gas pressure.

The injection should provide for a range of volumes to be injected at one of a selection of flow rates with the contrast heated to the correct temperature to be injected at a time and in a time to suit the physiological requirements of the part under examination; sometimes it is triggered by an ECG unit. In addition it must suit the timing of the X-ray series. The co-ordination of these events and others concerned with exposure, film changing and patient movement are integrated by the programming unit.

Many interlocks and safety devices are necessary to ensure that over pressure, excess volume or excess temperature contrast cannot be injected and that the sequence of events occurring in each piece of equipment is co-ordinated and safe.

The whole operation must be controlled for the injector (if one is in use) by a 'dead-man' type switch so that if the switch is released, the injection and radiation **stop** immediately and the film changer at the next 'null' point.

4. TOMOGRAPHIC UNITS

As the X-ray beam passes through the body, images formed by the various structures within it are shown overlying each other making it difficult to separate details occurring at different levels. In tomography objects at a se-lected plane are shown with good detail whilst those above and below are lost through blur-ring. The technique requires a system of co-ordinated movement of the film and focal spot about a fixed plane within the patient, or less commonly a movement of tube focus and pa-tient about the film. The principles of tom-ography are best explained by considering the simplest form, linear tomography by means of a tomographic attachment.

Linear tomography by a tomographic attachment

In tomography the X-ray tube and film move parallel to the plane of sharpness (see Fig. 16.14). Magnification is constant over the entire swing of the tube and film, but alters as the plane of sharpness is raised or lowered (Fig. 16.15). In practice this variation in the magnification of the image is too small to be significant. The plane of sharpness lies on the plane of the pivot point and runs parallel to the film.

Examination of Figure 16.16 shows that to obtain a tomograph it is necessary to couple the tube and bucky tray by a link pole and to pivot the pair about a point at the plane of sharpness required. The plane is sometimes termed the cut. The exposure is made as the tube and film move. The movement must be smooth and at a controllable speed coupled

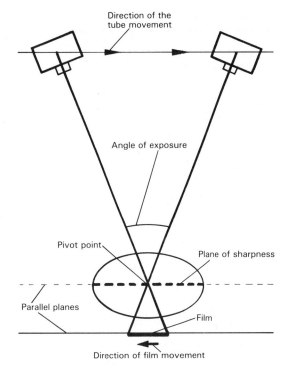

Fig. 16.14 Principles of linear tomography.

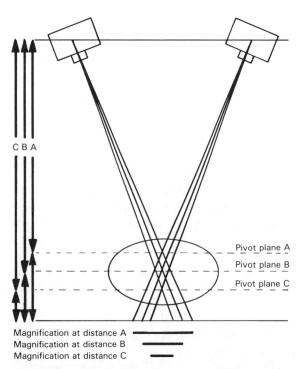

Magnification at distance A ──────
Magnification at distance B ────
Magnification at distance C ──

Fig. 16.15 Variation of the degree of magnification with different pivot levels set on a simple linear tomographic unit.

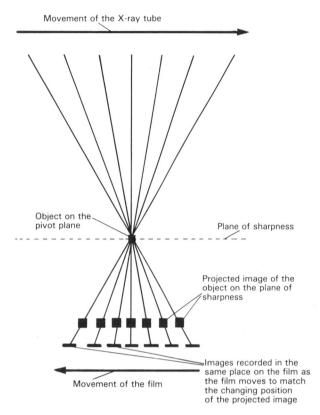

Fig. 16.16 Linear tomography.

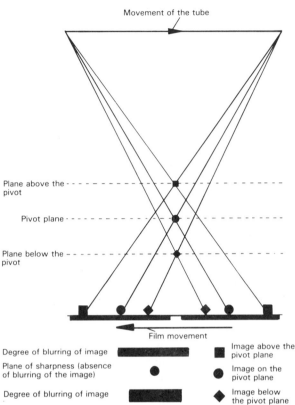

Fig. 16.17 Only objects on the pivot plane are recorded without blur.

with the exposure controls. The pivot point must be rigid, either on a pivot block which is firmly attached to the X-ray table top or sub-frame or in some dedicated tomographic units on a separate support. The height of the pivot in relation to the patient must be variable to allow a series of cuts to be obtained through the part to be examined. This is achieved by raising or lowering the pivot point or in some cases by raising the patient with respect to a fixed pivot point. Very recently equipment has been produced which, by the use of micro-processor control of tube and film movement, eliminates the need for a link pole and the sharpness level is controlled by the speed of travel of the film. This is a complicated concept and will not be considered further.

The thickness of the layer is determined by the amount of image unsharpness that is acceptable. Reference to Figure 16.17 shows that objects lying on the plane of the pivot are always projected on the same spot on the film and therefore appear sharp. Objects above or below this level are not projected on to the same spot as the tube moves across and so appear blurred. The degree of blurring depends upon the amount of movement that takes place. Therefore the greater the amount of movement, the thinner the layer remembering that it is the actual angle crossed by the tube during the exposure and not the angle of total tube travel. In Figure 16.18 the position of the micro-switches which control the exposure is shown along with how the exposure angle can be altered. The control of the exposure will be considered in greater detail on page 251.

The thickness of the layers having acceptable unsharpness obtained by the use of some typical exposure angles are as follows (see also Fig. 16.19):

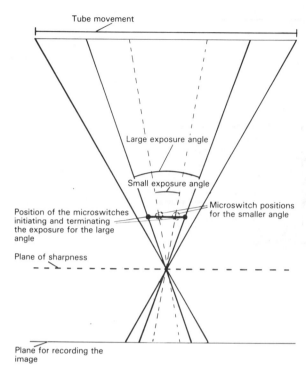

Fig. 16.18 Variation of the exposure angle by adjusting the position of the microswitch initiating the exposure, and the second terminating the exposure.

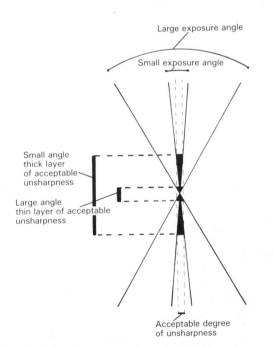

Fig. 16.19 Diagram to show how the thickness of a layer with acceptable unsharpness varies with different exposure angles.

60° angle	1.0 mm
30° angle	2.3 mm
10° angle	7.0 mm
5° angle	14.0 mm

The 5° and 10° angles give comparatively thick layers of acceptable sharpness and are used in zonography where the structures to be blurred are some distance in front or behind the part under examination and the sharp layer will display the part with the minimum number of tomographic cuts.

In the simple tomographic attachment, the layer height is adjusted by altering the pivot height by a knob which raises or lowers the point around which the link arm turns. Figure 16.20 shows the design of a very simple attachment which is secured to the patient support table. The link arm coupling the X-ray tube to the bucky tray must be telescopic or have some other means of altering its length to accommodate the changing focus to film distance as the tube moves from the exposure start position, across the vertical and on to the stop position. The link arm must also have a slot or some similar device to allow the pivot height to be raised or lowered (see Fig. 16.20a).

The control of exposure

In most units the exposure is started and stopped by the tomographic attachment. Selection of 'tomography' on the control panel transfer the control to the tomographic attachment. It is important that the mid-point of the exposure time is reached when the tube is at the mid-point of its travel. The simplest method of obtaining this is by placing a 'make' micro-switch and a 'break' micro-switch on the tomographic pivot attachment equidistant from the mid-point of the tube travel so that the link arm starts and ends the exposure by applying pressure on the micro-switches as it passes across them.

The speed of the tube's travel across the exposure angle also controls the length of the exposure time. Therefore to give greater exposure flexibility the motor which drives the tube support has a selector for slow and fast speed.

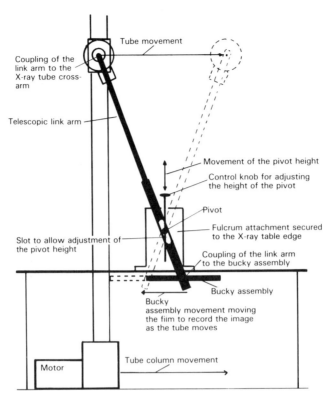

Fig. 16.20a Linear tomographic attachment fitted to the edge of the X-ray table (seen from the table side).

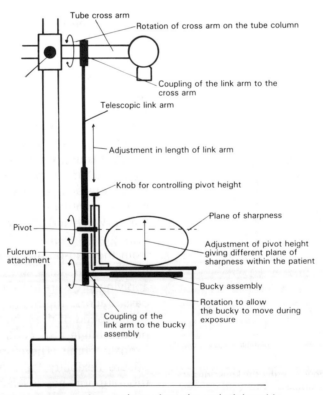

Fig. 16.20b Simple linear tomographic attachment shown from the end of the table.

Thus exposure time is controlled by the speed of the tube travel and the angle through which the exposure is made. The angle over which the exposure is made is selected on the attachment by setting the position where the 'make' and 'break' micro-switches operate. The angle determines the thickness of the layer.

There are units which employ automatic exposure control to ensure that the film density is optimum throughout the tube travel. Some sophisticated units even cut the exposure over the central part of the travel to reduce the dominance of this part caused by the reduced focus-to-film distance and the reduced blurring over this central area (see Fig. 16.21).

These techniques lead to an improved tomographic effect brought about by the increased emphasis on the image produced at the limits of the travel where the blurring of the unwanted shadows is at its maximum.

Other factors to be considered when selecting an exposure

In all tomography techniques the contrast of the radiograph is very low. This is due to the very thin layer in which the structures are sharply defined and each has contrast between adjacent structures. All the rest of the object's thickness above and below this layer is blurred by movement and forms an almost

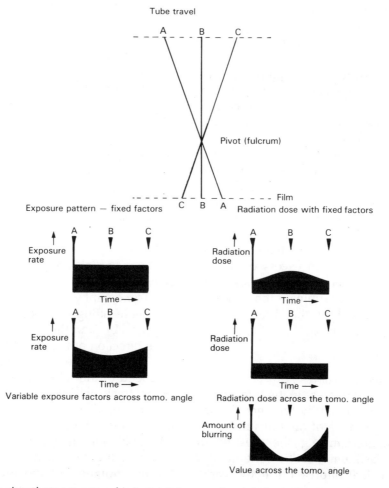

Fig. 16.21 Graphs to show how a tomographic image is improved and the radiation dose reduced if the exposure is varied as the tube crosses the exposure angle.

homogeneous non-image forming overall greyness. Therefore every means of increasing contrast must be used. These include low kVp, close collimation of the X-ray beam, an efficient grid aligned to the X-ray beam throughout its travel, high contrast intensifying screens and the use of displacement technique where practical.

Definition is also very important, so very smooth tube movement during the exposure is essential, for any random movement will effectively increase the focus size. Care must also be taken to secure the cassette in the bucky tray so that no movement can occur here during the travel of the bucky tray. In common with all radiographic techniques, the smallest possible focal spot size should be selected within the loading of the tube especially as in tomography the area of interest is on a plane well above the film giving a large object film distance.

Since the exposure is determined by the length of time the tube takes to cover the tomographic angle, a wide range of tube current must be available to allow the required mAs for the right film density to be fitted into the travel time selected. Many units provide for this by fitting a control which allows the free setting of very low tube currents, and if a very high mAs value is needed, a tube with very high rating will allow a high tube current to be used.

All units have an exposure time automatically set up by the unit in excess of the exposure time controlled by the tomographic attachment which will terminate the exposure in the unlikely event of the 'break' microswitch failing to operate.

The use of added filtration

There are a number of areas in the body where the part to be examined by tomography presents a very large range of densities to be displayed on a single film, e.g. the chest where the dense mediastinum must be penetrated to show the bronchial bifurcation at the carina and the radiolucent lung fields not over exposed in their peripheral areas. The most sat-

isfactory method is to add additional filtration to the beam so that the beam has an almost homogeneous spectrum of high energy X-ray photons. In this way contrast may be reduced to a level that can be recorded on a film and information in areas of low density seen as well as those of high density. Very high kVp or low contrast film will have the same effect.

Other desirable equipment features

1. Simple means of coupling the link arm to the tube and bucky tray through the pivot.
2. Simple rigid tomographic attachment easily and securely fitted on to the frame of the patient support table.
3. Easily set pivot point allowing the layer height to be varied from 0–25 cm above the table top.
4. Adjustable tomographic angles up to 60° and down to 5°.
5. Variable motor drive.
6. Floating table top to allow easy positioning of the area of examination beneath the X-ray beam.

All features must be designed for quick and easy assembly, accurate setting up of layer height and of the angle of travel, with smooth controllable movement.

Some manufacturers supply a bucky tray which will accept a multi-section cassette.

Problems and/or limitations of tomographic attachments

1. Tomography is restricted to a linear movement along the long axis of the patient support table and this movemenet may not be in the direction of the ideal blurring movement.
2. The exposure time, being controlled by the speed of the tube travel along the floor or ceiling track, will be lengthened or erratic if any dust or damage prevents the free movement of the tube along the track.
3. Reduction in definition or apparent increase in the thickness of the cut can arise through vibration of the tube or bucky tray during its travel from unevenness of the floor or track or wear in the tracks or bearings.

The problems are overcome by dedicated tomographic units. These are designed to perform tomography in the best possible manner. The needs of other radiographic techniques are not considered where they will detract from the operating efficiency of their tomographic function. As is the case with all dedicated units, their limitation to one function and their cost must be justified by their expected workload.

The dedicated tomographic unit

The dedicated tomographic unit has an integrated tube stand designed to provide a selection of tube movements (Fig. 16.22). Including:

Linear — longitudinal and transverse,
Circular — with alternative diameter lengths,
Eliptical — with the long axis along or across
the patient support table
Hypocycloidal
Spiral

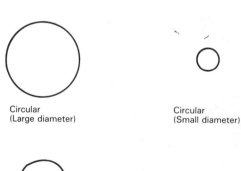

Linear
(Longitudinal and transverse)

Eliptical
(Longitudinal and transverse)

Circular
(Large diameter)

Circular
(Small diameter)

Hypocycloidal

Spiral

Fig. 16.22 Various types of tomographic movements.

The effectiveness of the blurring provided by these movements depends upon the angle through which the tube moves and the distance of the object from the plane of sharpness.

It is important in these units providing movements other than a simple linear movement to arrange for the grid to revolve in unison with the tube so that the X-radiation from the tube does not cut across the grid lines.

In these units the X-ray tube is fitted to one end of a strong column and the film holder to the other. The column is supported through a pivot to a heavy base (Fig. 16.23). The heavy base ensures stability as the tube and film support column are driven rapidly around a complex blurring path so preventing movement of the base, vibration of the tube or film holder or mechanical failure due to the strain of moving heavy components. The selection of a particular blurring path is made on the control unit and this action causes the motor-driven column to move the X-ray tube around the selected trajectory.

In dedicated units the patient is supported on a table which is independent of the tube support. By raising or lowering the patient on the table the desired plane of sharpness in the patient can be obtained by bringing it to the same level as the fixed pivot position. In this way the image magnification factor is constant at all levels of cut since the ratio of focus-object and object-film distances does not vary.

Magnification technique can generally be performed with these units since it is only necessary (a) to fit an additional cassette holder well below the normal holder, increasing further the object-film distance, and (b) to select a tube with a micro-focus. As a grid is not necessary in macro-radiography, the grid is removed to reduce the radiation needed to expose adequately the film and to avoid any problems associated with the alignment of the grid to the X-ray beam. The low position of this cassette holder also permits its angulation and makes inclined plane tomography a simple procedure, (Fig. 16.24).

An additional feature that may be supplied on request is an image intensifier and closed

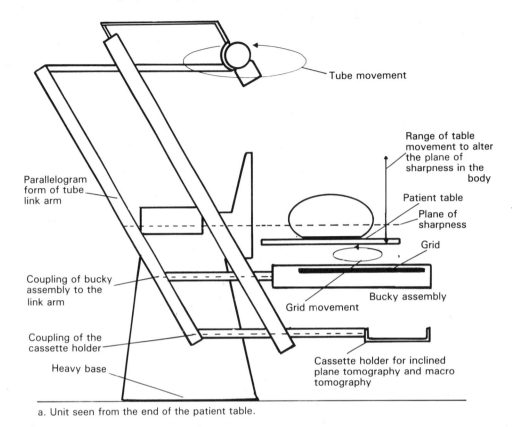

Tube movement

Range of table movement to alter the plane of sharpness in the body

Patient table

Plane of sharpness

Grid

Parallelogram form of tube link arm

Coupling of bucky assembly to the link arm

Grid movement

Bucky assembly

Coupling of the cassette holder

Heavy base

Cassette holder for inclined plane tomography and macro tomography

a. Unit seen from the end of the patient table.

Fig. 16.23A Dedicated tomographic unit seen from the end of the patient table.

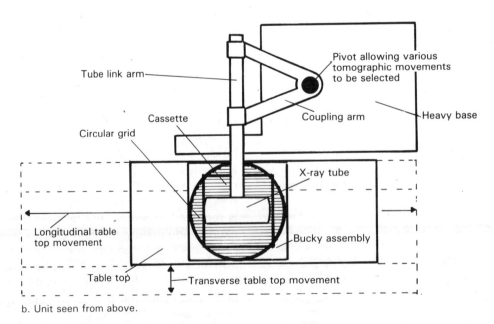

Tube link arm

Pivot allowing various tomographic movements to be selected

Cassette

Coupling arm

Heavy base

Circular grid

X-ray tube

Longitudinal table top movement

Bucky assembly

Table top

Transverse table top movement

b. Unit seen from above.

Fig. 16.23B Dedicated tomographic unit seen from above.

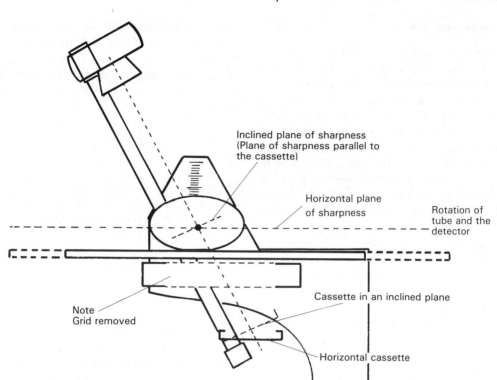

Fig. 16.24   Inclined plane tomography.

circuit TV system to simplify centering. The most sophisticated units may permit the unit to be used in the vertical as well as the horizontal position.

Advantages of a dedicated unit over a simple tomographic attachment

1. A range of blurring movements is available.

2. There is a constant magnification factor whatever plane is selected.

3. Image magnification techniques can be easy undertaken.

4. The fixed focus-to-film distance ensures a standard length of tube travel for the movement selected.

5. More accurate selection of layer thickness.

6. More effective blurring of unwanted shadows,

7. Inclined plane tomography is possible,

8. Very even stable tube and cassette movement.

Disadvantages

1. Price.

2. Function limited almost entirely to tomography.

3. Decision to use tomography must be made before the examination commences.

4. No chance of interposing some tomographic views during a procedure such as intra-venous urography.

5. Requires plenty of space for its installation and so may limit the accommodation available for more routine techniques which represent a very high percentage of the work of most departments.

6. Its sophistication requires very skilled maintenance.

Multisection tomography

Multisection tomography is the technique which enables a number of cuts to be obtained at different levels with a single exposure. Figure 16.25 shows the principle. To perform this technique it is only necessary to modify the bucky tray to hold a magazine containing the films and their intensifying screens in the correct position. The uppermost film in the magazine must be positioned at the level of the film in an ordinary cassette in the bucky tray. The films below this level will record planes of sharpness at lower levels.

The magazine, a light, tight box, holds the films between their intensifying screens and each set of screens separated by radiolucent compressible packing, polyfoam for example. The thickness of the packing controls the position of the films within the box, and so the level of cut they will record. Therefore the separation of the films must be calculated, taking into account the magnification factor for the exact location of the cuts within the patient to be known. The formula for this calculation is:

$$F1 = B1 \left(1 + \frac{d}{D}\right)$$

where: F1 = film spacing
B1 = cut spacing
d = pivot to top film distance
D = focus to pivot distance

The contents of the box must be compressed by the lid to ensure good film/screen contact. Figure 16.26(a) shows the arrangement of the magazine and its contents. Because of the absorption of each film/screen pair and the increasing focus-to-film distance, the exposure received by a film will be progressively lessened as the film is positioned for a lower cut. To compensate for this a series of intensifying screens with different intensifying factors will be needed.

Figure 16.26(b) shows the film/screen combinations of a five cut box selected to give each film the same exposure by increasing the speed of the screens so that when the five films are developed they will have the same density.

A similar multisection system can be used for the very close cuts required in tomography of the inner ear, but here no interspace material is used between the screens. Three films and their screens are placed one above the other in an ordinary deep cassette and when developed they will give three cuts separated only by the thickness of two screens.

For the best results it is unwise to expose too many films simultaneously. It is particularly important that there is very good screen contact and that the cassette is securely fixed during its movement. The X-ray beam must be closely collimated to eliminate the maximum amount of scatter.

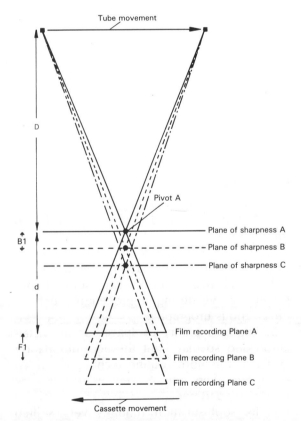

Fig. 16.25 Principles of multisection tomography.

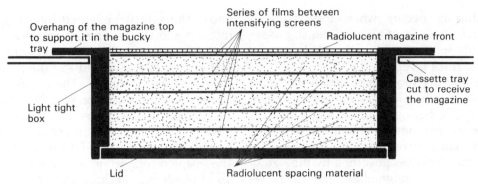

Overhang of the magazine top to support it in the bucky tray

Series of films between intensifying screens

Radiolucent magazine front

Cassette tray cut to receive the magazine

Light tight box

Lid

Radiolucent spacing material

a. Magazine showing features of the box and its support by the bucky tray.

Intensifying screens

High definition

Standard

Fast

Film

Packing material

b. Suggested set of film/screen combinations to give a series of five films of similar density.

Fig. 16.26 A multisection magazine.

Advantages of multisection tomography over single section tomography

1. Reduced patient dose.

2. All cuts taken at the same time, therefore all are at the same phase of physiological activity.

3. Less time taken for the examination, therefore less strain on the patient.

4. Less loading on the tube.

5. More accurate layer separation because of the fixed relationship between one cut and the one below.

Disadvantages

1. Some loss of image quality in the lower cuts.

2. Restriction in the choice of film/screen combinations.

3. Less flexibility in the kVp selected because of the change in the screens response to different kVp.

4. Identification of individual cuts is more difficult to arrange.

Tomography — procedure planning

In planning a tomographic examination it is important to have information on exactly what is to be demonstrated. Plain radiographs of the part are taken and examined to determine:

1. the patient position displaying the part most satisfactorily, remembering that maxi-

mum blurring occurs when the image is spread over the widest area, so dense images such as the spine should if possible be placed above the pivot level.

2. the blurring movement which will most effectively eliminate any unwanted dominant images, remembering that blurring is most effective when the tomographic movement cuts across dominant dense structures:

3. the cut thickness governed by the size of the part to be tomographed, the detail required and the separation of it from other structures above and below.

4. the number of cuts and their location within the body to ensure that all the part is examined.

It is important that the equipment is correctly assembled and the exposure factors selected to give maximum image information. Regular testing of the equipment is essential to ensure that it operates at maximum performance.

Care must be taken to ensure that all the cassettes and their contained film and intensifying screens are similar in absorption and speed, otherwise there will be differences in density in the cuts, unless a multisection box is to be used.

Computed tomography

The main components (Fig. 16.27) of the computed tomography unit are the X-ray tube, the collimator which reduces the X-ray beam to a fine rectangular beam, the wedge filter which compensates for the shape of the part being examined, the radiolucent patient support table, and the array of detectors. The detectors assess the radiation dose by means of a crystal or by a gas. The current generated by the detector in response to the radiation is amplified by a photomultiplier tube and passed to the computer.

The computer gathers the information as it scans around the patient either by simple rotation or by a linear movement followed by rotation. The scanning times for a complete rotation vary from a few seconds to 20 seconds. The rate is governed by the speed of rotation and the number of detectors.

At each position the attenuation of the beam by the patient is assessed and the information stored by the computer. The computer using all the stored information calculates the actual attenuation of every element within the part traversed. An element, described as a pixel, is a small block of tissue of 0.5 mm^2 or 1.8 mm^2. The image displayed on the TV monitor is built up of pixels, but because the eye can only appreciate between 20 and 30 shades of grey, the computer cannot at one time display all the information of the pixels it has stored. However, the computer can present its stored information in different ways. For instance only certain levels of attenuation can be displayed as shades of grey on an expanded scale by operating the controls or fewer shades of grey can be shown on the full scale. This alteration in the grey scale is spoken of as a change in band width. The information held on the computer can be shown straight away on the TV monitor or stored on floppy discs for showing at another time. Reconstruction techniques can be performed which amalgamate the information from several transverse cuts and reassemble them to give a longitudinal image of the area being examined.

The range of techniques and facilities available will not be discussed here nor will the detail of the operation of the different units be discussed, and readers are recommended to obtain the excellent technical information published by the manufacturers of the units.

MAMMOGRAPHIC EQUIPMENT

Mammography is the soft tissue radiography of the breast. The tissues forming the breast have very similar densities and so give very low subject contrast. The minimal differences in density must be amplified to allow the different tissues to be identified. In addition, very small discrete areas of calcification may be present within the breast tissue and these are of diagnostic significance, to see them the image must display very fine detail. It is also

a. Scanning movement around the patient

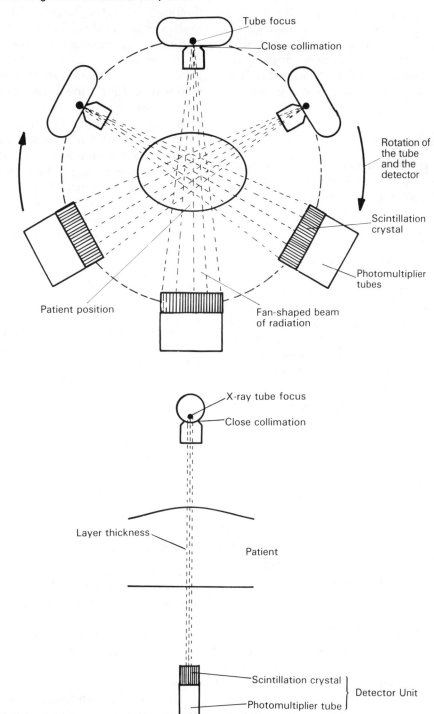

b. Narrowness of the beam across the long axis of the X-ray tube

Fig. 16.27 Principles of computed tomography.

important to limit the radiation dose to a minimum as breast tissue is very radio-sensitive. Therefore the equipment and radiographic technique must (1) improve image contrast, (2) minimise image unsharpness and provide for visualisation of very fine detail and (3) keep the dose low to satisfy these requirements.

1. Improve contrast

Maximum contrast between breast structures is produced by a kilovoltage between 20 and 30 kVp. The kilovoltage selected must be just adequate to penetrate the thickness of tissue. With such a low kV it is necessary to reduce the filtration of the X-ray beam to a minimum by removing all added filtration and by reducing the inherent filtration of the tube insert. The inherent filtration is reduced by grinding the glass of the envelope where the useful X-ray beam leaves the tube to reduce the thickness of the glass and to reduce the depth of oil between the insert and the shield. It is electrically safe to cut the amount of insulating oil as the kV is so low.

Reduction of scattered radiation will improve the contrast of the image, so very close collimation of the beam is provided by a diaphragm positioned very near to the insert to prevent the escape of off-focus radiation, or in some units the off-focus radiation is absorbed within the tube insert by placing a hood around the anode. Tissue compression will reduce the amount of scatter produced within the tissues. Compression is provided by a compression band or by a long cone whose end compresses the breast.

2. Minimise image unsharpness

The use of a fine focus, 0.6 mm or less, will reduce the geometric unsharpness made worse because some of the breast tissue is a distance from the film.

A tube with a steep angle anode, which the small field size permits, will allow the use of a higher tube current and a shorter exposure time to reduce the risk of patient movement.

Molybdenum is used as the X-ray tube target to take advantage of the increased X-ray production through characteristic radiation in molybdenum at 29 kVp. This increased X-ray output allows the exposure time to be reduced to minimise motional unsharpness. Molybdenum has a comparatively low melting point which would limit the tube loading at a high kV but does not produce significant limitation at the low operating kV. Figure 16.28 shows the spectrum of the X-radiation at 25–35 kVp from a molybdenum and a tungsten target.

The focal spot size is kept to its small size by reducing the filament to target distance to ensure close control of the electron beam which is not so well controlled at the normal distance by a low anode potential. It is electrically safe to reduce the gap between cathode and anode as the low potential will not produce a spark able to jump the gap.

The focus-to-film distance is as long as is practical to reduce the geometric unsharpness.

The film and intensifying screen combination is selected to give maximum detail, good contrast and have a speed which will allow a short exposure time to reduce the risk of motional unsharpness and to cut the radiation dose.

As image sharpness is affected by patient or equipment movement, the unit supporting the tube and film must be very stable and allow the patient to be positioned comfortably and so be able to keep still. Specially designed compression devices aid immobilisation.

3. Reduce radiation dose

The low energy beam required for mammography permits the use of a molybdenum target and this reduces the dose compared with that of a tungsten target. When a purpose built molybdenum target tube with a molybdenum filter is used the dose is cut to about one-third of the dose from a normal tungsten target tube.

The use of a long focus-to-film distance will reduce the dose to the skin especially in the part of the breast nearest to the radiation source.

Intensifying screens are used to enable the quantity of radiation to be greatly reduced.

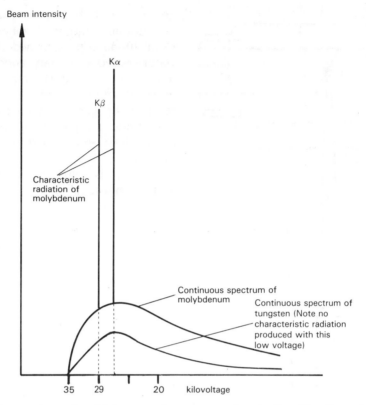

Fig. 16.28 The radiation spectrum of molybdenum and tungsten produced with a kilovoltage of 35.

The use of screens is the major factor in dose reduction.

The equipment used for mammography includes all or most of the features listed above and is designed to have a wide range of movement to allow the radiographic projections to be obtained easily without requiring the patient to hold an uncomfortable position even when they are standing, sitting or lying.

There are two types of unit available: the dedicated unit designed just for mammography having its own generator; and the unit with a special X-ray tube, tube column and cassette holder which is powered by a generator serving other tubes.

The dedicated mammography unit

Figure 16.29 shows the main features of a unit which has its generator enclosed in the casing which supports the tube and cassette. One of these units has a constant potential generator to provide a constant voltage to increase the

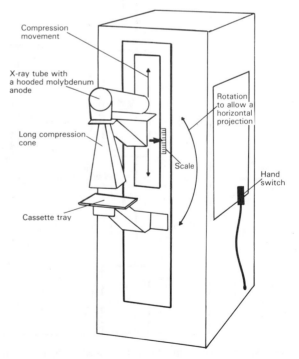

Fig. 16.29 Dedicated mammography unit.

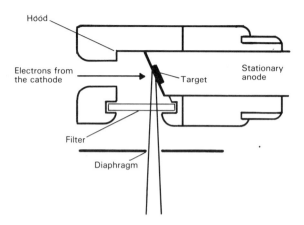

Fig. 16.30 A section through a hooded anode.

generation of characteristic radiation from the molybdenum target. A range of kilovoltages from 10–40 kVp is provided. The tube is a water-cooled stationary anode tube with the molybdenum target set in a copper block. The water is pumped up behind the target to remove the generated heat more effectively. The anode is hooded (Fig. 16.30) to eliminate as much off-focus (extra-focal) radiation as possible.

The tube is a dual focus tube with a 0.8 mm and 1.0 mm focal spot.

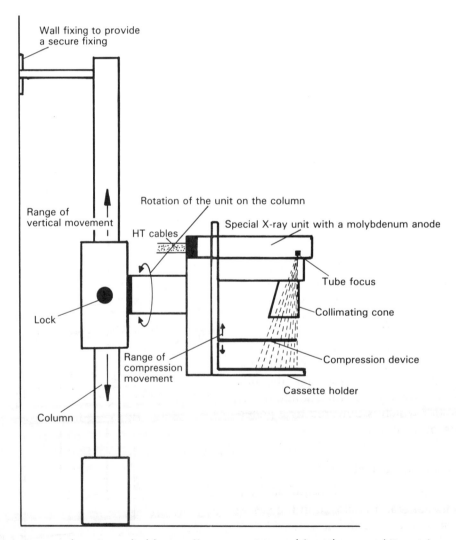

Fig. 16.31 A mammography unit supplied from an X-ray-generator supplying other normal X-ray tubes.

The special tube supplied by an ordinary generator

From Figure 16.31 it can be seen that the tube shield in this unit is specially designed to make alignment of the X-ray beam with the patient for this examination less difficult.

The tube is a rotating anode tube with a molybdenum target which allows 300 mA to be used at 30 kVp

For radiation protection — because of the absence of the required 2.5 mm Al eq. filter which is demanded for ordinary higher voltages used by the other tubes supplied by the same generator, and to prevent overloading of the mammography tube — a number of safety devices and interlocks are introduced into the circuit to make sure that the tube can only receive the exposure factors used for mammography.

Accessories available for both types include automatic exposure control, immobilising devices and a special chair for the patient which makes the setting up procedure more accurate. These together with an automatic exposure control reduces the risk of repeat exposures.

Recently specially low attenuating grids have been introduced to improve the image contrast.

DENTAL EQUIPMENT

Dental equipment can be considered in two groups: the simple dental unit found in most dental surgeries; and the sophisticated units required to provide information for orthodontic procedures.

1. The simple dental unit (Fig. 16.32)

The equipment for general dental work is designed to fulfil the needs of intra and extra oral radiography. The main requirements are that: the unit does not occupy too much space; it is simple, light, easy to manoeuvre and capable of maintaining a position without the need for locks and provide for very easy accurate angulation.

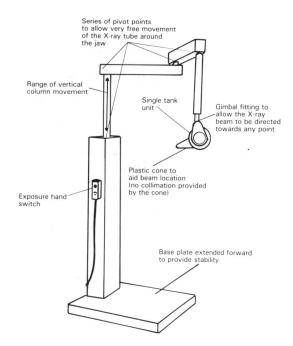

Fig. 16.32 Simple dental unit.

The radiographic output must be sufficient for all dental and some facio-maxillary examinations, and its must be able to operate from a low output electrical socket, 13 amp, 240 Volts.

It must be electrically safe and conform to radiation protection requirements.

The unit will be described in three parts: the tubehead, the tube support and the control unit.

The tubehead

The tubehead contains the X-ray tube, the high tension transformer, the filament transformer and the expansion bellows (Fig. 16.33). This single tank arrangement is possible because the output required is low and so does not require bulky insulation. The mA and kVp are fixed in value, or if adjustment is provided, it is limited to a choice of two kilovoltage settings. The limitation of the variables supplied reduces the space needed to house the components.

All of the tubehead contents are immersed in oil and because the high tension trans-

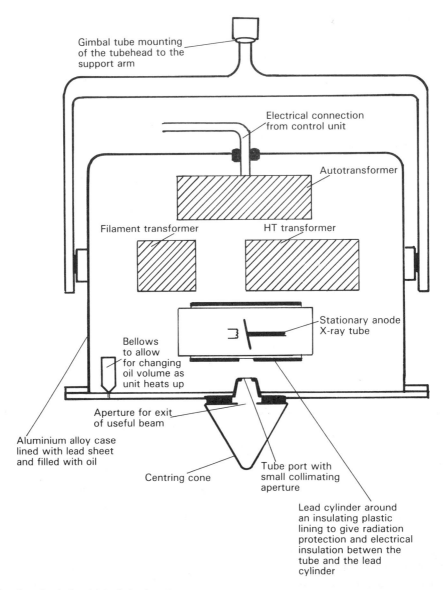

Fig. 16.33 The dental tubehead (single tank unit).

former is one of these components there are no external high tension cables. The absence of the heavy and relatively rigid high tension cables makes the tube head much easier to position. The only connections to the tubehead are those to the primary winding of the high tension transformer, the earthing conductor and sometimes the leads to a milli-ammeter positioned on the control panel.

The casing of the tubehead is made of aluminium alloy, lined where necessary with lead

sheet to ensure the required radiation protection level is reached. The useful radiation leaves the tubehead through a small tube port fitted with an additional collimating diaphragm to restrict the beam size to the smallest size which will cover the field size of dental films. There are two types of cone attached to the mounting plate surrounding the tube port. One is a conical plastic cone which serves only as a centring device and as a means of preventing the use of a too short focus-to-film distance. The other is a conventional type of cone made of metal which acts as an additional collimator and ensures the use of a much longer focus-to-film distance.

This longer focus-to-film distance has two advantages: it reduces the skin dose and improves the image quality by providing a more parallel X-ray beam (Fig. 16.34). The main disadvantages are that the positioning of the tube requires a greater range of movement around the patient to accommodate the siting of the focus further from the patient and the extra distance which requires a larger exposure. Figure 16.35 illustrates the two types of tubehead with their different types of cone.

There are also two types of X-ray tube in use. The more common is the simple stationary anode type which is found in most short focus-to-film units. In the more expensive sophisticated units a grid tube is used with a long focus-to-film distance.

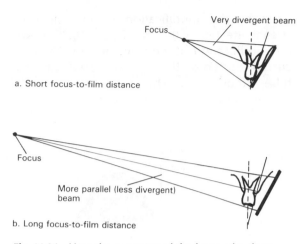

a. Short focus-to-film distance

b. Long focus-to-film distance

Fig. 16.34 How the geometry of the beam of a short focus-to-film dental unit differs from the more sophisticated long focus-to-film distance unit.

Simple stationary tube

The simple stationary anode tube has a single filament giving an effective focus of around 0.8 mm. The tube acts as its own rectifier. This is almost the only remaining form of self rectified unit marketed today. The only other unit where it is occasionally used is the very small, truly portable units.

To simplify the provision of radiation protection and to lessen the weight of the tubehead, it is common to find the tube invested in a lead sheet cylinder around its central area which has an aperture to allow the useful X-ray beam to emerge. By using this lead cylinder it is possible to reduce the amount of lead lining necessary for the housing to only those regions where additional protection is needed to ensure that the leakage radiation does not exceed the statutory limits.

The output from this type of tube is around 50–60 kVp and 7.5 mA with a range of times 0.1–1.0 seconds.

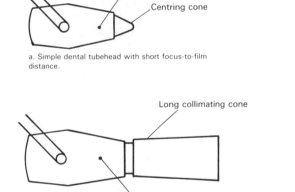

a. Simple dental tubehead with short focus-to-film distance.

b. Tubehead of sophisticated unit with long focus-to-film distance.

Fig. 16.35 Two types of dental tubehead.

The grid tube

The grid tube is a stationary anode tube with the cathode focusing cup separately biased to act as a grid. The effect of the grid is to prevent the passage of electrons across the tube until they are accelerated by the higher kilovoltage parts of the half cycles. This cut-off action gives an X-ray beam which contains more of the high energy photons which form the image, and fewer of the low energy photons which do not contribute to the image but do increase the skin dose. The output of this tube is greater than the simple stationary anode tube for the load on the target is lessened by the modification of the electron stream effected by the grid. Figure 16.36 shows the modification of the waveform of the tube current caused by the grid compared with the tube without a grid. The output of these units is around 65 kVp at 7.5 mA.

The tube support
The tubehead is connected to the tube support through a gimbal type of joint. The support has three or four other points of rotation which allow the X-ray beam to be pointed in any direction. The support system is well

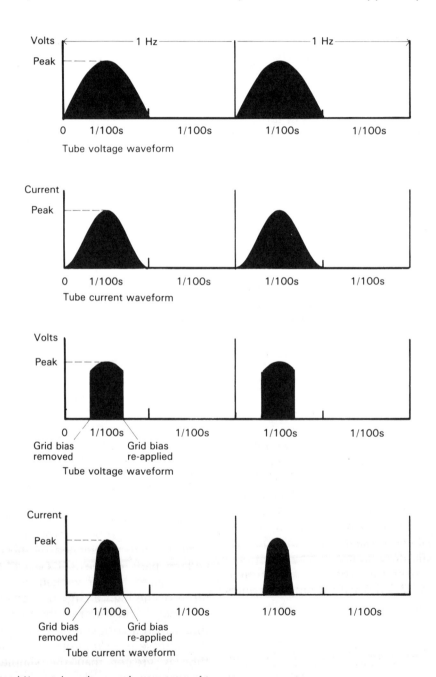

Fig. 16.36 Dental X-ray tube voltage and current waveform.

counter balanced and provided with locks which allow any tube position to be maintained. The support is either securely fixed to the wall or mounted on a very broad base so that the unit cannot tip over even when the tubehead is positioned well away from the central position. Floor mounted units are provided with castors to enable the unit to be moved out of the way when not required. The wall mounted unit is folded at its joints to a storage position close to the wall.

The control unit

The control unit is small and has a cable which connects it through a plug and socket to the mains supply. A multicore cable runs from the control unit to the tubehead where it supplies the primary of the HT transformer and the filament transformer. The tubehead is earthed by a lead within this multicore cable which passes through the control unit and the earth conductor of the mains cable to the earthed socket. A metre long cable connects an exposure switch to the exposure contactor in the control unit. This contactor is a simple type as the current to be switched on is quite small and the exposure times comparatively long. The exposure timer is generally a simple electronic unit although there are many units still in use which have clockwork mechanisms.

During the exposure a brightly lit indicator lamp is switched on to give anyone nearby a clear indication that X-rays are being generated. For radiation safety reasons, the type of push button switch used to make the exposure is recessed in a shallow socket so that there can be no risk of accidental exposure due to pressure on its surface. Additional safety precautions provided are to arrange the circuit so that the exposure switch must be compressed by the operator throughout the exposure, and to light automatically a different coloured indicator lamp as soon as the unit is switched on to show that the unit is ready to expose.

The cephalostat unit for orthodontic work

The cephalostat unit is designed to hold the head in a very precise position during radiog-

raphy in the antero-posterior and lateral position. By correct correlation between the patient's head, the focus of the X-ray tube and the film, it is possible to repeat accurately the radiographic projection on a series of visits. This allows the progress of orthodontic treatment to be assessed.

Figure 16.37 shows the essential features of the unit. It must be firmly attached either to an upright bucky or preferably to a base plate secured to the wall. The X-ray tube focus is centred to the unit by means of centring lamps or ideally by a mechanical link. The correct centring of the beam is verified by examination of the radiograph where two radio-opaque rings set in the head positioning device must be seen to be exactly superimposed.

The patient's head is held in a standard position by the use of ear plugs acting as ear locators and orbital and nasal positioners. Scales

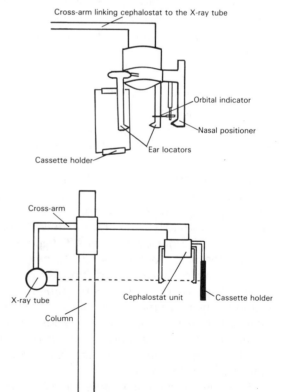

Fig. 16.37 Cephalostat.

are provided to allow the distance between the ear locators to be measured so that the magnification can be determined. The scales and equipment position adjusters allow the degree of head rotation to be fixed.

Image enlargement is reduced to a minimum by the use of a 180 cm focus-to-film distance. The distance between the head positioning device and the film is adjustable. This facility is rarely used once the technique has been agreed with the orthodontist.

The air gap between the patient and the film generally eliminates the need for an antiscatter grid. Should one be needed it must be of the parallel type to avoid cut-off at the long focus-to-film distance.

The radiograph must display both the soft tissue structures and the underlying bony framework. Therefore the contrast of the image must be low to ensure that all the different densities are adequately displayed by a single exposure. The techniques used are high kVp, low contrast films and sometimes the soft tissue profile of the face is outlined with opaque material, such as barium sulphate cream.

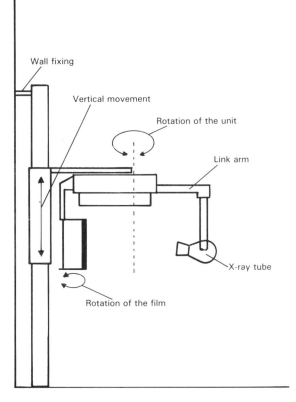

Fig. 16.38 Orthopantomograph unit.

Orthopantomographic equipment

Orthopantomographic equipment uses a system of synchronised rotary movements between the X-ray tube and an extra-oral film in a curved cassette as they move around the patient's head (Fig. 16.38). The tube follows the shape of the mandibular curve during the exposure and at the same time the curved cassette rotates on its own axis. The X-ray beam is closely collimated by a narrow vertical slit diaphragm at the tube port. As the cassette turns on its axis the narrow beam of radiation exposes a different section of the film as the tube moves round the head. In this way a full-mouth examination is possible with a single exposure. To eliminate scatter an additional slit diaphragm is fitted at the point where the X-ray beam emerges from the patient.

The tube movement is able to follow the mandibular arch by changing the fulcrum centre three times during the exposure. The position of the fulcrum centre is changed by causing the X-ray tube to trace a prefixed path in a plate which is fitted to the unit. A selection of plates is supplied to make the tube follow the shape of the various types of mandible. Figure 16.39 shows the site of the three fulcrum centres.

The success of this technique depends upon the very accurate positioning of the patient's head so head and chin supports are provided to immobilise the head in the exact position required. The tube is linked to the cassette by a support arm with the tube angled 10° to the head to avoid superimposition of the hard palate on the teeth. If the patient is incorrectly positioned, or the tube travel round the head does not closely follow the shape of the mandibular arch, there will be unsharpness in the image because the plane of sharpness of this tomographic procedure is not centered on the alveolar margin.

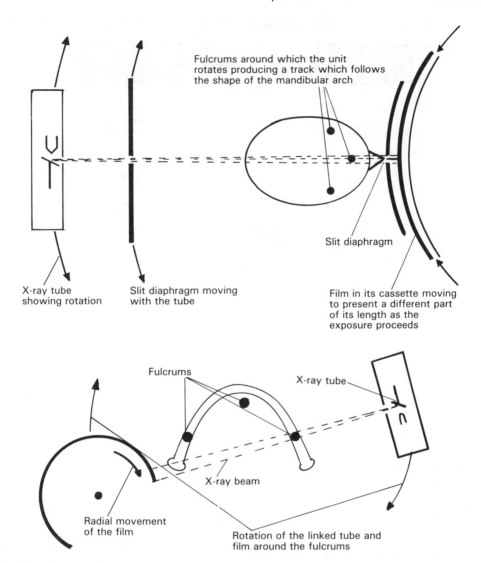

Fig. 16.39 Relationship of the X-ray tube and the film and their movements.

The X-ray tube must have a fine focus and is normally a stationary anode type with 0.6 mm focus with a 2 mm Al eq. filtration. The generator provides an output between 55–85 kVp and a tube current of 15 mA.

This unit is very useful for surveying the dental condition of a patient, and if the sharpness of the image does not reach the quality of an intra-oral, it enables the operator to select the intra oral films which must be taken. The examination of children and edentulous patients by intra-oral technique is very difficult and time consuming but this technique can prove of great value in these cases. Also the examination by pantomographic technique reduces the patient radiation dose to about one-third of the dose received from a full mouth series of 14 intra-oral films, and the upward angulation of the X-ray beam directs the beam away from the gonads.

The technique cannot be used for bedridden pateints or patients who cannot or will not co-operate.

There is an alternative way of displaying all the teeth with a single exposure on a single film. The technique is to introduce a very small

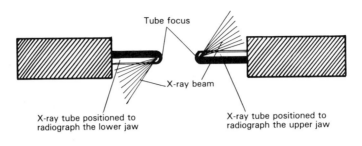

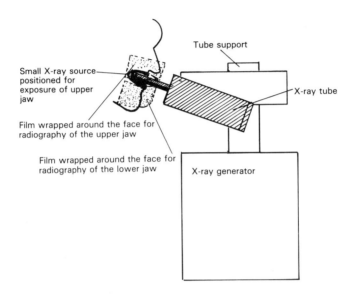

Fig. 16.40 Intra-oral X-ray source.

X-ray source into the mouth. The X-rays are generated in a specially designed X-ray tube in the mouth exposing a film wrapped around the face (Fig. 16.40). The technique, although appearing attractive, does not give good results every time as it is difficult to position the X-ray source accurately within the mouth. This is necessary as the radiation beam from the source must pass parallel to the spaces between the teeth, if overlap of one tooth's image on its neighbour is to be avoided.

17

Portable and mobile units

Portable and mobile units are units which can be moved from one place to another and used at the bedside or in the operating theatre where they are connected to the electrical supply through a plug and socket.

Their output is limited and their use restricted. They should not be used unless it is quite impossible to take the patient to a fixed unit where a more satisfactory examination can be undertaken.

Two types are available; the portable unit and the mobile unit. A portable unit can be carried in sections and reassembled by the operator at the site where it is to be used. A mobile unit is movable but, because of its weight, can only be wheeled along flat surfaces to the place where it is required. Both types will be considered.

PORTABLE X-RAY UNITS

A portable unit is designed to be divided into parts which make it possible for the operator to carry it to the place where it is required and then to reassemble it easily and quickly and make it ready for use. Its use is limited by low output, less stable design and less robust construction — all the result of making the unit transportable.

There are two types; the simple self-rectified unit with an output of about 80 kVp and 20 mA, and the capacitor discharge unit which provides a higher output by building up a

charge on a capacitor from a low output mains supply.

The portable unit is a single tank unit with a tubehead similar to those used for dental units. When it is divided into parts for transportation there is a tubehead, a control unit, a tube column, a cross arm and a base. The column is divided into convenient lengths for transportation. The base is mounted on castors.

The control unit has cables which connect it to the mains supply and to the tubehead by plugs and sockets. Figure 17.1 shows the unit assembled.

The tubehead is mounted on the cross arm which is moved up and down the vertical column by a rack and pinion type of drive (Fig. 17.2).

MOBILE X-RAY UNITS

The mobile unit is capable of higher output than the portable unit and being much heavier can in no way be described as portable. It is movable either manually or motor driven. The control table, high tension generator, tube column and the dual focus rotating anode tube are carried on a strong base plate. This base plate has wheels which by their size and mounting allows the unit to be moved forwards and backwards easily without drift from the desired path and able to turn in a small circle. Their tyres are made from hard plastic

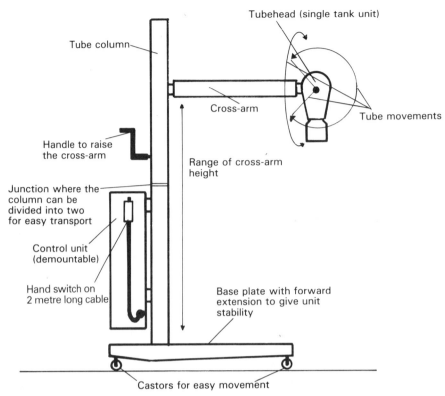

Fig. 17.1 Portable unit.

or rubber with anti-static properties making the unit safe for use in operating theatres. The weight of the units may be as great as 250 kilogrammes, so they are often driven by a battery-powered motor. When supplied, the batteries must be regularly charged and well maintained.

Two types of generators are used: the ordinary 2-pulse unit and the energy storage unit, either a condenser discharge or battery. powered type. The availability of solid-state rectifiers has allowed the use of full-wave rectification rather than self-rectification. This has greatly increased the X-ray output. Energy storage units provide a high X-ray output in sites where the mains supply is inadequate or where the type of work requires the delivery of a large quantity of radiation in a short time.

Mobile units are available in two forms based on the location of HT generator which may be either energy storage or 2-pulse. The unit in Figure 17.3a has the HT generator on

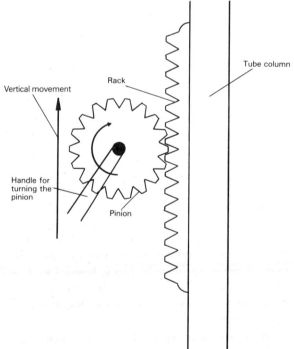

Fig. 17.2 Detail of the rack and pinion drive for raising the cross-arm.

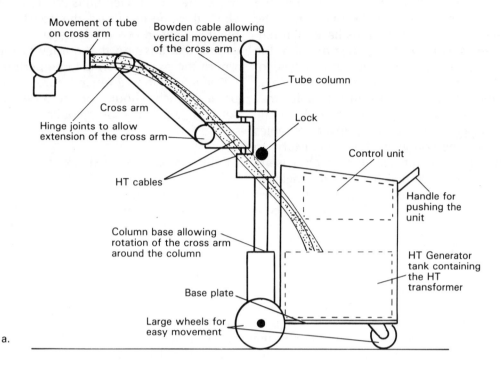

Movement of tube on cross arm

Bowden cable allowing vertical movement of the cross arm

Tube column

Cross arm

Lock

Hinge joints to allow extension of the cross arm

Control unit

HT cables

Handle for pushing the unit

Column base allowing rotation of the cross arm around the column

HT Generator tank containing the HT transformer

Base plate

Large wheels for easy movement

a.

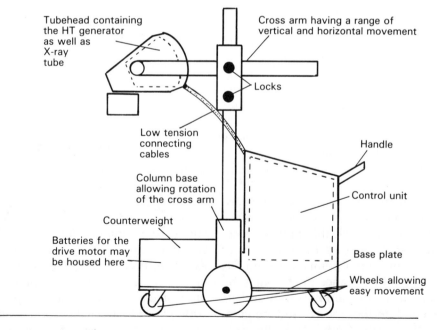

Tubehead containing the HT generator as well as X-ray tube

Cross arm having a range of vertical and horizontal movement

Locks

Low tension connecting cables

Handle

Column base allowing rotation of the cross arm

Control unit

Counterweight

Batteries for the drive motor may be housed here

Base plate

Wheels allowing easy movement

b.

Fig. 17.3 Two types of mobile unit.

the base plate; its weight helps to counter-balance the weight of the X-ray tube when the cross-arm support is extended away from the centre of the unit. These units have high tension cables linking the generator with the tube, a feature which identifies this type of unit. It has two disadvantages over the single tank unit: (1) the presence of HT cables may make tube positioning difficult and (2) the high voltage connection by external cables precluding the coupling of a second tube to the same control unit, a feature which is useful when two beams of radiation at right angles to each other are required. Figure 17.3b shows the alternative layout with the single tank containing the HT generator and the X-ray tube in the same housing, along with the other components which operate at high tension.

The design of these units must allow for their use at the bedside or in the theatre with minimal disturbance to the patient. They must by their design limit the radiation received by the patient, the operator or any others in the vicinity. The provision of a 2 metre cable for the hand switch connection allows the operator to stand in an area where the radiation level is low. It is important that the height and range of movement of the X-ray tube allow all the necessary techniques to be performed at an accepted focus-to-film distance and yet be able to be stowed very compactly during movement and storage. The height and weight limitations of any lift which may be encountered must never be exceeded. If the mobile's weight is within 80 kilogrammes of the lift maximum, the operator should not travel with the unit in the lift.

It is important that the mains supply is adequate for the unit and that the line resistance compensator is included in the mobile's electrical circuit to accommodate the variations in supply at different output points. Reference is made again to the importance of checking the condition of the mains supply cable and its plug top every time the unit is used, remembering that the earth conductor is the sole earthing provision for the unit. Mobile units require very frequent visual inspection of all locks, suspension cables and brakes for evidence of wear since these are subjected to more strain than fixed units due to the type of work they perform and the constant movement up and down corridors and in and out of lifts that arise on the journey to the place where the examination is to be performed.

The information given in Figure 17.4 lists the points which should be considered when selecting a portable or a mobile unit.

MOBILE IMAGE INTENSIFIER UNITS

Mobile image intensifiers are designed primarily for use in operating theatres and intensive care departments. Therefore they are used in the reduction and fixation of the fractured femoral neck, examination of the urinary and biliary system during surgery and any other surgical procedure aided by immediate X-ray visualisation. In intensive care departments the introduction of cardiac catheters and pace-makers is their main use.

The advantages of image intensification over mobile radiography include

1. Immediate localisation and manipulation of fractures, calculi and catheters under direct vision.
2. Fewer radiographs are needed to provide the required information, so reducing the patient dose and that received by the operator.
3. Reduced operating time can be achieved requiring less anaesthetic and more efficient use of theatre operating time.

The disadvantage is related to the management of the length of the fluoroscopy time. This may become extended when used by unskilled personnel. Fluoroscopy gives an accumulating radiation dose which must be kept to a minimum. The methods used to limit the exposure time include the use of fluoroscopic time display and, where justified by the volume of use, the provision of pulsed fluoroscopy with replay facility to give an apparently uninterrupted screening. Unauthorised use of the equipment is prevented by the fitting of a key operated switch.

There are two types of unit available: the

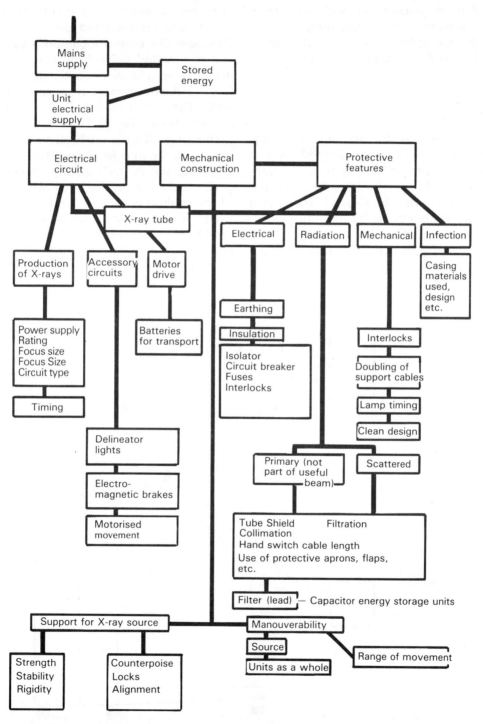

Fig. 17.4 Features to be considered when selecting a mobile unit.

'C'-arm with a single tube and intensifier, and a multiplane ring-stand unit with two tubes and two intensifiers set at right angles to each other. The multiplane unit can only conveniently be used for fixation of the femoral neck.

The 'C'-arm unit

The 'C'-arm unit has the tube and collimator mounted on one end of a C-shaped support with the intensifier on the other end. Counterweight is added if necessary to equal the weights of the ends. The C-arm is then fitted to a vertical column through a mounting which allows the tube and intensifier to be rotated around it. Somewhat limited rotation of the C-arm in the other plane is also provided

through the mounting. There is a vertical movement available on the column. The vertical column is mounted on a mobile base. This base like other mobile units has its generator mounted behind the column to make use of its weight as a counter balance for the C-arm. All movements have secure mechanical locks. The base is mounted on wheels for easy movement (see Fig. 17.5)

The X-ray tube is a dual focus rotating anode tube with 0.6 mm focal spot for fluoroscopy and a 1.2 mm for radiography. Radiography is performed by fitting the X-ray cassette in front of the intensifier face. A 2-pulse generator is used. The collimation fitted limits the radiation field to the size of the intensifier input phosphor and the added variable diaphragms can be adjusted to limit the field still further.

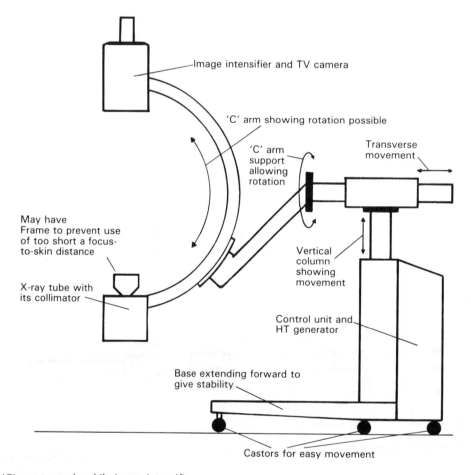

Fig. 17.5 'C' arm type of mobile image intensifier.

An integrated timer monitors the fluoroscopy time and may be supplemented by a dosimeter recording the total dose received by the patient. Fluoroscopy factors are usually automatically controlled.

The image is recorded by radiography using the cassette holder fitted to the intensifier face or by video. The video signal may be recorded on tape or on disc. The image is displayed on a TV monitor normally carried on a separate trolley which allows it to be positioned in the most convenient position for the surgeon.

The X-ray tube, collimator, image intensifier and closed circuit TV system are of normal design although the intensifier is restricted to a 15 cm field.

It is most important when using this C-arm unit that the tube is positioned as far away as possible from the patient. If the focus-to-skin distance is short, the skin dose received by the patient is very large and the quality of the image poor because of the increased patient-to-input phosphor distance causing increased geometric unsharpness and image enlarge-

ment. The image enlargement is a useful indicator of poor positioning. This possibility of poor positioning is a very serious danger which has been overcome in some units by fitting a guard to the front of the collimator to ensure a reasonable focus-to-skin distance.

The multi-plane ring-stand

The ring-stand is formed by two rings, one inside the other. The outer ring is supported on two posts which have some vertical movement. Each post is mounted on wheels with locking devices to enable the unit (Fig. 17.6) to be positioned and then secured in position. The inner ring carries two sets of X-ray tube and intensifier with TV camera at 90° to each other. Their X-ray beams intersect at the centre of the ring. The inner ring revolves inside the outer ring allowing the tubes to be positioned anywhere on the circumference. Once positioned the rings are locked together. The X-ray tubes with their collimators are fixed to the ring, and the intensifiers can

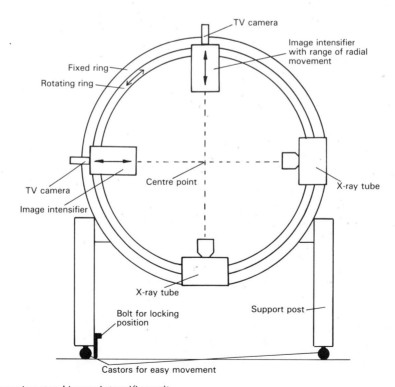

Fig. 17.6 Multiplane ring stand image intensifier unit.

be moved radially towards the centre of the ring to reduce the patient-to-phosphor distance so lessening the geometric unsharpness. By fixing the tube to the circumference and by making the two X-ray beams intersect at the centre of the ring, the part to be examined must be centrally placed to be seen in both planes. This ensures that there can be no possibility of a short focus-to-skin distance.

The selection of a particular X-ray tube/intensifier pair is made by operating a foot-switch to energise the appropriate pair.

Advantages of the multiplane ring-stand unit over the C-arm

1. With both projections at 90° to each other set up at the beginning of the operative procedure the operating time is shorter.

2. The patient receives less radiation as there is no need for fluoroscopy time to allow the tube to be repositioned between projections.

3. There is no risk of incorrectly positioning the tube with a short focus-to-skin distance.

4. There is less disturbance of theatre drapes as the unit once set up requires no further movement.

Disadvantages

1. The multiplane is very expensive to purchase and costs more to maintain.

2. The initial positioning of the unit is more difficult.

3. The surgeon may find the unit's ring an inconvenience.

4. The unit can only conveniently be used for a single purpose, the fixing of a fractured femoral neck.

18

Radio-nuclide imaging

Radio-nuclide images are produced by the gamma ray emission from an organ within the body containing a radio-active substance. The system requires the preparation of radio-pharmaceuticals which will be concentrated in the organ of interest by the normal physiological and metabolic pathways.

To produce useful images, it is necessary to collect information from very many small areas of the organ under investigation and record the number of radiation photons emitted from each of these areas as a level of density on a 'grey-scale'. On a 'grey-scale', a level of density represents a particular quantity of radiation.

The technique requires a wide understanding of the type of radio-pharmaceuticals available, their applications, their associated physiological and metabolic pathways and the method of recording the quantity and location of the radiation emission. This detail is outside the range of this book but the layout diagram (Fig. 18.1) shows the principal features of the system.

Central to the system is the gamma camera. In this unit the gamma rays, which are emitted in a direction so that they can pass through the small holes in a lead collimator, fall upon a scintillation crystal. The radiation photon causes the crystal to emit a light photon. This photon is collected by a photomultiplier tube placed immediately behind the crystal and aligned to the collimator hole. In this way an amplified electrical signal is produced proportional to the number of gamma photons it has received and projected on to the screen of the

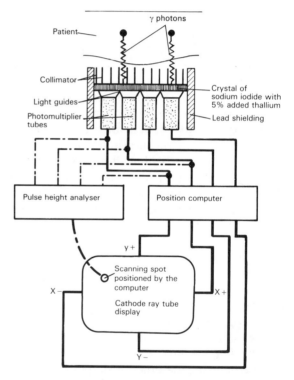

Fig. 18.1 Radio-nuclide imaging.

cathode ray tube. The signal from a particular location on the crystal is reproduced in the same position on the fluorescent screen by a positioning computer which records the position on an x-y axis on the crystal. The information is relayed to the horizontal and vertical deflecting coils of the cathode ray tube so that the position of each signal on the crystal is faithfully reproduced on the oscilloscope screen.

281

19
Ultrasound

Ultrasound units use the basic sound-echo principle to determine the depth of each echo-reflecting surface of a structure and by the amount of attenuation modifying the returning echoes, the nature of the tissues in the pathway of the beam can be determined.

The equipment needed for the production and recording of the ultrasound image comprises a generator of the ultrasound beam, a collector of the returning echoes registering their change in energy and a unit to measure the time interval between the originating pulses and the returning echoes and their intensity (Fig. 19.1). This information is computed to give the position of the reflecting surfaces and the nature of the tissue traversed. This is then displayed as an image on a cathode ray oscilloscope for immediate viewing or recording on hard-copy.

The pencil beam of ultrasound is generated by applying a voltage across the faces of a disc of piezo-electric material causing the electrical energy applied to it to be converted into pulses of ultrasound energy. This generator is called the probe or transducer.

The returning echoes are collected by the same probe or by separate detectors. In either case the returning sound energy interacts with the piezo-electric material changing the sound energy back into electrical energy. This electrical signal can be easily amplified and fed to a unit which projects it on to a cathode ray oscilloscope where an image of the tissues traversed by the sound waves is formed.

The cathode ray oscilloscope may have a short persistance phosphor screen which displays a real time image or it may have the long persistance phosphor of the storage type tube which builds up a static image that can be photographically recorded.

Only this brief description of ultrasound is given in this book as there are many very good books on the subject to which the student may refer and in addition it is such a rapidly advancing modality that it is better to obtain up-to-date information from journals and manufacturer's data sheets.

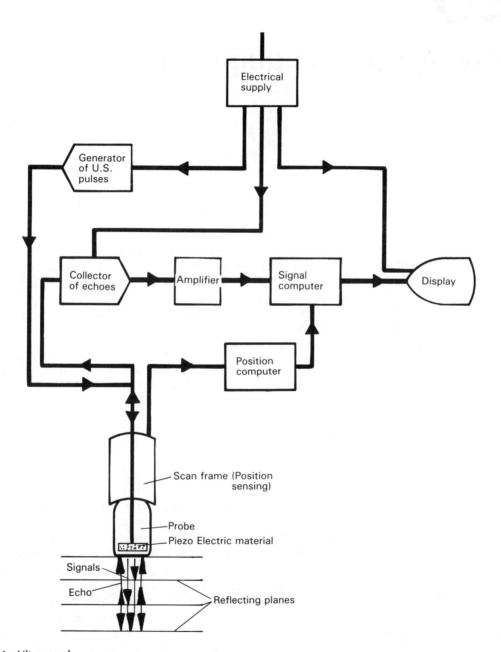

Fig. 19.1 Ultrasound.

20

General care of equipment

An operator cannot properly care for an X-ray unit without a good working knowledge of its function, its accessories and an underlying knowledge of the principles controlling its operation. Before, during and immediately after use the operator should be alert to any change from the normal in the feel, look and sound of the equipment or any unusual smell. All may indicate the malfunction of a component. The operator with knowledge will be able to identify the probable cause and the likely location of the fault. Any deviation from normal should be reported and recorded and if necessary the unit turned off until it has been checked and any fault cleared. This will avoid many breakdowns and costly repairs for finding minor or potential faults early may prevent serious faults occurring.

Regular maintenance by engineers should be arranged. The operator should undertake regular inspections and tests to reduce breakdowns. The operator can also help by taking care to handle the equipment correctly and see that it is kept clean and properly stowed when not in use. Some of the factors under the control of the user include:

1. Good equipment handling

Poor handling may cause brakes forced or worn to the point of failure because the equipment is moved before time has been allowed for them to become free. Knobs, screws, nuts and covers become lost if the operator fails to notice or if they do notice but do not see that they are secured back into place. Any screw found on the floor should be retained with a note stating where it was found so that when its location is found it can be replaced.

2. Tidiness and cleanliness of the working environment

It is essential for the efficient running of the department that the environment should be clean and tidy but in addition equipment damage can be avoided also by, for example:

a. Dusting — dust can prevent the free movement of trolley wheels making them difficult to move and this will cause more wear and may cause units to be pushed over. Dust or rubbish in floor tracks may cause tube columns to 'jump' the track or disturb the even travel of a tomographic run.

b. Failure to remove dirt from the TV monitor screen will reduce image quality, as will dirt on intensifying screens. Both may necessitate an increase in the load on the unit by requiring more exposure or a repeat film, quite apart from the unjustifiable increase in the radiation dose to the patient. On occasions contrast agents such as barium may trickle under the X-ray table and this has been known to interfere with the operation of a safety device. Dirt and spillage of liquids may also reduce electrical safety.

Regular dusting and cleaning of equipment give an opportunity for the unit to be inspected for damage or minor faults, for example, an oily patch on or around the X-ray tube indicating a failure of the oil seal in the tube. Finding this early will allow the leak to be repaired before the tube insert is in any danger. The inspection should extend to the fabric of the room, e.g. plaster dust on the floor may indicate loosening of the ceiling fixing.

3. Care with mechanical parts

Mechanical parts may suffer damage from overheating. The operator can avoid this by seeing that the equipment ventilating panels are kept clear of obstructions and any unit generating heat is not covered with articles like blankets or pillows which will delay the cooling process. Stationary grids can be severely damaged if they are placed on or near a radiator. These are just two examples of how heat can cause damage and how it may be avoided.

Mechanical damage may arise from many causes in addition to heat, e.g. trailing cables connecting units may be damaged by twisting, pulling, bending or crushing, if they are not carefully routed by the operator along a path which avoids these hazards. Pieces of equipment may collide with other pieces damaging one or both of them. The operator may prevent this by carefully positioning the equipment. Manufacturers fit safety devices in some sites to prevent damage through collision. Careless fitting of parts may damage connecting pins or threads. These are just a few causes of damage which the good operator will know about and be able to prevent.

4. Storage

Equipment must be stored carefully and correctly to avoid damage to equipment or injury to personnel. Units should be switched off after use, mechanical brakes applied and cables stored correctly when the unit is left or in the case of mobile units prepared for movement to another site. Containers should be labelled so that accessory equipment can be replaced after use in the correct place. Equipment such as anti-scatter grids require special storage arrangements to ensure that they will not be damaged. TV monitor and fluorescent screens should be protected from bright light as this will in time reduce the phosphor efficiency.

X-ray tubes and other equipment using a heated filament should be switched off after use to conserve their filament life. The anode rotor bearings will have a longer useful life if the anode is only rotated when needed, therefore the careful operator will keep the unit in the 'prepare' stage for the shortest possible time.

5. Good practice

The operator should take care when assembling equipment, avoiding the use of force when fitting the parts together and checking that they are properly coupled and are operating correctly before use.

X-ray tubes should be run-up before heavy loads are applied to a cold anode. Careful selection of exposure factors to avoid unnecessary heavy loading will extend the life of the unit.

The regular use of checking routines, using check lists, safety audits, and performing quality assurance tests, will assist the maintenance of an efficient unit. The value of checking systems can be enhanced by the recording of the findings and the values of the various parameters measured during the tests.

The training of operators in the use of equipment and the range of its facilities is essential to the care of equipment and this training should continue throughout the life of the equipment whenever the operator is not fully familiar with the equipment and its facilities. Staff must be trained to look, listen, act and report any untoward occurrences to reduce equipment faults and improve efficiency.

EQUIPMENT RECORDS

Equipment records are essential to the good management of an X-ray Department. They should be designed to give information on all pieces of equipment giving their history and highlighting any recurring problems, indicating reliability or unreliability. The record will show the amount of 'down-time' encountered and the efficiency of the servicing arrangements and the response time to a call. Information of this type is invaluable when arguing for an improvement in the servicing provision or for the need for replacement of a unit.

The record should be divided into two parts: the initial information and the service/maintenance log.

The initial information should include: details of the type of the equipment, the manufacturer, the servicing company responsible for it, the date of installation and the serial numbers of the parts of the equipment, such as the X-ray tube.

The service log should record the date and time a fault is found and the immediate action taken; the date and time of reporting the fault and to whom it was reported; the date and time of the engineers' attendance; the action taken by the engineer and a list of any parts used in the repair and any instructions on the future use of the equipment; the number of exposures recorded by each tube should be regularly recorded.

In addition a Quality Assurance Programme should be followed on all equipment.

QUALITY ASSURANCE PROGRAMMING

Quality assurance programmes will ensure that the equipment maintains a level of performance which will produce radiographic and fluoroscopic images with the maximum diagnostic information possible within the capability of the equipment. In addition the introduction of a Quality Assurance Programme will reduce running costs, keep the radiation dose received by the patient and the staff to a minimum and lead to improved departmental management.

To get the maximum advantage from such a programme, it must start at the time of the hand-over of the equipment by the manufacturer. The tests performed at this stage check that the equipment reaches the standard of performance specified by the manufacturer and also provides base-line measurements against which future values can be compared.

Therefore the objectives of a Quality Assurance Programme are:

1. to check the performance of the equipment on installation and make sure that it reaches the manufacturers specification
2. to provide base-line values so future checks can measure how well these values are maintained
3. to allow comparison between units
4. to make staff aware of the performance expected from the equipment and the effect on radiation dose of varying exposure factors and other parameters
5. to locate and detect faults which may give poor equipment performance resulting in poor image quality, sometimes even before the fault is bad enough to be obvious in the normal radiographic work
6. to provide the engineer with an indication of the likely cause of equipment failure.

To ensure that all tests and performance checks are undertaken systematically, a check list should be prepared. This check list should include a list of all the tests and checks to be performed and the frequency with which they are to be undertaken. Details of the standard test procedures should be kept with the list so that there is no variation in the method of performing the tests which could alter their results. The results from all the tests must be recorded in a way which enables their results to be easily compared with the result of the same test undertaken previously. The list must be amended when equipment is added or taken out of use. Details of any repairs or replacement of equipment or parts should be noted in the record.

Set out below is a list of the principal tests and checks that should be undertaken on equipment. It is by no means a complete list. The equipment checks and tests are grouped under radiographic equipment, fluoroscopic equipment tests and general performance and safety checks.

1. Radiographic equipment

a. kVp including half value thickness
b. Filtration
 — presence of required total filtration, any evidence of increasing inherant filtration through tungsten deposition on the inner wall of the glass insert
c. Radiation output over a range of kVp and mA
d. Evidence of an anode heel effect
e. Exposure time accuracy including
 — automatic exposure control, and operation of the guard time controls
 — accuracy and consistency of performance
f. Limit of resolution available from each focus
g. Reproducibility of exposure with varying tube currents
h. Consistency of film density over a series of exposures
i. X-ray beam alignment
j. Light-beam diaphragm — co-incidence of illuminated field and irradiated field in horizontal and vertical planes
k. Accuracy of collimator scales
l. Operation of delineator lamp time limiting control
m. Absence of leakage radiation from tube and collimator unit
n. Anti-scatter grid alignment to the X-ray beam
o. Uniform attenuation by the grid across the irradiated field
p. Smoothness of grid movement across its range
q. Shortest exposure time possible without grid lines obvious
r. On installation — the grid factor

s. Focus-to-film distances are as displayed on the scales provided
t. On installation — confirm the location of the fine and broad focal spots.

2. Fluoroscopic equipment

In addition to the appropriate tests from the list above the following should also be undertaken:

a. Accuracy and consistency of the automatic collimation of the beam to the image size of the recorded field
b. Conversion factor and contrast ratio of the fluoroscopic image
c. Degree of distortion present across the fluoroscopic image
d. Automatic brightness control operation and efficiency
e. Limiting resolution of the system
f. Radiation dose delivered to the input face of the image intensifier from a standard set of factors and parameters.

3. General performance and safety checks

General survey of the equipment to confirm that there is no evidence of damage, wear or absence of parts, screws etc. and that the equipment is in a safe working condition, paying particular attention to parts subjected to great wear and strain.

The full range of facilities should be tested and any associated interlocks and safety devices checked.

On installation, and after any changes in the equipment, the safety of the radiation protective barriers should be checked.

Radiation protective clothing, flexible aprons and flaps around the equipment must be checked to ensure their continuing effectiveness.

Other performance checks
A list of safety checks should be drawn up for all specialised equipment and accessories, e.g.

with a tomographic unit or attachment the following should be tested:

a. Accuracy of the layer indicated with the actual layer recorded
b. Thickness of the layer obtained with the range of settings provided
c. Uniformity and completeness of the tomographic movement
d. Angle over which the exposure is made
e. Smoothness of the movement throughout its travel
f. Uniformity of density obtained throughout the movement
g. Limit of resolution at the focal plane
h. Degree of image magnification.

The standard tests laid down by international and national organisations such as the British Standards Institute and World Health Organization should be used whenever possible.

21

Equipment selection and installation

EQUIPMENT SELECTION

Before equipment can be selected a number of questions must be asked and answered and these include the following:

1. What work is to be done?
2. What are the techniques the equipment will be required to perform?
3. Does the performance of these techniques require sophisticated equipment and/or accessories?
4. What accommodation is available:
   floor area and type of flooring
   finished room height and type of ceiling
   any weight limitation on the floor or ceiling
   access to the accommodation for delivery of the equipment?
5. Size of the department/hospital — any specialisation?
6. What other equipment is available in the department?
7. What workload may be expected?
8. What percentage of the workload is the new equipment expected to perform?
9. Are there any particular examinations which will predominate?
10. Are there any specific features and/or accessories necessary for the performance of the techniques required?
11. Are the majority of the patients in one particular category, e.g. paediatric, geriatric?

12. What are the cost limits for the installation?
13. Is there a particular delivery date to be adhered to and when is the unit required to be operational?
14. Are there any other constraints?
15. What arrangements will be made for servicing?
16. What is the line voltage and current available, is it single-or three-phase?
17. What is the minimum mains supply feeder cable (line) supply impedance at the equipment connecting point?
18. Are there any restraints on the revenue and/or staffing consequent upon the installation?
19. Are there staff available with the skills and knowledge to use the equipment to its full potential?
20. Is there or will there be a training programme made available to the operators and the local X-ray engineer?

With this information collected and a knowledge of the equipment necessary to perform the examinations to be undertaken on the equipment a specification can be drawn up for the equipment needed to meet the requirements. Once this is done the various manufacturer's equipment can be matched against the specification, or the list can be sent to the manufacturers for them to tender for the installation. The specification will include the relevant items from the following lists.

SPECIFICATION INCLUDES:

Generator

1. Physical dimensions
   maximum size _____
   weight of unit _____
2. Generator voltage supply
   single- or three-phase _____
   line resistance _____
   % line voltage regulation _____
   manual or automatic correction _____
3. Generator kilovoltage
   a. kW rating _____
      mA at 70 kVp _____
      mA at 100 kVp _____
      mA at 125 kVp _____
      mA at 150 kVp _____
   b. Maximum kV
      fluoroscopy _____
      radiography _____
   c. Minimum KV
      fluoroscopy _____
      radiography _____
   d. Number of kV steps
      fluoroscopy _____
      radiography _____
   e. kV accuracy over mA range _____
   f. Type of generator
      number of pulses _____
      method of smoothing _____
      falling load _____
      shared _____
4. Generator milliamperage
   a. Maximum setting
      fluoroscopy
         fine focus _____
         broad focus _____
      radiography
         fine focus _____
         broad focus _____
   b. Minimum setting
      fluoroscopy
         fine focus _____
         broad focus _____
      radiography
         fine focus _____ broad focus _____
   c. Number of mA settings
      radiography

      fine focus _____
      broad focus _____
   d. Fluoroscopy control
      manual/automatic _____
   e. Variable mA control control
      radiography _____
   f. mA accuracy over kV range _____
   g. mA reproducibility over a series of exposures _____
5. Timing controls
   a. Time selection range _____
   b. Maximum setting _____
   c. Minimum setting _____
   d. Type of contactor _____
   e. Switching
      primary _____
      secondary _____
   f. Timing
      electronic _____
      automatic _____
   g. Timer accuracy _____

5. *Control unit*
   a. Dimensions of the unit _____
   b. Layout of components
      one unit _____
      as two units _____
      remote control unit _____
   c. Form of display _____
   d. Layout of the controls _____
   e. Exposure control
      1 knob
      2 knobs
      3 knobs

X-ray tubes and collimators

X-ray tubes
a. Number of tubes
   fluoroscopic _____
   radiographic _____
b. Maximum kV rating
   fluoroscopic _____
   radiograph
      general _____
      mammographic _____
c. Rotational speed _____
d. Grid control _____

e. Anode heat storage capacity _____
f. Target heat storage capacity _____
g. Target disc diameter _____
h. Target angle
    fluoroscopic
        fine focus _____
        broad focus _____
    radiographic
        fine focus _____
        broad focus _____
i. Focal spot size
    fluoroscopic
        fine focus _____
        broad focus _____
    radiographic
        fine focus _____
        broad focus _____
j. Target angle
    fluoroscopic
        fine focus _____
        broad focus _____
    radiographic
        fine focus _____
        broad focus _____
k. Any additional heat dissipator
    fluoroscopic _____
    radiographic _____

Collimators
a. Type
    fluoroscopic tube _____
    radiographic tube _____
b. Diaphragms
    rectilinear _____
    iris _____
c. Automatic or manual
    fluoroscopic tube _____
    radiographic tube _____

Image intensifier, TV chain and image recording

Image intensifier
a. Diameter of input phosphor _____
b. Single, dual or triple field size _____
c. Image intensifier tube gain _____
d. Conversion ratio _____
e. Contrast ratio _____
f. Line pair resolution _____

Coupling system
a. Tandem lens _____
b. Fibre optic _____

Television camera
a. Standard vidicon _____
b. Plumbicon _____
c. Raster
    625 lines _____
    1249 lines _____
d. Resolution _____

Television monitor
a. Size (diagonal length) _____

Image recording system
a. Full-size film cassette sizes _____
b. Method of loading cassettes _____
c. Recording camera
    single shot camera _____
    cine camera _____
    video recorder
        tape _____
        disc _____
        disc storage _____
d. Exposure control _____
e. Parking position _____

Tube supports
a. Floor or ceiling mounted _____
b. Floor area covered by the X-ray beam
    longitudinal _____
    transverse _____
c. Minimum ceiling height required _____
d. Maximum height of focus above table top _____
e. Maximum height of focus above floor _____
f. Minimum height of focus above floor _____
g. Accuracy of measuring device for focus height _____
h. Movement manual or motor driven _____
i. Method of centring to the table and chest stand _____
j. Method of locking in position manual or electromagnetic _____
k. Degree of rotation
    about the tube transverse axis _____
    about the long axis of tube _____
    around the tube column _____

l. Convenience of controls _____
m. Facility for coupling of tomographic attachment _____

Radiographic/fluoroscopic tables

a. Table size _____
b. Height from the floor _____
c. Type of table
    flat _____
    tilting _____
d. If tilting
    range of movement _____
    indication of angle of tilt _____
    tilt speed-single/two speed _____
e. Table top
    attenuation factor _____
    dished or flat _____
    range of movement
        longitudinal _____
        transverse _____
    location of controls _____
f. Safety devices provided _____

Bucky assembly
g. Range of movement _____
h. Grid
    ratio _____
    factor _____
    movement _____
    minimum exposure time needed to blur grid lines _____
i. Cassette tray — cassette sizes accepted __
j. Any automatic collimation to cassette ____

Serial changer(explorator)
k. Method of support _____
l. Facilities provided _____
m. Range of movement
        longitudinal _____
        transverse _____
        compression _____
n. Transfer mechanism for cassettes _____
o. Delay caused by transfer of cassette ____

Safety devices provided
p. Against radiation
        primary _____
        secondary _____
q. Against electrical hazard _____

r. Against mechanical hazard _____

With the specification completed and having regard to the particular demands of the examinations to be performed, which include:

1. Image quality
   — degree of resolution required
2. Exposure factors
   — tube loading
   — single or serial exposures
3. Special problems related to the patients to be examined, including:

   a. their size — child or adult, incapacity
   b. any hazard in the examinations to be performed
   c. radiation dose limitations
   d. anatomical position of the part
   e. physiological factors
   f. tissue density
   g. subject contrast
   h. scatter production by the part.

The selection of a particular piece of equipment can then be made bearing in mind the following factors:

(i)   Is there any other equipment supplied by the proposed manufacturer in the same department, which would be of obvious advantage in the provision of servicing?
(ii) Is there any similar equipment is use locally that can be visited to find out, by discussion with a user, any limitations or difficulties experienced and give an opportunity to examine and handle the unit?
(iii) How will the equipment fit into the room? Will it be convenient to use and convenient for the patients?
(iv) What preinstallation work has to be done and how long will it take?
(v)   What training is provided by the manufacturer for the hospital staff engineer so that he is able to undertake first line repairs?
(vi) Is the unit designed to allow faulty circuits to be easily located and replaced?

THE INSTALLATION OF NEW EQUIPMENT

Following the selection of the equipment the purchaser is normally responsible for preparing the site to the unit installer's specification. This pre-installation work includes the connection of the electrical supply to a junction (connection) box, and supplying and fitting of a mains isolator so that the junction box can be completely cut off from the hospital mains supply. The trunking (metal channels) for the distribution of electrical cables connecting the various pieces of equipment must also be fitted in the positions shown on the manufacturer's room plan.

THE HAND-OVER PROCEDURES

Before accepting the equipment, the purchaser must:

1. check the equipment to see that it reaches the performance specified by the manufacturer and that it reaches safety standards;

2. perform quality assurance tests to check the actual level of the equipment's performance and provide a base-line against which future performance can be compared;

3. receive the operator and service manuals in English, with their accompanying circuit diagrams to enable the local engineer to undertake first-line repairs. In addition, some manufacturers provide a number of spare parts within the package. If this is the case, they should be checked against the manufacturer's list given with their tender.

4. receive adequate instruction by the supplier on the operation of the equipment and the use of the facilities and all its accessories. Training courses are sometimes provided by the manufacturer for the hospital staff engineer — the dates for these should be agreed at this stage.

Following acceptance the user should:

1. notify the Radiation Protection Advisor that the equipment is operational so that he can arrange to check on the radiation safety of the equipment and with the Radiation Protection Supervisor prepare the local rules appertaining to the equipment with which the user must comply;

2. set up the quality assurance programme for the unit, measuring and recording the unit's parameters;

3. compare the unit's radiation output against other units in the department, in terms of half value thickness and radiation dose per mAs as well as photographic comparison by the radiography of an aluminium step wedge under varying operating conditions;

4. set up training arrangements for all the staff who will use the equipment taking care to include all the facilities and accessories available and any particular safety arrangements, giving time for the staff to acquire a familiarity with the operation of the equipment so reducing the number of radiographs which will have to be rejected;

5. develop an exposure chart suggesting exposure factors and other technical information which will help the user to produce high quality radiographs.

Index